The Book of Nurse Saints
Are you a nurse who is Catholic or
a "Catholic nurse"?

Diana L. Ruzicka, RN

Diana L. Ruzicka Publisher
New Market, Alabama
Copies available at www.lulu.com

Cover Illustrations
(See specific saint for source of photo)

Front Cover:

St. Radegund (Thuringia [*modern Germany*]/France) (518-587).
  Patroness of the 1st Council of Catholic Nurses in the United States
  founded in Boston, Massachusetts in 1909.

St. Fabiola (Italy-Rome) (d. 399)
  The first nurse saint who founded the first hospital in Rome as recorded by
  St. Jerome in his letter to Oceanus.

St. Camillus de Lellis (Italy) (1550-1614)
  Founder, Ministers to the Sick (Camillians),
  Patron Saint of Nurses and Nurses Associations declared by Pope Pius XI.

St. John of God (Portugal/Spain) (1495-1550)
  Founder, Hospitallers of St. John of God
  Patron Saint of Nurses and Nurses Associations declared by Pope Pius XI.

Back Cover:

St. Catherine of Siena (Italy) (1347-1380)
  Doctor of the Church, Stigmatic and Mystic.

Please send recommended additions of any nurses who have been formally
declared Saints, Blessed, Venerable, Servants of God and/or Martrys to:
Diana.Ruzicka@gmail.com.

Diana L. Ruzicka Publisher
185 River Walk Trail
New Market, AL 35761
Telephone: 256-852-5519
Email: Diana.Ruzicka@gmail.com

Printed and bound in the United States of America
Copies of this publication are available at
www.lulu.com/spotlight/Ruzicka or
www.lulu.com (and search "Ruzicka")

This book is dedicated to all the nurses
who have gone before us leading the way,
those who have been canonized, beatified,
declared venerable, servants of God, martyrs,
and also to all nurses who are unnoticed and quietly
work to bring forth the Kingdom of God
on earth caring for Christ in the
sick, abandoned and lonely.

To the members and leadership of
the National Association of Catholic Nurses, U.S.A.
(NACN-USA) and the
International Catholic Committee of Nurses and
Medico-Social Assistants --- Comité International Catholique des
Infirmières et Assistantes Médico-Sociales (CICIAMS)
and all member associations around the world
for their example of what it means to be
A CATHOLIC NURSE.

Acknowledgments

There are many people across the world who made this endeavor possible in order for the timely release of the first edition at the International Catholic Committee of Nurses and Medico-Social Assistants (CICIAMS) XXI World Congress hosted by the National Association of Catholic Nurses, U.S.A. (NACN-USA), August 2-4, 2022, at the Shrine of Our Lady of Czestochowa in Doylestown, Pennsylvania, U.S.A.

Reverend Alban Butler's *Lives of the Saints* (1883), is the gold standard in books on saints. I wish to thank Douglas Bersaw of Loreto publications who promptly gave permission to include Rev. Butler's full text from the *original* works re-published in 2020. I thank Terry Jones, for allowing me liberal access to the content of his website "catholicsaints.info" on which he has an extensive list of saints who were nurses. When asked why he ever thought to list nurses as a category, he shared that he has *"always been a fan of nurses.."* and his *"mum was a nursing student when* [he] *came along to change her plans."* His list was instrumental in moving this project forward. Another excellent resource was Hagiography Circle. I thank Brother Reginald Cruz, CFX, General Coordinator, Hagiography Circle for their exceptional website and his explanation of the category "new martyrs" which His Holiness Pope St. John Paul II introduced in his Apostolic Letter *Tertio Millennio Adveniente* (10 November 1994). This resulted in several exemplary nurses being included in the text who would not have been otherwise.

I wish to also acknowledge all the religious orders who gave permission to include the biographies from their websites. I also thank, Dr. Patricia Sayers, DNP, RN, President Elect and Janet Munday, BSN, RN, Regional Director and Communications Chairman, NACN-USA; Dr. Margorita (Gosia) Brykczynska, PhD, RN, OCV, President, European Region, CICIAMS and English biographer for Blessed Hanna Chrzanowska, RN; and Helena Matoga, RN, MA, Vice Postulator for the Cause of the Canonization of Blessed Hanna Chrzanowska, RN, each shared names and brief summaries of several Catholic nurses. I thank Dr. Brykczynska for reviewing several summaries and assisting me in understanding the nuances in translation when the online translation was not clear. I specially thank Helena Matoga for sharing, for this publication, the immense work and collaboration that is required across disciplines in order to move forward a Cause for canonization.

PREFACE

This book provides a biography of nurses who have been declared saints, blessed, venerable, servants of God and martyrs. In this preface the history of the beatification and canonization process is described along with a brief outline of each step. Since nursing licensure did not begin until the early 1900's, the next section describes how it was determined that an individual was a nurse and therefore should be included in this text. Lastly the organization of the text is explained.

The History of Beatification and Canonization

Saints are persons who have lived an exemplary life, a life of heroic virtue, or persons who have been recognized as suffering martyrdom for the Christian faith. The early Church did not have an established concept of "saints" or "canonization." The veneration of deceased Christians developed quite spontaneously, when active persecution of Christians began in the Roman Empire in the first century A.D. Christians buried those martyred for the faith and began paying tribute to them on the anniversary of their deaths with annual liturgical commemorations. This began as a local practice for specified saints, but some of the better known ones, like the 3rd century deacon, St. Lawrence, spread to other areas in the Christian world.

Due to concerns about veracity, in 1234, His Holiness Pope Gregory IX issued *Decretals,* in which he declared that Rome alone had the exclusive right to declare the holiness of a departed member of the faithful and canonize saints. Over 200 years later, in 1588[1] Pope Sixtus V created the Congregation of Rites which was to conduct the formal beatification and canonization process.

In 1634, Pope Urban forbade any public veneration (*cultus*) for a purported saint unless the person's miraculous life and actions were formally recognized by the Holy See through the Congregation of Rites. Additionally, through the decree *Caelestis Hierusalem cives,* Pope Urban specifically wrote that the *cultus* of anyone regarded as a saint would not be licit unless a review proved that he/she had been the object of an immemorial public veneration for at least one hundred years before the publication of the decree.

In 1969, Pope St. Paul VI divide the Congregation of Rites into two separate offices and the Congregation for the Causes of Saints now has jurisdiction over all beatification and canonization proceedings. In the next section, the steps in the canonization process are very briefly described. Prior to each section is a more in-depth explanation of each phase.[2]

Process of Beatification and Canonization:[2]

Initiation of the Process - Usually 5 years has passed since the death, but this can and has been waived.

Servant of God - Once a Cause for Beatification and Canonization has been allowed to be initiated with the approval of the Holy See, the individual is titled "Servant of God" and testimony is gathered about the life and virtue of the person. The diocesan tribunal reviews the volumes of documentation called *Positio* and, if approved at the local level, forwards it to the Congregation for the Causes of Saints (CCS).

Venerable - Once the person's heroic virtues are recognized by the Holy Father, they receive the title, "Venerable" and may be called either: Venerable Servant of God or simply Venerable.

Blessed (beatification) - a miracle attributed to the intercessory power of the individual must be recognized by both scientific and theological commissions established by the CCS. The final determination is made by the Congregation in Rome and forwarded to the Holy Father for approval. In the case of martyrdom, the miracle may be waived — martyrdom is considered a miracle of grace.

Saint (canonization) - a second miracle attributed to the intercessory power of the individual is required for canonization using the same process described above. The Holy Father usually presides over a canonization declaring that the person is with God and is an example for imitation of the faithful of following Christ worthily. Now that the history of and canonization process has been described, how were individuals chosen to be in this text.

Only those servants of God may be venerated by public cult who have been numbered by ecclesiastical authority among the Saints or the Blessed (Canon 1187). Servants of God who have not yet been canonized or beatified may be venerated in private (Canon 1187 annotation).[10]

What is a nurse? Who is a nurse?

Nurses care for the sick. They treat patient's response to illness, promote health, educate, conduct research, and serve in administrative roles. They provide care to individuals, family, communities and populations independently and in collaboration with physicians and other health care professionals. Advanced Practice Nurses, also called Medico-Social Assistants in Asia, diagnose and treat illness. Across the world nurse midwives deliver infants and provide women's healthcare. In the mid-1900's, my grandmother, a licensed practical nurse, delivered anesthesia for in-office surgical procedures. Today, masters and doctoral prepared Certified Registered Nurse Anesthetists deliver a much more complicated regimen of anesthetics during childbirth, surgical procedures and to treat pain.

According to the International Catholic Committee of Nurses and Medico-Assistants (CICIAMS), Catholic nurses promote health, alleviate suffering, prevent illness and promote and defend the human dignity. They are concerned for and respect the sacredness of every human life from the moment of conception until natural death.

How was it determined which individuals to include in this first edition? Initially nurses were training within religious orders, families and by another experienced nurse on-the-job. For instance, St. Marianne Cope learned nursing from the religious sisters who came into her home to care for her ailing father. Standardized science-based professional education of nurses began when, following Florence Nightingale's experience in the Crimean War, she established "The Nightingale Training School for Nurses" at St. Thomas' Hospital in England in 1860. Nurses across the world established nursing programs following Florence's design and began sharing best practices. Licensure and registration of nurses soon followed at the turn of the 20th century.

Prior to the formal education and licensure of nurses, the easiest way to determine if an individual was a nurse, was if the individuals was specifically called a nurse or noted for providing nursing care. For example, St. Fabiola (d. 399), who established the first hospital in Rome was recognized by St. Jerome in his *Letter to Oceanus* as providing nursing care, *"She was the first person to found a hospital, into which she might gather sufferers out of the streets, and where she might nurse the unfortunate victims of sickness and want..."*

If an individual was described as doing the duties of a nurse in a hospital, home or community and/or serving as an infirmarian, they were included. Some provided nursing care for a short period. For example St. Bernadette of Lourdes provided care in and was in charge of the infirmary at the Mother House in Nevers. She also spent considerable time as a patient there. Many who served as nurses, were later appointed to other roles such as the Superior General of their order or to work in another field (e.g. teaching vocational life skills). Others dedicated their life to the care of the sick, established hospices-hospitals and started schools of nursing. If a nurse, expanded their scope of practice to include minor surgical procedures, they were still considered a nurse. However, if a person was trained by a barber/surgeon, such as St. Martin de Porres, they were considered to be trained as a physician-surgeon and was therefore not included.

Several nurses started religious orders to care for the sick. Two were declared by Pope Pius XI, in 1930, to be the patron saints of nurses and nurses associations: St. Camillus de Lellis and St. John of God. St. Camillus de Lellis established an order initially known as "Servants of the Sick" and then the "Order of the Ministers of the Infirm" and now members are simply called the "Camilians." St. John of God is the founder of the Brothers Hospitallers of St. John of God. Two additional nurses of the Brothers Hospitallers have been beatified. I leave it to you to discover who they are...

Ten nurses from the Congregation of St. Elizabeth founded by Blessed Maria Luisa Merkert (1817-1872) to nurse cholera and typhus patients and who take a fourth vow "to assist the sick and most needy" were all included. These ten represent the hundreds of religious sisters from the Congregation martyred in east bloc countries during the Soviet occupation. Their individual histories were very short though three specifically listed their nursing duties. Here I erred on the side of including all ten.

Organization of the Text. Traditionally a text on saints is usually ordered by the saint's Memorial day. The nurses who have been canonized or beatified have memorial days which are usually the date of their birth into eternal life (bodily death) but not always. Those who have the title Venerable, Servant of God and New Martyrs do not yet have an assigned memorial day. Therefore, the individuals in this text are ordered by the year of their birth except for the groups of martyrs, who are listed by the year of their death.

Though the plan for this book was to include all nurse who have been canonized (saints), beatified (blesseds), declared venerable, servants of God or martyrs, some many have inadvertently been omitted. Please assist this effort by sending a short biography with references for any nurses recognized as saints or in the canonization process.

May God enrich your life as you learn about the lives of these nurses who have helped manifest God's Kingdom here on earth. May we follow their example.

Diana Ruzicka, RN, MSN, MA, MA, PHN, RN
(Nursing Administration & Oncology, Strategic Studies,
Theology, Public Health Nursing, Registered Nurse)

SAINTS

Canonization

St. Fabiola (Italy-Rome) (d. 399)

She was the first person to found a hospital,
into which she might gather sufferers out of the streets,
and where she might nurse the unfortunate victims of sickness and want...
Often did she carry on her own shoulders persons
infected with jaundice or with filth.
Often too did she wash away the matter
discharged from wounds which others,
even though men, could not bear to look at.
She gave food to her patients with her own hand,
and moistened the scarce breathing lips of the dying with sips of liquid.
---St. Jerome, (399AD, Letter 77, 6)---

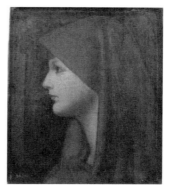

St. Fabiola (d 399) was a lay widow who divorced her husband for his dissolute life, and remarried. Estranged from the Church, upon the death of her second husband, she returned to the Church, devoted herself to charitable works and aiding churches. She built the first Christian public hospital in the West. There she personally tended the sick. According to her contemporary, St. Jerome, "She was the first person to found a hospital, where she might gather sufferers from the streets and where she might nurse the unfortunate victims of sickness and want."
(Memorial - December 27)

Letter LXXVII. To Oceanus:[1]
　　　　The eulogy of Fabiola whose restless life had come to an end in 399 A.D. Jerome tells the story of her sin and of her penitence (for which see Letter LV), of the hospital established by her at Portus, of her visit to Bethlehem, and of her earnestness in the study of Scripture. He relates how he wrote for her his account of the vestments of the high priest (Letter LXIV) and how, at the time of her death, he was at her request engaged upon a commentary on the forty-two halting-places of the Israelites in the wilderness (Letter LXXIX). This last he now sends along with this letter to Oceanus. Jerome also bestows praise upon Pammachius as the companion of all Fabiola's labours. The date of the letter is 399 A.D.

1. Several years since I consoled the venerated Paula, whilst her affliction was still recent for the falling asleep of Blaesilla (Letter XXXIX). Four summers ago I wrote for the bishop Heliodorus the epitaph of Nepotian, and expended what ability I possessed in giving expression to my grief at his loss (Letter LX). Only two years have elapsed since I sent a brief letter to my dear Pammachius on the sudden flitting of his Paulina (Letter LXVI). I blushed to say more to one so learned or to give him back his own thoughts: lest I should seem less the consoler of a friend than the officious instructor of one already perfect. But now, Oceanus my son, the duty that you lay upon me is one that I gladly accept and would even seek unasked. For when new virtues have to be dealt with, an old subject itself becomes new. In previous cases I have had to soften and restrain a mother's affection, an uncle's grief, and a husband's yearning; according to the different requirements of each I have had to apply from scripture different remedies.

2. Today you give me as my theme Fabiola, the praise of the Christians, the marvel of the gentiles, the sorrow of the poor, and the consolation of the monks. Whatever point in her character I choose to treat of first, pales into insignificance compared with those which follow after. Shall I praise her fasts? Her alms are greater still. Shall I commend her lowliness? The glow of her faith is yet brighter. Shall I mention her studied plainness in dress, her voluntary choice of plebeian costume and the garb of a slave that she might put to shame silken robes? To change one's disposition is a greater achievement than to change one's dress. It is harder for us to part with arrogance than with gold and gems. For, even though we throw away these, we plume ourselves sometimes on a meanness that is really ostentatious, and we make a bid with a saleable poverty for the popular applause. But a virtue that seeks concealment and is cherished in the inner consciousness appeals to no judgement but that of God. Thus the eulogies which I have to bestow upon Fabiola will be altogether new: I must neglect the order of the rhetoricians and begin all I have to say only from the cradle of her conversion and of her penitence. Another writer, mindful of the school, would perhaps bring forward Quintus Maximus, "the man who by delaying rescued Rome," (Ennius) and the whole Fabian family; he would describe their struggles and battles and would exult that Fabiola had come to us through a line so noble, shewing that qualities not apparent in the branch still existed in the root. But as I am a lover of the inn at Bethlehem and of the Lord's stable in which the virgin travailed with and gave birth to an infant God, I shall deduce the lineage of Christ's

16

handmaid not from a stock famous in history but from the lowliness of the church.

3. And because at the very outset there is a rock in the path and she is overwhelmed by a storm of censure, for having forsaken her first husband and having taken a second, I will not praise her for her conversion till I have first cleared her of this charge. So terrible then were the faults imputed to her former husband that not even a prostitute or a common slave could have put up with them. If I were to recount them, I should undo the heroism of the wife who chose to bear the blame of a separation rather than to blacken the character and expose the stains of him who was one body with her. I will only urge this one plea which is sufficient to exonerate a chaste matron and a Christian woman. The Lord has given commandment that a wife must not be put away "except it be for fornication, and that, if put away, she must remain unmarried" (Mt 19:9; 1 Cor 7:11). Now a commandment which is given to men logically applies to women also. For it cannot be that, while an adulterous wife is to be put away, an incontinent husband is to be retained. The apostle says: "he which is joined to an harlot is one body" (1 Cor 6:16). Therefore she also who is joined to a whoremonger and unchaste person is made one body with him. The laws of Caesar are different, it is true, from the laws of Christ: Papinianus[1] commands one thing; our own Paul another. Earthly laws give a free rein to the unchastity of men, merely condemning seduction and adultery; lust is allowed to range unrestrained among brothels and slave girls, as if the guilt were constituted by the rank of the person assailed and not by the purpose of the assailant. But with us Christians what is unlawful for women is equally unlawful for men, and as both serve the same God both are bound by the same obligations. Fabiola then has put away-they are quite right-a husband that was a sinner, guilty of this and that crime, sins-I have almost mentioned their names-with which the whole neighbourhood resounded but which the wife alone refused to disclose. If however it is made a charge against her that after repudiating her husband she did not continue unmarried, I readily admit this to have been a fault, but at the same time declare that it may have been a case of necessity. "It is better," the apostle tells us, "to marry than to burn" (1 Cor 7:9). She was quite a young woman, she was not able to continue in widowhood. In the words

---

[1]A Roman jurist of great renown who held high legal office first under Marcus Aurelius and afterwards under Severus. He was put to death by Caracalla.

17

of the apostle she saw another law in her members warring against the law of her mind; (Rm 7:23) she felt herself dragged in chains as a captive towards the indulgences of wedlock. Therefore she thought it better openly to confess her weakness and to accept the semblance of an unhappy marriage than, with the flame of a monogamist, to ply the trade of a courtesan. The same apostle wills that the younger widows should marry, bear children, and give no occasion to the adversary to speak reproachfully (1 Tim 5:14) And he at once goes on to explain his wish: "for some are already turned aside after Satan" (1 Tim 5:15). Fabiola therefore was fully persuaded in her own mind: she thought she had acted legitimately in putting away her husband, and that when she had done so she was free to marry again. She did not know that the rigour of the gospel takes away from women all pretexts for re-marriage so long as their former husbands are alive; and not knowing this, though she contrived to evade other assaults of the devil, she at this point unwittingly exposed herself to a wound from him.

4. But why do I linger over old and forgotten matters, seeking to excuse a fault for which Fabiola has herself confessed her penitence? Who would believe that, after the death of her second husband at a time when most widows, having shaken off the yoke of servitude, grow careless and allow themselves more liberty than ever, frequenting the baths, flitting through the streets, shewing their harlot faces everywhere; that at this time Fabiola came to herself? Yet it was then that she put on sackcloth to make public confession of her error. It was then that in the presence of all Rome (in the basilica which formerly belonged to that Lateranus who perished by the sword of Caesar[2]) she stood in the ranks of the penitents and exposed before bishop, presbyters, and people-all of whom wept when they saw her weep-her disheveled hair, pale features, soiled hands and unwashed neck. What sins would such a penance fail to purge away? What ingrained stains would such tears be unable to wash out? By a threefold confession Peter blotted out his threefold denial (Jn 18:15-27; Jn 21:15-17), If Aaron committed sacrilege by fashioning molten gold into the head of a calf, his brother's prayers made amends for his transgressions (Ex 32:30-35). If holy David, meekest of men, committed the double sin of murder and adultery, he atoned for it by a fast of

---

[2] A senator who having conspired against Nero was by that emperor put to death. His palace on the Aelian Hill was long afterwards bestowed by Constantine upon pope Silvester who made it a church which it has ever since remained.

seven days. He lay upon the earth, he rolled in the ashes, he forgot his royal power, he sought for light in the darkness (2 Sam 12:16). And then, turning his eyes to that God whom he had so deeply offended, he cried with a lamentable voice: "Against thee, thee only, have I sinned, and done this evil in thy sight," and "Restore unto me the joy of thy salvation and uphold me with thy free spirit" Ps. 101:4; Ps 101:12). He who by his virtues teaches me how to stand and not to fall, by his penitence teaches me how, if I fall, I may rise again. Among the kings do we read of any so wicked as Ahab, of whom the scripture says: "there was none like unto Ahab which did sell himself to work wickedness in the sight of the Lord"? (1 Kings 21:25). For shedding Naboth's blood Elijah rebuked him, and the prophet denounced God's wrath against him: "Hast thou killed and also taken possession? ...behold I will bring evil upon thee and will take away thy posterity" (1Kgs 21:19, 1 Kgs 21:21) and so on. Yet when Ahab heard these words "he rent his clothes, and put sackcloth upon his flesh, and fasted ...in sackcloth, and went softly" (1 Kgs 21:27). Then came the word of God to Elijah the Tishbite saying: "Seest thou how Ahab humbleth himself before me? Because he humbleth himself before me, I will not bring the evil in his days" 1Kgs 21:28; 1Kgs21:29). O happy penitence which has drawn down upon itself the eyes of God, and which has by confessing its error changed the sentence of God's anger! The same conduct is in the Chronicles (2 Chr. 33:12; 2 Chr 33:13) attributed to Manasseh, and in the book of the prophet Jonah (Jon 3:5-10) to Nineveh, and in the gospel to the publican (Lk 18:13). The first of these not only was allowed to obtain forgiveness but also recovered his kingdom, the second broke the force of God's impending wrath, while the third, smiting his breast with his hands, "would not lift up so much as his eyes to heaven." Yet for all that the publican with his humble confession of his faults went back justified far more than the Pharisee with his arrogant boasting of his virtues. This is not however the place to preach penitence, neither am I writing against Montanus and Novatus.[3] Else would I say of it that it is "a sacrifice ...well pleasing to God," (Ph 4:18) I would cite the words of the psalmist: "the sacrifices of God are a broken spirit," (Ps. 101:17) and those of Ezekiel "I prefer the repentance of a sinner rather than his death," (cf. Ez 18:23) and those of Baruch, "Arise, arise, O Jerusalem," (Bar 5:5, cf. Is 110:1) and many other proclamations

---

[3]Rigourists who denied the power of the Church to absolve persons who had fallen into sin.

19

made by the trumpets of the prophets.

5. But this one thing I will say, for it is at once useful to my readers and pertinent to my present theme. As Fabiola was not ashamed of the Lord on earth, so He shall not be ashamed of her in heaven (Lk 9:26). She laid bare her wound to the gaze of all, and Rome beheld with tears the disfiguring scar which marred her beauty. She uncovered her limbs, bared her head, and closed her mouth. She no longer entered the church of God but, like Miriam the sister of Moses, (Nu 12:14) she sat apart without the camp, till the priest who had cast her out should himself call her back. She came down like the daughter of Babylon from the throne of her daintiness, she took the millstones and ground meal, she passed barefooted through rivers of tears (Is 47:1-2). She sat upon the coals of fire, and these became her aid (Is 47:14 Vulgate). That face by which she had once pleased her second husband she now smote with blows; she hated jewels, shunned ornaments and could not bear to look upon fine linen. In fact she bewailed the sin she had committed as bitterly as if it had been adultery, and went to the expense of many remedies in her eagerness to cure her one wound.

6. Having found myself aground in the shallows of Fabiola's sin, I have dwelt thus long upon her penitence in order that I might open up a larger and quite unimpeded space for the description of her praises. Restored to communion before the eyes of the whole church, what did she do? In the day of prosperity she was not forgetful of affliction; (Ecc. 11:25) and, having once suffered shipwreck she was unwilling again to face the risks of the sea. Instead therefore of re-embarking on her old life, she broke up and sold all that she could lay hands on of her property (it was large and suitable to her rank), and turning it into money she laid out this for the benefit of the poor. She was the first person to found a hospital, into which she might gather sufferers out of the streets, and where she might nurse the unfortunate victims of sickness and want. Need I now recount the various ailments of human beings? Need I speak of noses slit, eyes put out, feet half burnt, hands covered with sores? Or of limbs dropsical and atrophied? Or of diseased flesh alive with worms? Often did she carry on her own shoulders persons infected with jaundice or with filth. Often too did she wash away the matter discharged from wounds which others, even though men, could not bear to look at. She gave food to her patients with her own hand, and moistened the scarce breathing lips of the dying with sips of liquid. I know of many wealthy and devout persons who, unable to overcome their natural repugnance to such sights, perform this work of mercy by the agency of others, giving money instead of personal aid. I do not

blame them and am far from construing their weakness of resolution into a want of faith. While however I pardon such squeamishness, I extol to the skies the enthusiastic zeal of a mind that is above it. A great faith makes little of such trifles. But I know how terrible was the retribution which fell upon the proud mind of the rich man clothed in purple for not having helped Lazarus (Lk 16:19-24). The poor wretch whom we despise, whom we cannot so much as look at, and the very sight of whom turns our stomachs, is human like ourselves, is made of the same clay as we are, is formed out of the same elements. All that he suffers we too may suffer. Let us then regard his wounds as though they were our own, and then all our insensibility to another's suffering will give way before our pity for ourselves.

Not with a hundred tongues or throat of bronze, could I exhaust the forms of fell disease (Virg. Aen. 6, 625-627) which Fabiola so wonderfully alleviated in the suffering poor that many of the healthy fell to envying the sick. However she showed the same liberality towards the clergy and monks and virgins. Was there a monastery which was not supported by Fabiola's wealth? Was there a naked or bedridden person who was not clothed with garments supplied by her? Were there ever any in want to whom she failed to give a quick and unhesitating supply? Even Rome was not wide enough for her pity. Either in her own person or else through the agency of reverend and trustworthy men she went from island to island and carried her bounty not only round the Etruscan Sea, but throughout the district of the Volscians, as it stands along those secluded and winding shores where communities of monks are to be found.

7. Suddenly she made up her mind, against the advice of all her friends, to take ship and to come to Jerusalem. Here she was welcomed by a large concourse of people and for a short time took advantage of my hospitality. Indeed, when I call to mind our meeting, I seem to see her here now instead of in the past. Blessed Jesus, what zeal, what earnestness she bestowed upon the sacred volumes! In her eagerness to satisfy what was a veritable craving she would run through Prophets, Gospels, and Psalms: she would suggest questions and treasure up the answers in the desk of her own bosom. And yet this eagerness to hear did not bring with it any feeling of satiety: increasing her knowledge she also increased her sorrow, (Eccl. 1:18) and by casting oil upon the flame she did but supply fuel for a still more burning zeal. One day we had before us the book of Numbers written by Moses, and she modestly questioned me as to the meaning of the great mass of names there to be found. Why was it, she inquired, that single tribes were

21

differently associated in this passage and in that, how came it that the soothsayer Balaam in prophesying of the future mysteries of Christ (Nu. 24:15-19) spoke more plainly of Him than almost any other prophet? I replied as best I could and tried to satisfy her enquiries. Then unrolling the book still farther she came to the passage (Nu. 33) in which is given the list of all the halting-places by which the people after leaving Egypt made its way to the waters of Jordan. And when she asked me the meaning and reason of each of these, I spoke doubtfully about some, dealt with others in a tone of assurance, and in several instances simply confessed my ignorance. Hereupon she began to press me harder still, expostulating with me as though it were a thing unallowable that I should be ignorant of what I did not know, yet at the same time affirming her own unworthiness to understand mysteries so deep. In a word I was ashamed to refuse her request and allowed her to extort from me a promise that I would devote a special work to this subject for her use. Till the present time I have had to defer the fulfilment of my promise: as I now perceive, by the Will of God in order that it should be consecrated to her memory. As in a previous work (Letter LXIV) I clothed her with the priestly vestments, so in the pages of the present (Letter LXXVIII on the Mansions or Halting-places of Israel in the Desert) she may rejoice that she has passed through the wilderness of this world and has come at last to the land of promise.

8. But let me continue the task which I have begun. Whilst I was in search of a suitable dwelling for so great a lady, whose only conception of the solitary life included a place of resort like Mary's inn; suddenly messengers flew this way and that and the whole East was terror-struck. For news came that the hordes of the Huns had poured forth all the way from Maeotis (The Sea of Azov) (they had their haunts between the icy Tanais (The Don) and the rude Massagetae (An Asiatic tribe to the East of the Caspian Sea) where the gates of Alexander keep back the wild peoples behind the Caucasus); and that, speeding hither and thither on their nimble-footed horses, they were filling all the world with panic and bloodshed. The Roman army was absent at the time, being detained in Italy on account of the civil wars. Of these Huns Herodotus (Hdt. 1:106 of the Scythians) tells us that under Darius King of the Medes they held the East in bondage for twenty years and that from the Egyptians and Ethiopians they exacted a yearly tribute. May Jesus avert from the Roman world the farther assaults of these wild beasts! Everywhere their approach was unexpected, they outstripped rumour in speed, and, when they came, they spared neither religion nor rank nor age, even for wailing infants they had

22

no pity. Children were forced to die before it could be said that they had begun to live; and little ones not realizing their miserable fate might be seen smiling in the hands and at the weapons of their enemies. It was generally agreed that the goal of the invaders was Jerusalem and that it was their excessive desire for gold which made them hasten to this particular city. Its walls uncared for in time of peace were accordingly put in repair. Antioch was in a state of siege. Tyre, desirous of cutting itself off from the land, sought once more its ancient island. We too were compelled to marl our ships and to lie off the shore as a precaution against the arrival of our foes. No matter how hard the winds might blow, we could not but dread the barbarians more than shipwreck. It was not, however, so much for our own safety that we were anxious as for the chastity of the virgins who were with us. Just at that time also there was dissension among us,[4] and our intestine struggles threw into the shade our battle with the barbarians. I myself clung to my long-settled abode in the East and gave way to my deep-seated love for the holy places. Fabiola, used as she was to moving from city to city and having no other property but what her baggage contained, returned to her native land; to live in poverty where she had once been rich, to lodge in the house of another, she who in old days had lodged many guests in her own, and-not unduly to prolong my account-to bestow upon the poor before the eyes of Rome the proceeds of that property which Rome knew her to have sold.

9. This only do I lament that in her the holy places lost a necklace of the loveliest. Rome recovered what it had previously parted with, and the wanton and slanderous tongues of the heathen were confuted by the testimony of their own eyes. Others may commend her pity, her humility, her faith: I will rather praise her ardour of soul. The letter (Letter XIV) in which as a young man I once urged Heliodorus to the life of a hermit she knew by heart, and whenever she looked upon the walls of Rome she complained that she was in a prison. Forgetful of her sex, unmindful of her frailty, and only desiring to be alone she was in fact there[5] where her soul lingered. The counsels of her friends could not hold her back; so eager was she to burst from the city as from a place of bondage. Nor did she leave the distribution of her alms to others; she distributed them herself. Her wish was that, after equitably

---

[4]The Origenistic controversy in which Jerome, Paula and Epiphanius took one side, John bishop of Jerusalem, Rufinus, and Melania the other.
[5]i.e. in the desert where many women lived as solitares.

dispensing her money to the poor, she might herself find support from others for the sake of Christ. In such haste was she and so impatient of delay that you would fancy her on the eve of her departure. As she was always ready, death could not find her unprepared.

10. As I pen her praises, my dear Pammachius seems suddenly to rise before me. His wife Paulina sleeps that he may keep vigil; she has gone before her husband that he remaining behind may be Christ's servant. Although he was his wife's heir, others-I mean the poor-are now in possession of his inheritance. He and Fabiola contended for the privilege of setting up a tent like that of Abraham[6] at Portus. The contest which arose between them was for the supremacy in showing kindness. Each conquered and each was overcome. Both admitted themselves to be at once victors and vanquished for what each had desired to effect alone both accomplished together. They united their resources and combined their plans that harmony might forward what rivalry must have brought to nought. No sooner was the scheme broached than it was carried out. A house was purchased to serve as a shelter, and a crowd flocked into it. "There was no more travail in Jacob nor distress in Israel" (Num 23:21). The seas carried voyagers to find a welcome here on landing. Travelers left Rome in haste to take advantage of the mild coast before setting sail. What Publius once did in the island of Malta for one apostle and-not to leave room for gainsaying-for a single ship's crew, (Acts 28:7). Fabiola and Pammachius have done over and over again for large numbers; and not only have they supplied the wants of the destitute, but so universal has been their munificence that they have provided additional means for those who have something already. The whole world knows that a home for strangers has been established at Portus; and Britain has learned in the summer what Egypt and Parthia knew in the spring.

11. In the death of this noble lady we have seen a fulfilment of the apostle's words:-"All things work together for good to them that fear God" (Rm 8:28).[7] Having a presentiment of what would happen, she had written to several monks to come and release her from the burthen under which she labored;[8] for she wished to make to herself friends of the mammon of

---

[6]Like that in which Abraham entertained the angels. See Letter LXVI. 11.
[7]Note that Jerome substitutes fear for love.
[8]The remnant of her fortune.

24

unrighteousness that they might receive her into everlasting habitations (Lk 16:9). They came to her and she made them her friends; she fell asleep in the way that she had wished, and having at last laid aside her burthen she soared more lightly up to heaven. How great a marvel Fabiola had been to Rome while she lived came out in the behavior of the people now that she was dead. Hardly had she breathed her last breath, hardly had she given back her soul to Christ whose it was when Flying Rumor heralding the woe (Virg. A. 11:139) gathered the entire city to attend her obsequies. Psalms were chanted and the gilded ceilings of the temples were shaken with uplifted shouts of Alleluia.

The choirs of young and old extolled her deeds and sang the praises of her holy soul (Virg. A. 8:287, 288). Her triumph was more glorious far than those won by Furius over the Gauls, by Papirius over the Samnites, by Scipio over Numantia, by Pompey over Pontus. They had conquered physical force, she had mastered spiritual iniquities (Eph. 6:12). I seem to hear even now the squadrons which led the van of the procession, and the sound of the feet of the multitude which thronged in thousands to attend her funeral. The streets, porches, and roofs from which a view could be obtained were inadequate to accommodate the spectators. On that day Rome saw all her peoples gathered together in one, and each person present flattered himself that he had some part in the glory of her penitence. No wonder indeed that men should thus exult in the salvation of one at whose conversion there was joy among the angels in heaven (Lk 15:7; Lk 15:10).

12. I give you this, Fabiola, (Letter LXXVIII) the best gift of my aged powers, to be as it were a funeral offering. Oftentimes have I praised virgins and widows and married women who have kept their garments always white (Eccl 9:8; Rev 3:4) and who follow the Lamb whithersoever He goeth (Rev 14:4). Happy indeed is she in her encomium who throughout her life has been stained by no defilement. But let envy depart and censoriousness be silent. If the father of the house is good why should our eye be evil? (Mt 20:15) The soul which fell among thieves has been carried home upon the shoulders of Christ (Lk 10:30; Lk 15:5). In our father's house are many mansions (Jn 14:2). Where sin hath abounded, grace hath much more abounded (Rm 5:20). To whom more is forgiven the same loveth more (Lk 7:47).

Reference:

1) The Letter of St. Jerome (399 AD). Letter 77 to Oceanus (article 6). https://www.tertullian.org/fathers2/NPNF2-06/Npnf2-06-03.htm#P3201_835203 (accessed January 19, 2022).

St. Radegund (Thuringia [*modern Germany*]/France) (518-587)

Queen of France Radegund cared for the poor, the sick and captives.
She founded a hospital for lepers, whom she waited on herself,
and was one day seen kissing their diseased bodies.
(Patroness of the 1st Council of Catholic Nurses in the United States
founded in Boston in 1909)

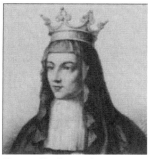

Queen Radegund
Source: catholicculture.org

St. Radegund (also known as [aka] Radegundes) was born in 518, probably in Erfurt, Thuringia, current day, Germany. She was a princess and the daughter of the King of Thuringia, Berthaire, a pagan, who was assassinated by his brother, Hermenefrid. In 531 Theodoric, King of Austrasia, and his half-brother, Clotaire I, King of Neustria, attacked Hermenefrid, vanquished him, and carried home a great booty. Among the prisoners was Radegund, who was twelve years old. King Clotaire received her as his booty, caused her to have a Christian education and had her baptized.

From the time of her baptism, she exhibited Christian virtue: fed the poor whom she personally served, and had a dedicated prayer and penitential life. She desired to remain a virgin but was required to marry King Clotaire. She fulfilled her duties of state while continuing her pious exercises. Her piety upset the king who stated he had married a nun rather than a queen, who had converted his court to a monastery. She bore these criticisms with patience and humility. She cared for the sick, poor and captives. She founded a hospital for lepers, whom she waited on herself.[1] When King Clotaire had Radegund's brother assassinated, in an effort to seize his holding in Thuringia, Queen Radegund begged his leave to retire from court, which he granted.

Radegund moved to Sais, an estate of the king's in Poitou. She lived an austere life and gave almost her whole income to serve the poor. She had a monastery built in Poitiers, funded by the King, and overseen by a holy virgin, Agnes, the first abbess. When King Clotaire repented of having allowed his wife to leave court, he went, with his son, Sigebert, to retrieve her. Queen Radegund wrote the bishop of Paris, St. Germanus requesting his assistance. He

27

interceded and the King repented of his intent and returned to court without Queen Radegund. She collaborated with Abbess Agnes to establish the rule of St. Caesarius of Arles at the monastery of the Holy Cross, where she lived with over 200 nuns, some of whom where daughters of senators and some of royal blood.

In the year 560 AD, Clotaire, who was the fourth son of Clovis the great (466-511), became the sole king of France. He repented at the tomb of St. Martin in Tours in the last year of his life. He is reported to have said at the last moments before his death, "How powerful is the heavenly king, by whose command the greatest monarchs of the earth resign their life!" King Clotaire died in 561 AD after reigning fifty years. His four sons divided the kingdom and Childebert, her grandson, following the death of his father and two uncles, served as a protector of his grandmother, Radegund, until her death on August 13, 587 AD. St. Gregory, Archbishop of Tours performed the funeral Holy Sacrifice of the Mass and interment.

At her funeral a blindman recovered his sight and many miracles occurred at her tomb. Her bones were enshrined in the Church of Our Lady in Poitiers, France until they were dispersed by the Huguenots. (Memorial - August 13).

St. Radegundes, Queen of France, from Rev. Alban Butler's (1883) Lives of Saints (*with permission* from Loreto Publications):

> She was daughter of Bertaire, a pagan king of part of Thuringia in Germany, who was assassinated by his brother Hermenfred. Theodoric, or Thierry, king of Austrasia, or Metz, and his brother Clotaire I, then king of Soissons, fell upon Hermenfred, vanquished him, and carried home a great booty. Among the prisoners, Radegundes, then about twelve years old, fell to the lot of king Clotaire, who gave her an education suitable to her birth, and caused her to be instructed in the Christian religion and baptized. The great mysteries of our holy faith made such an impression on her tender soul, that, from the moment of her baptism, she gave herself to God with her whole heart, abridged her meals to feed the poor, whom she served with her own hands, and made prayer, humiliations, and austerities her whole delight. It was her earnest desire to serve God in the state of perpetual virginity; but was obliged at length to acquiesce in the king's desire to marry her. Being by this exaltation become a great queen, she

28

continued no less an enemy to sloth and vanity then she was before, and she divided her time chiefly between her oratory, the church, and the care of the poor. She also kept long fasts, and during Lent wore a hair-cloth under her rich garments. Clotaire was at first pleased with her devotions, and allowed her full liberty in them; but afterward, by ambition and other passions, his affections began to be alienated from her, and he used frequently to reproach her for her pious exercises, saying, he had married a nun rather than a queen, who converted his court into a monastery. His complaints were unjust; for she made it one of the first points of her devotion never to be wanting in any duty of her state, and to show the king all possible complaisance. She repaid injuries only with patience and greater courtesy and condescension, doing all the good in her power to those who were her declared enemies in prepossessing her husband against her. Clotaire at length caused her brother to be treacherously assassinated, that he might seize on his dominions in Thuringia. Radegundes, shocked at this base act of inhumanity, asked his leave to retire from court, which she easily obtained. Clotaire himself sent her to Noyon, that she might receive the religious veil from the hands of St. Medard. The holy prelate scrupled to do it for some time, because she was a married woman; but was at length prevailed upon to consecrate her a deaconess.

Radegundes first withdrew to Sais, an estate which the king had given her in Poitou, living wholly on bread made of rye and barley, and on roots and pulse, and never drinking any wine; and her bed was a piece of sackcloth spread upon ashes. She employed almost her whole revenue in alms, and served the poor with her own hands. She wore next to her skin a chain which had been given her by St. Junian, a holy priest in that country, whom she furnished with clothes worked with her own hands. St. Radegundes went some time after to Poitiers, and there, by the orders of king Clotaire, built a great monastery of nuns, in which she procured a holy virgin, named Agnes, to be made the first abbess, and paid to her an implicit obedience in all things, not reserving to herself the disposal of the least thing. Not long after, king Clotaire, repenting that he had consented to her taking the veil, went as far as Tours with his son Sigebert, upon a religious pretense, but intending to proceed to Poitiers, and carry her again to court. She was alarmed at the news, and wrote to St. Germanus of Paris, desiring him to divert so great an evil. The bishop having received her letter, went to the king, and throwing himself at his feet before the tomb of St. Martin, conjured him, with tears, in the name of God, not to go to Poitiers. The king, at the same time, prostrated himself before St. Germanus, beseeching him that

29

Radesgundes would pray that God would pardon that wicked design, to which he said he had been prompted by evil advice. The same lively faith which made the saint pass with joy from the court to a cloister, and from the throne to a poor cell, filled her with alarms when she heard of her danger of being called again to a court. Her happiness seemed complete when she saw herself securely fixed in her solitude.

Being desirous to perpetuate the work of God, she wrote to a council of bishops that was assembled at Tours in 566, entreating them to confirm the foundation of her monastery, which they did under the most severe censures. She had already enriched the church she had built with the relics of a great number of saints; but was very desirous to procure a particle of the true cross of our Redeemer, and sent certain clerks to Constantinople, to the emperor Justin, for that purpose. The emperor readily sent her a piece of that sacred wood adorned with gold and precious stones; also a book of the four gospels beautified in the same manner, and the relics of several saints. They were carried into Poitiers, and deposited in the church of the monastery by the archbishop of Tours in the most solemn manner, with a great procession, wax tapers, incense, and singing of psalms. It was on that occasion that Venantius Fortunatus composed the hymn, *Vexilla regius prodeunt*. St. Radesgundes had invited him and several other holy and learned men to Poitiers; was herself a scholar, and read both the Latin and Greek fathers. She established in her monastery of the Holy cross the rule of St. Caesarius of Arles, a copy of which she procured from St. Caesaria II, abbess of St. John's at Arles. She probably took that name from St. Caesesaria, sister of St. Caesesarius, first abbess of that house, who died in 524. She was her worthy successor in all her great virtues, no less than in her dignity; and her admirable sanctity is much extolled by Fortunatus. She excelled particularly in holy prudence, which, as St. Ambrose remarks, must be, as it were, the salt to season all other virtues, which cannot be perfect or true without it. St. Caesaria sent to St. Radegundes, together with the copy of this rule, an excellent letter of advice, most useful to all superiors and others, which has been lately published by Don. Martenne. In it she says that persons who desire sincerely to serve God, must apply themselves earnestly to holy prayers, begging continually of God that he be pleased to make known to them his holy will, and direct them to follow it in all things; that they must, in the next place, diligently hear, read, and meditate on the word of God, which is a doctrine infinitely more precious than that of men, and a mind which can never be exhausted; that they must never cease praising God, and giving him

30

thanks for his mercies; that they must give alms to the utmost of their abilities, and must practice austerities according to the rules of obedience and discretion. She prescribes that every nun shall learn the psalter by heart, and be able to read; and she gives the strictest caution to be watchful against all particular fond friendships or familiarities in communities. St. Radegundes, not satisfied with these instructions, took with her Agnes, the abbess of her monastery, and made a journey to Arles, more perfectly to acquaint herself with the obligations of her rule. Being returned to Poitiers, she assisted Agnes in settling the discipline of her house.

In the year 560, Clotaire, who was the fourth son of Clovis the Great, became sole king of France, his three brothers and their sons being all dead. In the last year of his reign he went to the tomb of St. Martin at Tours, carrying with him very rich gifts. He there enumerated all the sins of his past life, and with deep groans, besought the holy confessor to implore God's mercy in his behalf. He founded St. Medard's abbey at Soissons, and gave great marks of a sincere repentance. Yet during his last illness, he showed great alarm and disturbance of mind at the remembrance of the crimes he had committed, and said in his last moments:"How powerful is the heavenly king, by whose command the greatest monarchs of the earth resign their life!" He died in 561, having reigned fifty years. His four sons divided his kingdom; Charibert, who reigned at Paris, had the Isle of France, Anjou, Maine, Touraine, Poitou, Guienne, and Languedoc. Chilperic resided at Soissons, and enjoyed Picardy, Normandy, and all the Low Countries. Gontran was king of Orleans, and his dominions were extended to the source of the Loire, and comprised also Provence, Dauphine, and Savoy. Austrasia fell to Sigebert, and comprehended Lorraine, Champagne, Auvergne, and some provinces in Germany. Charibert lived but a short time; and the civil wars between Sigebert, married to Brunehault, and Chilperic, whose concubine was the famous Fredegonda, distracted all France. Childebert, son of Sigebert and Brunehault, after the death of his father, and two uncles Chilperic and Gontran, became sovereign of Austrasia, Orleans, and Paris and continued, as his father had always been, a great protector of St. Radegundes, and her monastery of the Holy Cross, in which she had assembled two hundred nuns, among whom were several daughters of senators, and some of royal blood. The holy foundress, amidst all the storms, that disturbed the kingdom, enjoyed a perfect tranquility in her secure harbor, and died in the year 587, the twelfth of king Childebert, on the 13th of August, on which day the Church honors her memory. St. Gregory, archbishop of Tours, went to Poitiers upon the news of her death, and, the

31

bishop of Poitiers being absent, performed the funeral office at her interment.

The nun Baudonivia, who had received her education under St. Radegundes, and was present at her burial, relates that during it a blind man recovered his sight. Many other miracles were performed at the tomb of this saint. Her relics lay in the church of our Lady at Poitiers till they were dispersed by the Huguenots, together with those of St. Hilary, in 1562. See her life written by Fortunatus of Poitiers, her chaplain; and a second book added to the same by the nun Baudonivia, her disciple. See also St. Gregory of tours, Hist. Fr. 1. 3, c. 4, 7, etc.. and 1. De Glor. Conf. C. 23. On her life compiled by Hildebert, bishop of Mans, afterward archbishop of Tours, who died in 1134, see Mabillon, Annual. At. 1, p. 298. Hildebert has borrowed every part of this history from Fortunatus and Baudonivia, but given a more elegant turn tot he style. Obscure passages he has passed over. (Butler, Vol 5, p164-169)

References:

1) Herbert J. Thurston, S.J. & Donald Attwater (1956), *Butler's Lives of the Saints*, Vol III. Notre Dame, Indiana, Christian Classics, 318-320.

2) Father Alban Butler (1883). *Lives of the Saints*. V.5. Re-published by Loreto Publications, Fitzwilliam, New Hampshire (2020). Vol 5. p 164-169.

3) New Advent Catholic Encyclopedia. Accessed 20 May 2022. https://www.newadvent.org/cathen/04070a.htm

St. Bertille (France) (d. 703)
Infirmarian[1]

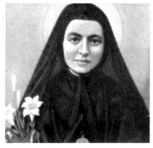

St. Bertille was a Benedictine nun at the convent in Jouarre, Brie, France. Born of one of the most illustrious families in the territory of Soissons (modern day France) She served as the infirmarian (nurse) and convent school headmistress. She was the first Prioress of the Abbey at Chelles after St. Bathildis, the wife of King Clovis II (Reigned 638-656). She refounded the convent-abbey around 646 AD. Several Merovingian princesses and many Anglo-Saxon noble women entered the convent including: St. Bathildis and Queen Hereswith,[2] the widow of the king of the East Angles.

St. Bertille, Abbess of Chelles (November 5), from the *original* Rev. Alban Butler's (1883) Lives of Saints:

> St. Bertille was born of one of the most illustrious families in the territory of Soissons, in the reign of Dagobert I, and by her piety acquired the true nobility of the children of God. From her infancy she preferred the love of God to that of creatures , shunned as much as possible the company and amusements of the world, and employed her time in serious duties, and chiefly in holy prayer. As she grew up, by relishing daily more and more the sweetness of conversing with God, she learned perfectly to despise the world, and earnestly desired to renounce it. Not daring to discover this inclination to her parents, she first opened herself to St. Ouen, by whom she was encouraged in her resolution; but they both took some time to pray to the Father of lights, that He would guide her according to his holy will, and manifest by what spirit she was directed; knowing that every impulse is not from the Holy Ghost. Self-love early disguises itself in every shape, and the devil often transforms himself into an angel of light. Not to be deceived through precipitation and rashness, in so important a choice as that of a state of life, impartial advice, prayer, careful self-examination and mature deliberation are necessary. These means having been employed, the saint's parents were made acquainted with her desire, which God inclined them not to oppose. They conducted her to Jouarre, a great monastery in Brie, four leagues from Meaux, founded not long before, about the year 630, by Ado, the elder

brother of St. Ouen, who took the monastic habit there with many other young noblemen, and established a nunnery in the neighborhood, which became the principal house. St. Thelchildes, a virgin of noble descent, who seems to have been educated or first professed in the monastery of Faremoutier, was the First abbess of Jouarre, and governed that house till about the year 660. By her and her religious community St. Bertille was received with great joy and trained up in the strictest practice of monastic perfection. Our saint looking upon this solitude as a secure harbor, never ceased to return thanks to God for his infinite mercy in having drawn her out of the tempestuous ocean of the world; but was persuaded she could never deserve to become the spouse of Jesus Christ, unless she endeavored to follow him in the path of humiliation and self-denial. By her perfect submission to all her sisters she seemed everyone's servant and in her whole conduct was a model of humility, obedience, regularity and devotion. Though she was yet young, her prudence and virtue appeared consummate, and the care of entertaining strangers, of the sick, and of the children that were educated in the monastery, was successively committed to her. In all these employments she had acquitted herself with great charity and edification when she was chosen prioress to assist the abbess in her administration. In this office her tender devotion, her habitual sense of the divine presence, and her other virtues shone forth with new luster, and has a wonderful influence in the direction of the whole community. Everyone, by her example, was ashamed to fail in any part of the practice of the like devotion, or in the most punctual and scrupulous observance of the least rule of monastic discipline.

When St. Bathildes, wife of Clovis II, munificently re-founded the abbey of Chelles, which St. Clotildis had instituted near the Marne, four leagues from Paris, she desired St. Thelchildes to furnish this new community with a small colony of the most experienced and virtuous nuns of Jouarre, who might direct the novices in the rule of monastic perfection. Bertille was sent at the head of this holy company and was appointed first abbess of Chelles, in 646, or thereabouts. The reputation of the sanctity and prudence of our saint, and the excellent discipline which she established in this house, drew several foreign princesses thither. Among others Bede mentions Hereswith, queen of the East-Angles. She was daughter of Hereic, brother, or brother-in-law to St. Edwin, king of Northumberland, and married the religious king Annas, with whose consent she renounced the world, and passing into France in 646, became a nun at Chelles, and there happily finished her earthly pilgrimage. In Wilson's English martyrology she is placed among the saints on the 20th of September. Queen Bathildes, after the death of her husband, in 655, was left regent of the kingdom during the minority of her son Clotaire III, but as soon as he was of age to govern, in 665, she retired hither, took the religious habit from the hands of St. Bertille, obeyed her as if she had been the last sister in the house, and passed to the glory of the angels in 680. In this numerous family of holy queens, princesses, and virgins, no contests arose but those of humility and charity; no strife was ever known but who should first submit, or humble herself lowest, and who should outdo the rest in meekness, devotion, penance, and in all the exercises of monastic discipline. The holy abbess, who saw two great queens every day at her feet, seemed the most humble and the most fervent among her sisters, and showed by her conduct that no one commands well or with safety who has not first learned, and is not always ready, to obey well. This humble disposition of soul extinguishes pride, and removes the fatal pleasure of power which that vice inspires, and which is the seed of tyranny, the worst corruption of the human heart. This virtue alone makes command sweet and amiable in its very severity, and renders us patient and firm in every observance and duty. St. Bertille governed this great monastery for the space of forty-six years with equal vigor and discretion. In her old age, far from abating her fervor, she strove daily to redouble it both in her penances and in her devotions; as the courser exerts himself with fresh vigor when he sees himself almost touching the goal, or as the laborer makes the strongest efforts in his last strokes to finish well his task. In these holy dispositions of fervor the saint closed her penitential life in 695.

One who has truly in spirit renounced the world, sees its figure pass before his eyes contemns the smoke of its enjoyments, shudders at the tragical scenes of its ambition, dreads its snares, and abhors its cheating promises, magnificent impostures, and poisonous pleasures by which it ceases not to enchant many unhappy souls. With the security and tranquility of a man who is in the harbor, he beholds the boisterous raging and the violent tosses of this tempestuous sea, in the midst of which the unhappy Egyptian struggle against the fury of the waves, and after toiling for some time sink on a sudden one after another, and are buried in the abyss. Those only escape this ruin whose souls soar above it, so that their affections are no way entangled or engaged [34].
(Memorial November 5)

References:

1) "Saint Bertille". CatholicSaints.Info. 6 November 2021. Web. 10 December 2021. <https://catholicsaints.info/saint-bertille/>

2) EWTN Library. St. Bertille. (Accessed 17 Oct 2021) https://www.ewtn.com/catholicism/saints/bertille-499

3) Reverend Alban Butler (1883). *The Lives of the Saints* as republished by Loreto Publications: Fitzwilliam, New Hampshire, 2020. Book Six, Vol. X & XI, 635-638.

4) St Bertille, Abbess of Chelles. *e-Catholic 2000*. (Accessed 12/14/2021) https://www.ecatholic2000.com/butler/vol11/november23.shtml

36

St. Juliana of Mont-Cornillon (Belgium) (1192-1258)
Worked with the sick and in the convent's hospital.[1]
Promoted a feast dedicated to the Blessed Sacrament
which became known at the Feast of Corpus Christi

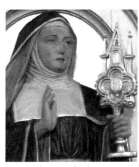

St. Juliana of Liege
http://catholicsaints.info/

Saint Juliana of Mont-Cornillon was also known as **St. Juliana of Liege**. Juliana was an Augustinian nun and is known as the nun who gave us the feast of Corpus Christi. Juliana was born in 1192 at Retinnes, Flanders, Belgium. At this time in Liege there were many people dedicated to the Blessed Sacrament. Juliana was orphaned at the age of five and she and her sister Agnes were entrusted to the care of the Augustinian nuns at the convent and leprosarium of Mont-Cornillon. Juliana was taught mainly by Sister Sapienza [her name meaning wisdom]. She was in charge of Juliana's spiritual development to the time Juliana received the religious habit of an Augustinian nun at Liege, Belgium in 1206. Sister Juliana worked with the sick, and in the convent hospital. She became the Prioress of the convent at Mount Cornillon in 1225.

Saint Juliana received a vision from Christ, who pointed out that there was no feast in honor of the Blessed Sacrament. She promoted a feast which became known as the Feast of Corpus Christi for which St. Thomas Aquinas composed several beautiful hymns. She was branded "a visionary" and accused of mismanagement of hospital funds. An investigation by the bishop exonerate her and she was returned to her position. The bishop introduced the Feast of Corpus Christi in Liege, Belgium in 1246. Upon his death two years later, Juliana was driven from Mount Cornillon. She fled to the house of the Cistercian nuns at Salzinnes until it was burned by Henry II of Luxembourg. She then withdrew from the world becoming an anchoress at Fosses. She died on April 5, 1258 from natural causes and is buried at Villiers, France.

Blessed Eva of Liege, a friend to St. Juliana, also promoted the new feast and it was sanctioned for the universal Church by Pope Urban IV in 1264. The feast became mandatory in the Roman Church in 1312.[2] Pope Blessed Pius IX canonized St. Juliana in 1869. (Memorial - April 6).[3]

"And lo, I am with you always, to the close of the age"
(Mt 28:20).

From November 17, 2010 General Audience of Pope Benedict XVI:[4]
Dear Brothers and Sisters,

This morning too I would like to introduce a female figure to you. She is little known but the Church is deeply indebted to her, not only because of the holiness of her life but also because, with her great fervour, she contributed to the institution of one of the most important solemn Liturgies of the year: Corpus Christi.

She is St Juliana de Cornillon, also known as St Juliana of Liège. We know several facts about her life, mainly from a Biography that was probably written by a contemporary cleric; it is a collection of various testimonies of people who were directly acquainted with the Saint.

Juliana was born near Liège, Belgium between 1191 and 1192. It is important to emphasize this place because at that time the Diocese of Liège was, so to speak, a true "Eucharistic Upper Room." Before Juliana, eminent theologians had illustrated the supreme value of the Sacrament of the Eucharist and, again in Liège, there were groups of women generously dedicated to Eucharistic worship and to fervent communion. Guided by exemplary priests, they lived together, devoting themselves to prayer and to charitable works.

Orphaned at the age of five, Juliana, together with her sister Agnes, was entrusted to the care of the Augustinian nuns at the convent and leprosarium of Mont-Cornillon.

She was taught mainly by a sister called "Sapienza" [wisdom], who was in charge of her spiritual development to the time Juliana received the religious habit and thus became an Augustinian nun.

She became so learned that she could read the words of the Church Fathers, of St Augustine and St Bernard in particular, in Latin. In addition to a keen intelligence, Juliana showed a special propensity for contemplation from the outset. She had a profound sense of Christ's presence, which she experienced by living the Sacrament of the Eucharist especially intensely and by pausing frequently to meditate upon Jesus' words: "And lo, I am with you always, to the close of the age" (Mt 28:20).

When Juliana was 16 she had her first vision which recurred subsequently several times during her Eucharistic adoration. Her vision presented the moon in its full splendour, crossed diametrically by a dark stripe. The Lord made her

38

understand the meaning of what had appeared to her. The moon symbolized the life of the Church on earth, the opaque line, on the other hand, represented the absence of a liturgical feast for whose institution Juliana was asked to plead effectively: namely, a feast in which believers would be able to adore the Eucharist so as to increase in faith, to advance in the practice of the virtues and to make reparation for offences to the Most Holy Sacrament.

Juliana, who in the meantime had become Prioress of the convent, kept this revelation that had filled her heart with joy a secret for about 20 years. She then confided it to two other fervent adorers of the Eucharist, Blessed Eva, who lived as a hermit, and Isabella, who had joined her at the Monastery of Mont-Cornillon. The three women established a sort of "spiritual alliance" for the purpose of glorifying the Most Holy Sacrament.

They also chose to involve a highly regarded Priest, John of Lausanne, who was a canon of the Church of St Martin in Liège. They asked him to consult theologians and clerics on what was important to them. Their affirmative response was encouraging.

What happened to Juliana of Cornillon occurs frequently in the lives of Saints. To have confirmation that an inspiration comes from God it is always necessary to be immersed in prayer to wait patiently, to seek friendship and exchanges with other good souls and to submit all things to the judgement of the Pastors of the Church.

It was in fact Bishop Robert Torote, Liège who, after initial hesitation, accepted the proposal of Juliana and her companions and first introduced the Solemnity of Corpus Christi in his diocese. Later other Bishops following his example instituted this Feast in the territories entrusted to their pastoral care.

However, to increase their faith the Lord often asks Saints to sustain trials. This also happened to Juliana who had to bear the harsh opposition of certain members of the clergy and even of the superior on whom her monastery depended.

Of her own free will, therefore, Juliana left the Convent of Mont-Cornillon with several companions. For 10 years — from 1248 to 1258 — she stayed as a guest at various monasteries of Cistercian sisters.

She edified all with her humility, she had no words of criticism or reproach for her adversaries and continued zealously to spread Eucharistic worship.

She died at Fosses-La-Ville, Belgium, in 1258. In the cell where she lay the Blessed Sacrament was exposed and, according to her biographer's account, Juliana died contemplating with a last effusion to love Jesus in the Eucharist whom she had always loved, honoured and adored. Jacques Pantaléon of Troyes was also won over to the good cause of the Feast of Corpus Christi during his ministry as Archdeacon in Liège. It was he who, having become Pope with the name of Urban IV in 1264, instituted the Solemnity of Corpus Christi on the Thursday after Pentecost as a feast of precept for the universal Church.

In the Bull of its institution, entitled *Transiturus de hoc mundo* (11 Aug. 1264),[5] Pope Urban even referred discreetly to Juliana's mystical experiences, corroborating their authenticity. He wrote: "Although the Eucharist is celebrated solemnly every day, we deem it fitting that at least once a year it be celebrated with greater honour and a solemn commemoration.

"Indeed we grasp the other things we commemorate with our spirit and our mind, but this does not mean that we obtain their real presence. On the contrary, in this sacramental commemoration of Christ, even though in a different form, Jesus Christ is present with us in his own substance. While he was about to ascend into Heaven he said 'And lo, I am with you always, to the close of the age' (Matthew 28:20)".

The Pontiff made a point of setting an example by celebrating the solemnity of Corpus Christi in Orvieto, the town where he was then residing. Indeed, he ordered that the famous Corporal with the traces of the Eucharistic miracle which had occurred in Bolsena the previous year, 1263, be kept in Orvieto Cathedral — where it still is today.

While a priest was consecrating the bread and the wine he was overcome by strong doubts about the Real Presence of the Body and Blood of Christ in the sacrament of the Eucharist. A few drops of blood began miraculously to ooze from the consecrated Host, thereby confirming what our faith professes.

Urban IV asked one of the greatest theologians of history, St Thomas Aquinas — who at that time was accompanying the Pope and was in Orvieto — to compose the texts of the Liturgical Office for this great feast. They are masterpieces, still in use in the Church today, in which theology and poetry are fuse. These texts pluck at the heartstrings in an expression of praise and gratitude to the Most Holy Sacrament, while the mind, penetrating the mystery with wonder, recognizes in the Eucharist the Living and Real Presence of Jesus, of his Sacrifice of love that reconciles us with the Father, and gives us salvation.

Although after the death of Urban iv the celebration of the Feast of Corpus Christi was limited to certain regions of France, Germany, Hungary and Northern Italy, it was another Pontiff, John XXII, who in 1317 re-established it for the universal Church. Since then the Feast experienced a wonderful development and is still deeply appreciated by the Christian people.

I would like to affirm with joy that today there is a "Eucharistic springtime" in the Church: How many people pause in silence before the Tabernacle to engage in a loving conversation with Jesus! It is comforting to know that many groups of young people have rediscovered the beauty of praying in adoration before the Most Blessed Sacrament.

I am thinking, for example, of our Eucharistic adoration in Hyde Park, London. I pray that this Eucharistic "springtime" may spread increasingly in every parish and in particular in Belgium, St Juliana's homeland.

Venerable John Paul II said in his Encyclical *Ecclesia de Eucharistia*:[6] "In many places, adoration of the Blessed Sacrament is also an important daily practice and becomes an inexhaustible source of holiness. The devout participation of the faithful in the Eucharistic procession on the Solemnity of the Body and Blood of Christ is a grace from the Lord which yearly brings joy to those who take part in it. Other positive signs of Eucharistic faith and love might also be mentioned" (n. 10).

In remembering St Juliana of Cornillon let us also renew our faith in the Real Presence of Christ in the Eucharist. As we are taught by the Compendium of the Catechism of the Catholic Church, "Jesus Christ is present in the Eucharist in a unique and incomparable way. He is present in a true, real and substantial way, with his Body and his Blood, with his Soul and his Divinity. In the Eucharist, therefore, there is present in a sacramental way, that is, under the Eucharistic Species of bread and wine, Christ whole and entire, God and Man" (n. 282).[7]

Dear friends, fidelity to the encounter with the Christ in the Eucharist in Holy Mass on Sunday is essential for the journey of faith, but let us also seek to pay frequent visits to the Lord present in the Tabernacle! In gazing in adoration at the consecrated Host, we discover the gift of God's love, we discover Jesus' Passion and Cross and likewise his Resurrection. It is precisely through our gazing in adoration that the Lord draws us towards him into his mystery in order to transform us as he transforms the bread and the wine.

The Saints never failed to find strength, consolation and joy in the Eucharistic encounter. Let us repeat before the Lord present in the Most Blessed Sacrament the words of the Eucharistic hymn "*Adoro te devote*": [Devoutly I adore Thee]: Make me believe ever more in you, "Draw me deeply into faith, / Into Your hope, into Your love".   Thank you.

References:

1) "Blessed Juliana of Mont Cornillon". CatholicSaints.Info. 11 November 2021. Web. 8 December 2021.
<https://catholicsaints.info/blessed-juliana-of-mont-cornillon/>

2) "Blessed Juliana of Mont Cornillon". CatholicSaints.Info. 11 November 2021. Web. 17 February 2022.
<https://catholicsaints.info/blessed-juliana-of-mont-cornillon/>

3) Norbertine History, O. Praem Saints and Beati. Corpus Christi & St. Juliana of Liege. May 25, 2008. Accessed 17Feb2022.
https://norbertinevocations.wordpress.com/2008/05/25/corpus-christi-st-juliana-of-liege/

4) Pope Benedict XVI. (17Nov2010). General Audience. St. Juliana de Cornillon (St. Juliana of Liege). Accessed 25 May 2022.
https://www.vatican.va/content/benedict-xvi/en/audiences/2010/documents/hf_ben-xvi_aud_20101117.html

5) Pope Urban IV. (11Aug1264). Transiturua de hoc mundo.
https://www.vatican.va/content/urbanus-iv/es/documents/bulla-transiturus-de-mundo-11-aug-1264.html. Accessed 14 June 2022.

6) Pope St. John Paul II. (17Apr2003). Ecclesia de Eucharistia (On the Eucharist and Its relationship to the Church). Accessed 14 June 2022.
https://www.vatican.va/content/john-paul-ii/en/encyclicals/documents/hf_jp-ii_enc_20030417_eccl-de-euch.html

7) Libreria Edditrice Vaticana (2006). Compendium of the Catechism of the Catholic Church, 282.

St. Elizabeth of Hungary (Slovakia/Hungary) (1207-1231)

Erected a hospital at the base of the steep rock on which their castle was built where she often fed the infirmed with her own hands, made their beds and attended them even in the heat of the summer[1]

Saint Elizabeth was born in 1207 in present-day Bratislava, Slovakia to Andrew II, the pious and brave, King of Hungary and Queen Gertrude, daughter of the duke of Carinthia. As an infant, she was promised in marriage to the infant Lewis [Louis], son of Herman, the landgrave of Thuringia (Germany). She was sent to Herman's court at the age of four where she was brought up under the care of a virtuous lady.

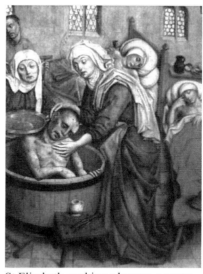

When Elizabeth was nine years old, Herman died and the government fell into the hands of his wife who persecuted Elizabeth for her piety. Elizabeth "learned to take up her cross and follow Christ

St Elisabeth washing a beggar, a scene from the main altar of St Elisabeth Cathedral in Košice, Slovakia

by the exercise of meekness, humility, patience, and charity, toward unjust persecutors; and to unite her soul to God by resignation, love and prayer."[1] When she was fourteen years old Lewis returned home from a long absence to further his education. He appreciated her great piety and soon after solemnized his marriage with her.

With her pious husband's consent Elizabeth continued her pious practices. She often arose in the night to pray. When she was not spending time in prayer or pious reading, she performed acts of charity and many austere practices. During the severe famine in Germany in 1225, she distributed to the poor her whole crop of corn. Since her residence, the castle of Marpurg, was located on a steep rock, Elizabeth built a hospital at its based in which she cared for the infirm. "She often fed them with her own hands, made their beds, and attended them even in the heat of the summer." She provided for helpless children, especially orphans. She built a second hospital which house 28. She fed 900 daily at her own gates.

43

Lewis and Elizabeth had three children. Herman, Sophia, who married the duke of Brabant, and Gertrude who became a nun and died abbess of Aldemburg. When Herman was yet an infant, Lewis left the family to accompany emperor Frederic Barbarossa on the holy war (crusades) to Palestine. He fell ill of a fever at Otranto near the kingdom of Naples and died after having received the last sacraments from the patriarch of Jerusalem. Lewis died on September 11, 1227.

Lewis' younger brother Henry took over government of the estate and dominions of the langraviate. He turned out of the castle of Marpurg, Elizabeth, followed by her three children. He forbid any persons to support her in away way. She lived in poverty for some time. She was assisted by the Franciscan friars. Her aunt, sister of her mother, was the abbess of Kitzingen in the diocese of Wurtzburg. She invited her to the monastery in Kitzingen and seeing her condition sent her to Elizabeth's uncle who was the bishop of Bamberg. He recommended she remarry use that alliance to recover her rights. She preferred to remain in God's service in a chaste state.

Her husband's body, which had been buried at Otranto, Italy, had been exhumed, the bones placed in a rich chest and carried by procession home accompanied by great retinue of princes, dukes, counts, barons and knights. When they approached the castle of Marpurg, following the wishes of Elizabeth, they only remonstrated Henry for his poor treatment of Elizabeth. He repented and restored her position.

She continued her pious practice and became a third order Franciscan. Eventually she left the castle and lived on the boundary of her husband's dominion. She died on November 19, 1231 at the age of twenty-four in Hesse, Germany (previously Marburg, Landgraviate of Thuringia). She was buried in the chapel near the hospital she founded near the Marpurg castle. Many miracles occurred at her tomb and are described below. St. Elizabeth of Hungary was canonized on Whit-Sunday, May 27, 1235 by His Holiness Pope Gregory IX.[2] Her relics were removed from the grave in 1236 and placed in a rich vermilion case upon the altar in the church of the hospital with over 200,000 people present. Emperor Frederic II took up the first stone from her grave and he also placed on the shrine a crown of gold. Her children also participated in the ceremony. (Memorial - November 17)

The following is a quote from *the Legends of the Breviary* which is the Roman history of the saints as they appeared in the Breviary as of the mid-1800's.[3]

> "The Church keeps an official register of the actions, and maxims, and virtues of the saints, who are her glory; there she has chronicled through all these eighteen hundred years, the wonders which God has wrought in them and by them, and the blessings she has received through their intercession"[4]
>
> Elizabeth, a daughter of Andrew king of Hungary, feared God from her infancy, and increased in piety as she advanced in age. She was married to Lewis, landgrave of Hesse and Thuringia, and devoted herself to the service of God and of her husband. She used to rise in the night and spend a long time in prayer; and, moreover, she devoted herself to works of mercy, diligently caring for widows and orphans, the sick and the poor. In time of famine she freely distributed her store of corn. She received lepers into her house and kissed their hands and feet; she also built a splendid hospital where the poor might be fed and cared for. On the death of her husband, she, in order to serve God with greater freedom, laid aside all worldly ornaments, clothed herself in a rough tunic and entered the Order of Penance of St. Francis. She was very remarkable for her patience and humility. Being despoiled of all her possessions and turned out of her own house and abandoned by all, she bore insults, mockeries, and reproaches with undaunting courage, rejoicing exceedingly to suffer thus for God's sake. She humbled herself by performing the lowest offices for the poor and sick and procured them all they needed, contenting herself with herbs and vegetables for her only food. She was living in this holy manner, occupied with these and many other good works when the end of her pilgrimage drew nigh, as she had foretold to her companions. She was absorbed in divine contemplation, with her eyes fixed on heaven; and after being wonderfully consoled by God, and strengthened with the Sacraments, she fell asleep in our Lord. Many miracles were immediately wrought at her tomb; and on her being duly proved, Gregory IX enrolled her among the saints.

The following is a letter by Conrad of Marburg, spiritual director of Saint Elizabeth:[5]

> "From this time onward Elizabeth's goodness greatly increased. She was a lifelong friend of the poor and gave herself entirely to

45

relieving the hungry. She ordered that one of her castles should be converted into a hospital in which she gathered many of the weak and feeble. She generously gave alms to all who were in need, not only in that place but in all the territories of her husband's empire. She spent all her own revenue from her husband's four principalities, and finally she sold her luxurious possessions and rich clothes for the sake of the poor. Twice a day, in the morning and in the evening, Elizabeth went to visit the sick. She personally cared for those who were particularly repulsive; to some she gave food, to others clothing; some she carried on her own shoulders, and performed many other kindly services. Her husband, of happy memory, gladly approved of these charitable works. Finally, when her husband died, she sought the highest perfection; filled with tears, she implored me to let her beg for alms from door to door. On Good Friday of that year, when the altars had been stripped, she laid her hands on the altar in a chapel in her own town, where she had established the Friars Minor, and before witnesses she voluntarily renounced all worldly display and everything that our Savior in the gospel advises us to abandon. Even then she saw that she could still be distracted by the cares and worldly glory which had surrounded her while her husband was alive. Against my will she followed me to Marburg. Here in the town she built a hospice where she gathered together the weak and feeble. There she attended the most wretched and contemptible at her own table. Apart from those active good works, I declare before God that I have seldom seen more contemplative woman. When she was coming from private prayer, some religious men and women often saw her face shining marvelously and light coming from her eyes like the rays of the sun. Before her death I heard her confession. When I asked what should be done about her goods and possessions, she replied, that anything which seemed to be hers belonged to the poor. She asked me to distribute everything except one worn out dress in which she wished to be buried. When all this had been decided, she received the body of our Lord. Afterward, until vespers, she spoke often of the holiest things she had heard in sermons. Then, she devoutly commended to God all who were sitting near her, and as if falling into a gentle sleep, she died."

St. Elizabeth of Hungary, Widow (November 19), from the *original* Rev. Alban Butler's (1883) *Lives of Saints*:[1]

Elizabeth, daughter to Alexander II, the valiant and religious king of Hungary, and his queen, Gertrude, daughter to the duke of

Carinthia, was born in Hungary in 1207. Herman, landgrave of Thuringia and Hesse, had a son born about the same time, and named Lewis [Louis]. This prince obtained, by ambassadors, a promise from the king of Hungary that his daughter should be given in marriage to his newborn son and, to secure the effect of this engagement, at the landgrave's request, the princess, at four years of age, was sent to his court, and there brought up under the care of a virtuous lady. Five years after, Herman died, and Lewis became landgrave. Elizabeth, from her cradle, was so happily prevented with the love of God, that no room for creatures could be found in her heart; and though surrounded, and, as it were, besieged by worldly pleasures in their most engaging shapes, she had no relish for them, prayed with an astonishing recollection, and seemed scarce to know any other use of money than to give it to the poor; for her father allowed her, till her marriage was solemnized, a competent yearly revenue for maintaining a court suitable to her rank. This child of heaven, in her very recreations, studied to practice frequent humiliations and self-denials; and stole often to the chapel, and there knelt down and said a short prayer before every altar, bowing her body reverently, or, if nobody was there, prostrating herself upon the ground. If she found the doors of the chapel in the palace shut, not to lose her labor, she knelt down at the threshold, and always put up her petition to the throne of God. Her devotion she indulged with more liberty in her private closet. She was very devout to her angel guardian and the saints, particularly St. John the Evangelist. She was educated with Agnes, sister to the young landgrave, and upon their first appearing together at church, they were dressed alike, and wore coronets set with jewels. At their entering the house of God, Sophia, the landgrave's mother, observing our saint take off her coronet, asked why she did so; to which the princess replied, that she could not bear to appear with jewels on her head, where she saw that of Jesus Christ, crowned with thorns. Agnes and her mother, who were strangers to such kind sentiments, and fond of what Elizabeth trampled upon, conceived an aversion for the young princess, and said, that since she seemed to have so little relish for a court, a convent would be the properest place for her. The courtiers carried their reflections much further, and did all in their power to bring the saint into contempt, saying that neither her fortune not her person were such as the landgrave had a right to expect, that he had no inclination for her, and that she would either be sent back to Hungary, or married to some nobleman in the country. These taunts and trials were more severe and continual, as the landgrave, Herman, dying when Elizabeth was only nine years old, the government fell into the hands of his widow in the name of her son till he should be of age. These persecutions and injuries were, to the saint, occasions of the greatest spiritual advantages; for by them she daily learned a more perfect contempt of all earthly things, to which the heavenly lover exhorts his spouse, saying: "Hearken, daughter, forget thy people." She learned also the evangelical hatred of herself, and crucifixion of self-love; by which she was enabled to say with the apostles Behold, we have left all things. In this entire disengagement of her heart, she learned to take up her cross and follow Christ by the exercise of meekness, humility, patience, and charity, towards unjust persecutors; and to cleave to God by the closest union of her soul to Him by resignation, love and prayer, contemning herself, and esteeming the vanity of the world as filth and dung. She desired to please God only, and in this spirit she was wont to pray: "O sovereign spouse of my soul, never suffer me to love anything but in Thee, not to Thee, be bitter and painful, and Thy will alone sweet. May Thy will be always mine: as in heaven Thy will is punctually performed, so may it be done on earth by all creatures, particularly in me and by me. And as love requires a union, and entire resignation of all things into the hands of the beloved, I give up my whole self to thee without reserve. In my heart I renounce all riches and pomp: if I had many worlds I would leave them all to adhere to Thee; alone in poverty and nakedness of spirit, as Thou madest Thyself poor for me. O Spouse of my heart, so great is the love I bear Thee, and holy poverty for thy sake, that with joy I leave all that I am, that I may be transformed into Thee, and that abandoned state so amiable to Thee."

The saint was in her fourteenth year when Lewis, the young landgrave, returned home after a long absence, on account of his education. Address in marital exercises and other great accomplishments introduced the young prince into the world with a mighty reputation: but nothing was so remarkable in him as a sincere love of piety. The eminent virtue of Elizabeth gave him the highest esteem for her person. However, he seldom saw or spoke to her, even in public, and never in private, till the question was one day put to him, what his thoughts were with regard to marrying her, and he was told what rumors were spread in the court to her disadvantage. Here at he expressed much displeasure, and said, that he prized her virtue above all the mountains of gold and rubies that the world could afford. Forthwith he sent her by a nobleman a glass garnished with precious stones of inestimable value, with two crystals opening on each side, in the one of which was a looking-glass: on the other figure of Christ crucified was most curiously wrought. And not long after he solemnized his marriage with her, and the ceremony was performed with the utmost pomp, and with extraordinary public rejoicings. The stream of public applause followed the favor of the prince; the whole court expressed the most profound veneration for the saint, and all the clouds which had so long hung over her head were at once dispersed. Conrad of Marpurg, a most holy and learned priest, and an eloquent pathetic preacher, whose disinterestedness, and love of holy poverty, mortified life, and extraordinary devotion and spirit of prayer, rendered him a model to the clergy of that age, was the person whom she chose for her spiritual director, and to his advice she submitted herself in all things relating to her spiritual concerns. This holy and experienced guide, observing how deep root the seeds of virtue had taken in her soul, applied himself by cultivating them to conduct her to the summit of Christian perfection, and encouraged her in the path of mortification and penance, but was obliged often to moderate her corporal austerities by the precept of obedience. The landgrave also reposed an entire confidence in Conrad, and gave this holy man the privilege of disposing of all ecclesiastical benefices in the prince's gift. Elizabeth, with her pious husband's consent, often rose in the night to pray, and consecrated great part of her time to her devotions, insomuch that on Sundays and holidays she never allowed herself much leisure to dress herself. The rest of her time which was not spent in prayer or reading, she devoted to works of charity, and to spinning, or carding wool, in which she would only work very coarse wool for the use of the poor, or of the Franciscan friars. The mysteries of the life and sufferings of our Savior were the subjects of her most tender and daily meditation. Weighing of what importance prayer and mortification, or penance are in a spiritual life, she studied to make her prayer virtually continual, by breaking forth into fervent acts of compunction and divine love amidst all her employments. The austerity of her life surpassed that of recluses. When she sat at table, next to the landgrave, to dissemble her abstinence from flesh and savory dishes, she used to deceive the attention of others by discoursing with the guests, or with the prince, carving for others, sending her maids upon errands, often changing her plates, and a thousand other artifices. Her meal frequently consisted only of bread and honey, or a dry crust, with a cup of the smallest wine, or the like; especially when she dined privately in her chamber, with two maids, who voluntarily followed her rules as to diet. She never ate but what came out of her own kitchen, that she might be sure nothing was mixed contrary to the severe rules she had laid down; and this kitchen she kept out of her own private purse, not to be the least charge to her husband. She was a great enemy to rich apparel, though in compliance to the landgrave, she on certain public occasions conformed in some degree to the fashions of the court. When ambassadors came from her father, the king of Hungary, her husband desired her not to appear in that homely apparel which she usually wore; but she prevailed upon him to suffer it; and God was please to give so extraordinary a gracefulness to her person, that the ambassadors were exceedingly struck at the comeliness and majesty of the appearance she made. In the absence of her husband she commonly wore only coarse cloth, not dyed, but in the natural color of the wool, such as the poor people used. She so strongly recommended to her maids of honor simplicity of dress, penance, and assiduous prayer, that several of them were warmed into an imitation of her virtues but they could only follow her at a distance, for she seemed inimitable in her heroic practices, especially in her profound humility, with which she courted the most mortifying humiliation. In attending the poor and the sick, she cheerfully washed and cleansed the most filthy sores, and waited on those that were infected with the most loathsome diseases.

Her alms seemed at all times to have no bounds; in which the good landgrave rejoiced exceedingly, and gave her full liberty. In 1225, Germany being severely visited by a famine, she exhausted the treasury and distributed her whole crop of corn amongst those who felt the weight of that calamity heaviest. The landgrave was then in Apulia with the emperor; and at his return the officers of his household complained loudly to him of her profusion in favor of the poor. But the prince was so well assured of her piety and prudence, that without examining into the mater, he asked if she had alienated his dominions. They answered: "No." "As for her charities," said he, "they will entail upon us the divine blessings and we shall not want so long as we suffer her to relieve the poor as she does." The castle of Marpurg, the residence of the landgrave, was built on a steep rock, which the infirm and weak were not able to climb. The holy margravine therefore built an hospital at the foot of the rock for their reception and entertainment; where she often fed them with her own hands, made their beds, and attended them even in the heat of the summer, when the place seemed insupportable to all those who were strangers to the sentiments of her generous and indefatigable charity. The helpless children, especially all orphans, were provided for at her expense. Elizabeth was the foundress of another hospital, in which twenty-eight persons were constantly relieved; she fed nine hundred daily at her own gate, besides an incredible number in the different parts of the dominion, so that the revenue in her hands was truly the patrimony of the distressed. But the saint's charity was tempered with discretion; and instead of encouraging in idleness such as were able to work, she employed them in a way suitable to their strength and capacity. Her husband, edified and charmed with her extraordinary piety, not only approved of all she did, but was himself an imitator of her charity, devotion, and other virtues; insomuch that he is deservedly styled by historians, the Pious Landgrave. He had by her three children, Herman, Sophia, who was afterwards married to the duke of Brabant, and Gertrude, who became a nun, and died abbess of Aldemburg. Purely upon motives of religion, the landgrave took the cross to accompany the emperor Frederic Barbarossa, in the holy war, to Palestine. The separation of this pious and loving couple was a great trial; though moderated by the heroic spirit of religion with which both were animated. The landgrave joined the emperor in the kingdom of Naples; but as he was going to embark, fell ill of a malignant fever at Otranto, and having received the last sacraments at the hands of the patriarch of Jerusalem, expired in great sentiments of piety, on the 11th of September, 1227. Many miracles are related to have been wrought by him, in the history of Thuringia, and in that of the crusades. Elizabeth, who at his departure had put on the dress of a widow, upon hearing this melancholy news, wept bitterly, and said: "If my husband be dead, I promise to die henceforth to myself, and to the world with all its vanities." God himself was pleased to complete this her sacrifice by a train of other afflictions into which she fell, being a sensible instance of the instability of human things, in which nothing is more constant then an unsteadiness of fortune: the life of man being a perpetual scene of interludes, and virtue being his only support, a check to pride in prosperity, and a solid comfort in adversity.

Envy, jealousy, and rancor, all broke loose at once against the virtuous landgravine, which during her husband's life, for the great love and respect he bore her, had been raked up and covered over as fire under the ashes. As pretenses are never wanting to cloak ambition, envy, and other passions, which never dare show themselves barefaced, it was alleged that the saint, had squandered away the public revenue upon the poor; that the infant Herman being unfit for the government of the estate, it ought to be given to one who was able to defend and even extend the dominions of the landgraviate; and that therefore Henry, younger brother to the landgrave, ought to be advanced to the principality. The mob being soothed by the fine speeches of certain powerful factious men, Henry got possession, and turned Elizabeth out of the castle without furniture, provision, or necessaries for the support of nature, and all persons in the town were forbid to let her any lodgings. The princess bore this unjust treatment with a patience for transcending the power of nature, showing nothing in her gestures which was not as composed as if she had been the greatest tranquility possible. And rejoicing in her heart of see herself so ill treated, she went down the castle hill to the town, placing her whole confidence in God, and with her damsels and maids went into a common inn, or, as others say, a poor woman's cottage, where she remained till midnight, when the bell ringing to matins at the church of the Franciscan friars, she went thither, and desired the good fathers to sing a Te Deum with solemnity to give God thanks for his mercies to her in visiting her with afflictions. Though she sent about the next day, and used all her endeavors to procure some kind of lodging in the town, no one durst afford her any for fear of the usurper and his associates. She stayed the whole day in the church of the friars, and a evening had the additional affliction to see her three children, whom their barbarous uncle had sent out of the castle coming down the hill. She received them in the church porch, with undaunted fortitude, but could not refrain from tenderly weeping to see the innocent babes so insensible of their condition as to smile upon her, rejoicing that they had recovered their mother. Reduced to the lowest ebb she applied to a priest for relief, who received her into his little house, where she had but one straight poor chamber for herself, her maids, and children. Her enemies soon forced her from thence, so that with thanks to those who had given her and hers some kind of shelter from the severities of a very sharp winter season, she returned to the inn or cottage. Thus she, who had entertained thousands of poor, could find no entertainment or harbor; and she, who had been a mother to so many infants and orphans of others, was glad to beg an alms for her own, and to receive it from her enemies. God failed not to comfort her in her distress, and she addressed herself to Him in raptures of love, praying that she might be wholly converted into His love, and that His pure love might reign in her. Melting in the sweetness of divine love she poured forth her soul in inflamed ejaculations, saying, for example: "Ah, my Lord and my God, may Thou be all mine, and I all Thine. What is this, my God and my love? Thou all mine and I all Thine. Let me love Thee, my God, above all things, and let me not love myself but for Thee, and all other things in Thee. Let me love Thee, with all my soul, with all my memory." etc. In these fervent aspiration, overflowing with interior joy, she sometimes fell into wonderful raptures, which astonished Hentrude, a lady of honor, particularly beloved by her, and her companion in her devotions and mortifications.

52

The abbess of Kitzingen, in the diocese of Wurtzburg, our saint's aunt, sister to her mother, hearing of her misfortunes, invited her to her monastery, and being extremely moved at the sight of her desolate condition and poverty, advised her to repair to her uncle, the bishop of Bamberg, a man of great power, charity, and prudence. The bishop received her with many tears, which compassion drew from his eyes, and from those of all the clergy that were with him; and provided for her a commodious house near his palace. His first views were, as she was young and beautiful, to endeavor to look out for a suitable party, that, marrying some powerful prince, she might strengthen her interest, and that of her family, by a new alliance, which might enable her to recover her right: but such projects she entirely put a stop to, declaring it was her fixed resolution to devote herself to the divine service in a state of perpetual chastity. In the mean time the body of her late husband, which had been buried at Otranto, was taken up, and, the flesh being entirely consumed, the bones were put into a rich chest, and carried into Germany. The hearse was attended by a great many princes and dukes, and by counts, barons, and knights without number, marching in martial order, with ensigns folded up, the mournful sound of drums all covered with black, and other warlike instruments in like manner. Where some of these princes left the corpse to return home, the nobility of each country through which it passed took their place and every night it was lodged in some church or monastery where masses and dirges were said, and gifts offered. When the funeral pomp approached Bamberg, the bishop went out with the clergy and monks in procession to meet it, having left the nobility and knights with the disconsolate pious margravine. At the sight of the hearse her grief was inexpressible; yet, while there was not a dry eye in the church, she showed by restraining her sorrow how great command she had of her passions. Yet, when the chest was opened, her tears burst forth against her will. But, recollecting herself in God, she gave thanks to His divine majesty for having so disposed of her honored husband, as to take him into His eternal tabernacles, so seasonably for himself, though to her severe trial. The corpse remained several days at Bamberg, during which the funeral rites were continued with the utmost solemnity, and it was then conducted with great state into Thuringia. The princess entreated the barons and knights that attended it to use their interest with her brother-in-law to do her justice, not blaming him for the treatment she had received, but imputing it to evil counselors. Fired with indignation at the indignities she had received, they engaged to neglect no means of restoring her to her right: so that it was necessary for her to

53

moderate their resentment, and to beg they would only use humble remonstrances. This they did, reproaching Henry I for having brought so foul a blot and dishonor upon his house, and having violated all laws divine, civil, and natural, and broke the strongest ties of humanity. They conjured him by God, who beholds all things, and asked him in what point a weak woman, full of peace and piety, could offend him and what innocent princely babes, who were his own blood, could have done, the tenderness of whose years made them very unfit to suffer such injuries. Ambition strangely steals a heart to all sentiments of justice, charity, or humanity. Yet these remonstrances, made by the chief barons of the principality, softened the heart of Henry, and he promised them to restore to Elizabeth her dower and all the rights of her widowhood, and even to put the government of the dominions into her hands. This last she voluntarily chose to renounce, provided it was reserved for her son. Hereupon she was conducted back to the castle out of which she had been expelled, and from that time Henry began to treat her as princess, and obsequiously executed whatever she intimated to be her pleasure. Yet her persecutions were often renewed till her death.

The devout priest Conrad had attended her in great part of her travels, and returned to Marpurg, which was his usual residence. Elizabeth loathing the grandeur and dreading the distractions of the world, with his advice, bound herself by a vow which she made in his presence, in the church of the Franciscans, to observe the third rule of St. Francis, and secretly put on a little habit under her clothes. Her confessor relates that, laying her hands on the altar in the church of the friars minor, she by vow renounced the pomps of the world, she was going to add the vow of poverty, but he stopped her, saying she was obliged, in order to discharge many obligations of her late husband, and what she owed to the poor, to keep in her own hands the disposal of her revenues. Her dower she converted to the use of the poor; and as her director Conrad, in whom she reposed an entire confidence, was obliged to live in the town of Marpurg, when she quitted her palace she made that which was on the boundary of her husband's dominion, her place of residence, living first in a little cottage near the town, while a house was building for her, in which she spent the last three years of her life in the most fervent practices of devotion, charity, and penance. In her speech she was so reserved and modest that if she affirmed or denied anything, her words seemed to imply a fear of some mistake. She spoke little always with gravity, and most commonly of God; and never let drop anything that tended to her own praise. Out of a love of religious silence she shunned tattlers:

54

in all things she praised God, and being intent on spiritual things was never puffed up with prosperity, or troubled at adversity. She tied herself by vow to obey her confessor Conrad, and received at his hands a habit made of coarse cloth of the natural color of the wool without being dyed. Whence pope Gregory IX, who had corresponded with her, says she took the religious habit, and subjected herself to the yoke of obedience. Thus she imitated the state of nuns, though, by the advice of her confessor, she remained a secular, that she might better dispose of her alms for the relief of the poor. Conrad having observed that her attachment to her two principal maids, Iserurude and Guta, seemed too strong, and an impediment to her spiritual progress, proposed to her to dismiss them: and, without making any reply, she instantly obeyed him, though the sacrifice cost mutual tears. The saint, by spinning coarse wool, earned her own maintenance, and, with her maids, dressed her own victuals, which were chiefly herbs, bread, and water. While her hands were busy, in her heart she conversed with God. The king of Hungary, her father, earnestly invited her to his court but she preferred a state of humiliation and suffering. She chose by preference to do every kind of service in attending the most loathsome lepers among the poor. Spiritual and corporal works of mercy occupied her even to last moments, and by her moving exhortations many obstinate sinners were converted to God. It seemed, indeed, impossible for anything to resist the eminent spirit of prayer with which she was endowed. In prayer she found her comfort and her strength in her mortal pilgrimage, and was favored in it with frequent raptures, and heavenly communications. Her confessor, Conrad, assures us, that when she returned from secret prayers, her countenance often seemed to dart forth rays of light from the divine conversation. Being forewarned by God of her approaching passage to eternity, which she mentioned to her confessor four days before she fell ill, as he assured us, she redoubled her fervor, by her last will made Christ her heir in his poor, made a general confession of her whole life on the twelfth day, survived yet four days, received the last sacraments, and, to her last breath, ceased not to pray, or to discourse in the most pathetic manner on the mysteries of the sacred life and sufferings of our Redeemer, and on his coming to judge us. The day of her happy death was on the 19th of November, in 1231, in the twenty-fourth year of her age. Her venerable body was deposited in a chapel near the hospital which she had founded. Many sick persons were restored to health at her tomb an account of which miracles Siffrid, archbishop of Mentz, sent to Rome, having first caused them to be authenticated by a juridical examination before himself and others. Pope Gregory IX, after a long and mature discussion, performed the ceremony of her canonization on Whit-Sunday in 1235, four years after her death. Siffrid, upon news hereof, appointed a day for the translation of her relics, which he performed at Marpurg in 1236. The emperor Frederic II would be present, took up the first stone of the saint's grave, and gave and place on the shine with his own hands a rich crown of gold. St. Elizabeth's son, Herman, then landgrave, and his two sisters, Sophia and Gertrude, assisted at this August ceremony; also the archbishop of Cologne and Bremen, and an incredible number of other princes, prelates, and people, so that the number is said to have amounted to above two hundred thousand persons. The relics were enshrined in a rich vermilion case, and placed upon the altar in the church of the hospital. A Cistercian monk affirmed upon oath that, a little before this translation, praying at the tomb of the saint, he was cured of a palpitation of the heart and grievous melancholy, with which he had been grievously troubled for forty years, and had in vain sought remedies from physicians and every other means. Many instances are mentioned by Montanus, and by the archbishop of Mentz, and the confessor Conrad, of persons afflicted with palsies, and other inveterate diseases, who recovered their health at her tomb, or by invoking her intercession as, of a boy blind from is birth, by the mother's invocation of St. Elizabeth at her sepulcher, applying some of the dust to his eyes, upon which a skin, which covered each eye, burst, and he saw, as several witnesses declared upon oath, and Master Conrad saw the eyes thus healed of a boy three years old, dead, cold, and stiff a whole night, raised to life the next morning by a pious grandmother praying to God through the intercession of St. Elizabeth, with a vow of an alms to her hospital, and of dedicating the child to the divine service; attested in every circumstance by the depositions of the mother, father, grandmother, uncle, and others, recorded by Conrad of a boy dead and stiff for many house, just going to be carried to burial, raised by the invocation of St. Elizabeth: of a youth drowned, restored to life by the like prayer; of a boy drawn out of a well, dead, black, etc., and a child stillborn, brought to life: others cured of palsies, falling-sickness, fevers, madness, lameness, blindness, the bloody flux, etc., in the authentic relation. A portion of her relics is kept in the church of the Carmelites at Brussels; another in the magnificent chapel of La Roche-Guyon, upon the Seine, and a considerable part in a precious shrine is in the electoral treasury of Hanover. Some persons of the third order of St. Francis having raised that institute into a religious order long after the death of our saint, (without prejudice to the secular state of this order, which is still embraced by many who live in the world.) The religious women of this order chose her for their patroness, and are sometimes called the nuns of Saint Elizabeth.

Perfection consists not essentially in mortification, but in charity: and he is most perfect who is most united to God by love. But humility and self-denial remove the impediments to this love, by retrenching the inordinate appetites and evil inclinations which wed the heart to creatures. The affections must be united by mortification, and the heart set at liberty by an entire disengagement from the slavery of the senses, and all irregular affections. Then will a soul, by the assistance of grace, easily raise her affections to God, and adhere purely to him and his holy love will take possession of them. A stone cannot fall down to its center so long as the lets which hold it up are not taken away. So neither can a soul attain to the pure love of God while the strings of earthly attachment hold her down. Hence the maxims of the gospel and the example of the saints strongly inculcate the necessity of dying to ourselves by humility, meekness, patience, self-denial, and obedience. Nor does anything so much advance this interior crucifixion of the old man as the patient suffering of afflictions.

Her life compiled by Cresarius, monk of Heisterbach, is lost. Theodoric of Thuringia, a Dominican, (who seems to be the famous Theodoric of Apoldo, in 1289, author of the life of St. Dominic) wrote that of St. Elizabeth in eight books, extant in Canisius, (Lect. Antiq. t. 5) Lambecius (t. 2, Bibl. Vind.) Published an additional fragment, with several pieces relative to her canonization. Her life by James Montanus of Spire, published by Sedulius, abridged by D'Andilly, etc., is taken from the work of Theodoric. The letter of the holy priest, Conrad of Marpurg, the saint's confessor, to pope Gregory IX soon after her death, bears authentic testimony to her heroic virtues. Conrad's letter is published in an Appendix to the supplement of the Byzantine Historians, printed at Venice in 1723. It is accompanied with the authentic relation of miracles examined before Sifrid, archbishop of Mentz, Reymund, the Cistercian abbot of Eberbac, and master, or doctor Conrad, preacher of the ord of God, by commission of the holy see, who jointly sent the relation to the pope. See also St. Bonaventure, Serm. De S. Elizabetha, t. 5 A.D. 1231.

References:

1) Reverend Alban Butler (1883). *The Lives of the Saints*. Loreto Publications: Fitzwilliam, New Hampshire, 2020. Book Six, 811-823.

2) Hagiography Circle. Papal Canonizations before 1588 (2). Accessed 16 May 2022. http://newsaints.faithweb.com/Premodern_Canonizations2.htm

3) Dom Prosper Gueranger, O.S.B. (1805-1875). (2013). *The Liturgical Year: Volume XV - Time after Pentecost Book Six*. Fitzwilliam, New Hampshire: Loreto Publication, 289-299.

4) Dom Prosper Gueranger, O.S.B. (1805-1875). (2013). *The Liturgical Year*. Vol I - Advent. Fitzwilliam, New Hampshire: Loreto Publication, 266.

5) *The Liturgy of the Hours* Volume IV. (1975). English translation prepared by the International Commission on English in the Liturgy. New York: Catholic Book Publishing, 1567-1569

St. Amato Ronconi (Italy) (1238-1304)

*Rose to great heights of sanctity by serving God as a
hermit, pilgrim and nurse.
He founded the Hospital for Poor Pilgrims of Saludecio
and spent the last years of his life as a nurse[1]*

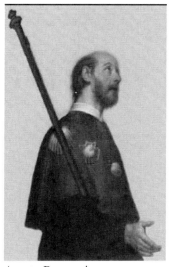

Amato Ronconi
Source: zivotopisysvatych.sk

Amato Ronconi was a layman, a Franciscan tertiary who followed the rule of 1221. Amato was born in 1225 (some text date his birth to 1238) in Saludecio, near Rimini (current day Italy). He lost his parents when he was young and was raised by his older brother, Giacomo, and worked on his farm. His brother's wife, Lansberga, wanted Amato to marry her younger sister in order to keep the family estate intact. However, Amato felt that God was calling him to a life of prayer and penance and instead joined the Third Order of St. Francis. He adopted a penitential lifestyle, living like a hermit at times, augmented by extravagant generosity to the poor. Many thought him a fool but God revealed miraculous signs. For example, a mysterious light was seen shining over the hut which served as his shelter and heavenly songs were heard to issue from it.

He went on pilgrimage to several shrines including making four pilgrimages to Santiago de Compostela in Spain, the site of the tomb of St. James the Great, Apostle. He also left his hermitage to take care of the poor and sick.

Lansberga was concerned about his extravagant giving to the poor and feared that he would literally give the farm away. Giacomo then divided the family estate and gave Amato a portion. This he converted to a hospital-hospice for the indigent, the sick and the many pilgrims on their way to Rome. (Hospice for Poor Pilgrims of Saludecio). It is now known as the Beato Amato Ronconi Nursing Home.[2]

On his fifth Camino trip, an angel appeared to Amato and urged him to head back. This, he believed, was a sign of his pending

59

death. He therefore deeded his property to the Benedictines so they could continue to serve the poor and ill. St. Amato Ronconi died in 1304 at the age of sixty-six. A home for the elderly continues to operate on the site of the hospital he founded.[3]

Many miracles were attributed to the intercession of Amato Ronconi. Pope Pius VI approved his beatification through the process of confirmation of cultus[4] on April 17, 1776.

In 1634 Pope Urban VIII forbade the public veneration of any purported saint unless the Congregation of Rites (now called the Congregation for the Causes of Saints [CCS]) proved that the person had been the object of an immemorial public veneration *(cultus ab immemorabili tempore]* at least one hundred years before the decree *Caelestis Hierusalem Cives.*

A formal diocesan inquiry was opened for Blessed Amato Ronconi on November 12, 1997. The decree of heroic virtue was promulgated on October 9, 2013 by Pope Francis and Pope Francis presided over his canonization at St. Peter's Square on November 23, 2014,[5] the Feast of Christ the King. (Memorial - May 15).

References:
1) Fr. Marion Habig, OFM. Franciscan Book of Saints. Accessed 19 April 2022. https://www.roman-catholic-saints.com/blessed-amatus-ronconi.html

2) Charles G. Braganza. Hagiography Circle. News 2014: Ordinary Public Consistory-Amato Ronconi. Accessed 19 April 2022. http://newsaints.faithweb.com/news_archives_2014.htm

3) Rick Becker. (25Oct2015). St. Amato Ronconi. Accessed 19 April 2022. https://clingingtoonions.blogspot.com/2015/10/saint-amato-ronconi-1225-1292.html.

4) Hagiography Circle. Confirmation of Cultus (1). Accessed 19 April 2022. http://www.newsaints.faithweb.com/confirmation_cultus.htm

5) Hagiography Circle. 13th century (12-Amato Ronconi). Accessed 19 April 2022. http://newsaints.faithweb.com/confirmation_cultus2.htm

St. Margaret of Cortona (Italy) (1247-1297), Incorrupt
*Initially provided nursing care to sick ladies, then
served the sick poor without recompense, subsisting solely on alms
Established a hospital in Cortona.
Founded Confraternity of Our Lady of Mercy to care for sick[1]
Franciscan Tertiary and Mystic*

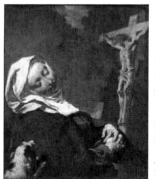

St. Margaret of Cortona by Giovanni Battista Piazzetta (fineartamerica.com)

Saint Margaret of Cortona was born in Laviano, Tuscany (Italy) in 1247. Her father was a farmer. In 1254, when she was seven years old, her mother died. She found it difficult to live with her step-mother.

At the age of 14, she left home and lived with a young 16-year old son of a local baron from Montepulciano named Arsenio, with whom she bore a son. She lived with him in the family castle as his mistress for nine years. Arsenio was murdered. This she discovered when his dog returned home without him and then led her to the forest to his decaying corpse.

The crime shocked Margaret into a life of penance. She returned with her son to Laviano but was not welcomed by her father or stepmother. She then moved to Cortona where she received asylum from the Friars Minor of Cortona. Margaret still had difficulty overcoming the temptations of the flesh. One Sunday she returned to Laviano with a cord around her neck. At Mass, she asked for pardon for her past scandal. She attempted to mutilate her face but was prevented by Friar Giunta.

She earned a living proving nursing care to sick ladies. She then began serving the sick poor without recompense and subsisted solely on alms. She became such a skilled midwife that many women insisted that only Margaret deliver their infants.[2]

In 1277, at the age of 30, Margaret became a Franciscan tertiary and pursued a life of prayer and penance at Cortona. Her son became a Franciscan Friar a few years later.

Margaret was a mystic and received messages from God some of which were recorded by Friar Giunta. She was said to be in direct contact with Jesus and received frequent ecstacies.

There around 1286 A.D., she received a charter allowing her to work for the sick poor on a permanent basis. She founded a hospital in 1288 and worked there as a nurse, preferring to serve those with the most repulsive diseases. She formed a group of tertiaries called The Poverelle or "Little Poor Sisters" to care for the ill serving in the hospital she had established in Cortona. She also founded the confraternity of Our Lady of Mercy,[3] composed of people, like herself, who were penitent over past sexual sins, to serve the City's poor.

Some people accused Margaret of having illicit relations with Friar Giunta. However, this she disregarded and continued to teach against vice, and through her, many returned to the sacraments. Sinners were drawn to her for advise and inspiration. She was devoted to the Eucharist and to the Passion of Jesus Christ.

She was divinely infused with the knowledge of the day and hour of her death. She died peacefully on February 22, 1297 after having spent 29 years performing acts of penance. Many miracles occurred at her grave including the raising of twelve persons. Her body is incorrupt and visible beneath the main altar of the Basilica of Cortona.[3]

Canonized in 1728 by Pope Benedict XIII. Patron saint of falsely accused, hoboes, homeless, insane, orphaned, mentally ill, midwives, penitents, single mothers, reformed prostitutes, third children, tramps.[4] (Memorial February 22)

St. Margaret of Cortona, Penitent, (February 22), from Rev. Alban Butler's (1883) Lives of Saints, Loreto Publications:[5]

> Margaret was a native of Alviano, in Tuscany. The harshness of a stepmother, and her own indulged propension to vice, cast her headlong into the greatest disorders. The sight of the carcass of a man, half putrefied, who had been her gallant, struck her with so great a fear of the divine judgments, and with so deep a sense of the treachery of this world, that she in a moment became a perfect penitent. The first thing she did was throw herself at her father's feet, bathed in tears, to beg his pardon for her contempt of his authority and fatherly admonitions. She spent the days and nights in tears; and to repair the scandal she had given by her crimes, she went to the parish church of Alviano, with a rope about her neck, and there asked public pardon for them. After this she repaired to Cortona, and made her most penitent confession to a father of the

order of St. Francis, who admired the great sentiments of compunction with which she was filled, and prescribed her austerities and practices suitable to her fervor. Her conversion happened in the year 1274, the twenty-fifth of her age. She was assaulted by violent temptations of various kinds, but courageously overcame them, and after a trial of three years, was admitted to her profession among the penitents of the third order of St. Francis, in Cortona. The extraordinary austerities with which she punished her criminal flesh soon disfigured her body. To exterior mortification she joined all sorts of humiliations; and the confusion with which she was covered at the sight of her own sins, pushed her on continually to invent many extraordinary means of drawing upon herself all manner of confusion before men. This model of true penitents, after twenty-three years spent in severe penance, and twenty of them in the religious habit, being worn out by austerities, and consumed by the fire of divine love, died on 22nd of February, in 1297. After the proof of many miracles, Leo X granted an office in her honor to the city of Cortona, which Urban VIII extended to the whole Franciscan order, in 1623; and she was canonized by Benedict XIII in 1728.

From her life written by her confessor, in the Acta Sanctorum; by Bollandus, p. 298. Wadding, Annal. FF. Minorum ad an. 1297; and the Lives of the SS. of Third Ord. Barb. T. 1, p. 508. A. D. 1297.

References:
1) Catholic Online. St. Margaret of Cortona. Accessed 9 May 2022.
https://www.catholic.org/saints/saint.php?saint_id=234

2)Thomas Craughwell. St. Margaret of Cortona: A saint for single mothers. Accessed 26 May 2022.
https://www.simplycatholic.com/st-margaret-of-cortona/

3) Confraternity of Our Lady of Mercy. Accessed 9May2022.
http://confraternityofourladyofmercy.org/

4) Francois Mauriac. Saint Margaret of Cortona. Accessed 26 May 2022.
https://www.goodreads.com/book/show/1828786.Saint_Margaret_of_Cortona

5) Reverend Alban Butler (1883). *The Lives of the Saints* as republished by Loreto Publications: Fitzwilliam, New Hampshire, 2020. Book Two, Vol. II & III, 184-185.

63

St. Elzear of Sabran (1295-1323) & Bl. Delphina Glandeves (1293-1369) (France/Italy)

He visited hospitals, especially those of lepers, whose loathsome sores he frequently kissed, cleansed and dressed with his own hands
Nursed the sick with such charity & reverence as if he were actually performing these services to Christ Himself
Performed miracles - Cured lepers & godson who became Pope Urban V
Only Franciscan couple to be formally canonized/beatified

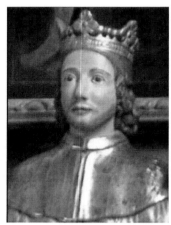

St. Elzear of Sabran
Source: saints.sqpn.com

Saint Elzear of Sabran was born in 1295 to Hermengaud of Sabran and Lauduna of Albes in the castle of Saint-Jean de Robians, at Ansois in the Diocese of Apt, in Provence, France. Both families were distinguished for their nobility. In addition to being the head of the House of Sabran in southern France, his father was created Count of Arian in the Kingdom of Naples. Elzear's mother, known as "the good countess" was a woman of great piety known for her charity work.

Upon his baptism, his mother consecrated him to God, asking that God to preserve him from ever staining his soul with sin. As he grew, he was friendly towards everyone and particularly devoted to the poor. Elzear was well educated in the eternal and human sciences and the use of weapons by his Uncle William of Sabran, Abbot of St. Victor at Marseilles.

At the age of 10, Charles II, King of Sicily and Count of Provence, caused Elzear to be affianced to Delphina of Glandeves. She was 12 at the time and two years his senior.

Delphina of Glandeves was born in 1293 the wealthy Count William of

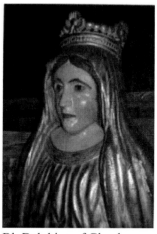

Bl. Delphina of Glandeves
melanierigney.com

64

Glandeves in southern France, the Lord of Chateau Pui-Michel, Languedoc, France. She was orphaned at a young age and raised by her aunt, the abbess at St. Catherine's Monastery in Sorbo. There she received an excellent education in both piety and everything pertaining to her eminent rank.

Elzear and Delphina had their marriage solemnized in 1308 at the castle of Pui-Michel. Both were in their early teens. At Delphina's suggestions, they both secretly agreed to live as brother and sister. Though not common in married couples, a celibate marriage was practice by many of the Essenes, a sect of Judaism; St. Joseph and the Blessed Virgin Mary; by some Third Order Franciscans and others. Sometimes the celibate union is for a few years, as was the case of the parents of St. Therese of Lisieux who subsequently had nine children, or for a lifetime as was the case between Elzear and Delphina.

With the brother of the King of Naples, Elzear commanded an army against Emperor Henry VII, who led the anti-papist Ghibelline party in Italy. After two battles, Elzear defeated the German sovereign, who died soon afterward in 1313. Count Elzear received many honors and prizes as reward for his victories.

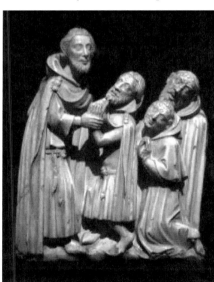

With great solicitude towards the poor, every day at noon he and the countess dined with the poor. He was calm and self-possessed. When people attempted to insult him, he would respond , "Worse things were said about Christ." St. Elzear often visited the hospitals, especially those of lepers, whose loathsome sores he frequently kissed, cleansed and dressed with his own hands. He every day washed the feet of twelve poor men and often served them himself, performing the office of a carver and cup-bearer.

St. Elzear Curing the Lepers - 1373
Walters Art Museum
ipernity.com

65

When Elzear was 23 years old, his father died and he inherited the County of Ariano and went to Italy to assume the government. Elzear considered it his sacred duty to care for the welfare of his people. They were initially opposed to his rule but through meekness and goodness he won their favor. He continued to observe the laws of God and his Church serving as an example to his people. He required those in his household to follow a Christian rule of life.

Returning to France, the couple joined the Third Order of St. Francis to be more intimately united to God. Elzear increased his pious exercises. He prayed the divine office daily, mortified his body and exhibited great acts of charity, nursing the sick with such charity and reverence as if he were actually performing these services to Christ himself. He was given the gift of miracles and cured several lepers and restored health to the son of the count of Grimoard, his godchild. He had prescient knowledge that his child would be elected to the office of the Holy Father and indeed he later became Pope Urban V.[1]

Elzear died at age 28 while on diplomatic mission to Paris, France. Meditating on Christ's passion gave him much solace amidst his pains. After receiving holy viaticum and extreme unction (now called the Sacrament of the Anointing of the Sick), Elzear died on September 27, 1323 in Paris. He was buried in Apt at the church of the Franciscan Friars.

His wife remained in the court of the King Robert and Queen Sancia of Naples. When King Robert died in 1343, Queen Sancia donned the habit of the Poor Clares in a nunnery she had founded in Naples where she lived for 10 years. Delphina accompanied the Queen and, then after her death, returned to Provence and led the life of a recluse in the castle of Ansois practicing penance, charity, assiduous prayers and other virtues. Delphina died on September 26, 1369 at age 76. She was buried with Elzear in Apt, France.

The miracles attributed to Elzear were recorded by order of His Holiness Pope Clement VI (1342-1352). Pope Urban V (1362-1370) signed the decree of his canonization on April 15, 1369, 46 years after Elzear's death.[2] Numerous miracles were also attributed to Delphina. His Holiness Pope Urban V approved her veneration. (Memorial September 26).

It is no great matter for a lion to tear lambs;
but for a lamb to pull a lion in pieces is admirable.
Now by God's assistance, you will shortly see this miracle.
If I receive any affront, or feel any movement of impatience begin to
arise in my breast, I turn all my thoughts towards Jesus Christ
crucified and say to myself: Can what I suffer bear any comparison
with what Jesus Christ was pleased to undergo for me?"
Thus to triumph over injuries was not want of courage,
but the most heroic greatness of soul, and true Christian generosity.

Writing out of Italy to St. Delphina who was in France, he said:
You desire to hear often of me. Go often to visit our amiable Lord
Jesus Christ in the holy sacrament. Enter in spirit His Sacred Heart.
You know that to be my constant dwelling. You will always find me
there.

When you are angry, speak not a word; otherwise you undo yourself.
More princes are ruined by their tongues and anger,
than by the edge of the sword.

The following is from *the original* Reverend Alban Butler's *Lives of Saints* (1883) republished in 2020 by Loreto Publications[3]:

St. Elzear Count of Arian and Delphina
        St. Elzear was descended of the ancient and illustrious family of Sabran in Provence; his father, Hermengaud of Sabran, was created count of Arian in the kingdom of Naples, his mother was Lauduna of Albes, a family no less distinguished for its nobility. The saint was born in 1295 at Ansois, a castle belonging to his father in the diocese of Apt. Immediately after his birth, his mother, whose great piety and charity to the poor had procured her the name of The Good Countess, taking him in her arms, offered him to God with great fervor, begging that he might never offend his divine majesty, but might rather die in his infancy than live ever to be guilty of so dreadful an evil. The child seemed formed from his cradle to piety and virtue; nor could he by any means be satisfied if he saw any poor beggar, till he was relieved; for which reason his nurses and governess were obliged to have their pockets always furnished with bread and small money, in order to give something to every poor person they met when they took him abroad; and it was his delight to divide his dinner with poor

children. The first impression of virtue he received from his mother, but these were perfected by his religious uncle, William of Sabran, abbot of St. Victor's at Marseilles, under whom he had his education in that monastery. In his tender age he wore a rough knotty cord, armed with sharp pricks, which galled his flesh, so that it was discovered by blood issuing from the wounds. The abbot severely chid him for this and some other extraordinary austerities which he practiced calling him a self-murderer; yet secretly admired so great fervor in a tender young lord.

The saint was only ten years old when Charles II, king of Sicily, and count of Provence, caused him to be affianced to Delphina of Glandeves, daughter to the lord of Pui-Michel, she being no more than twelve years of age. Three years after, in 1308, the marriage was solemnized at the castle of Pui-Michel; but at the suggestion of the young lady, they both secretly agreed to live together as brother and sister. The austerity with which they kept Lent, revived the example of the saints of the primitive ages and they fasted almost in the same manner Advent and many other days in the year. They lived seven years at Ansois; after which they removed to the castle of Pui-Michel. Elzear had til that time lived with his parents in the most dutiful and respectful subjection to them. He left them, with their consent, only for the sake of greater solitude, and that he might be more at liberty to pursue his exercises of devotion and piety. The saint was twenty-three years old when, by their deaths, he inherited his father's honors and estates; but these advantages he looked merely upon as talents and instruments put into his hands to be employed for the advancement of piety, the support of justice, and the relief and protection of the poor. By fervent and assiduous prayer and meditation on heavenly things, he fortified his soul against the poison of all inordinate love of creatures; he perfectly understood the falsehood and illusion of all those things which flatter and dazzle the senses, and he had a sovereign contempt and distaste for all that can only serve to feed self-love. Eternal goods were the sole object of his desires. He recited every day the office of the Church, with many other devotions, and he communicated almost every day, striving to do it every time with greater devotion. He said one day to Delphina: "I do not think a man on earth can enjoy any pleasure equal to that which I feel in the holy communion. It is the greatest delight and comfort of a soul in her earthly pilgrimage, to receive most frequently this divine sacrament." In prayer he was often favored with raptures and heavenly graces. By the constant habitual union of his soul with God he never found any difficulty in keeping it recollected in all places and at all times. He often watched great part of the nights on his knees in prayer. His devotion was not morose, because it was true and perfect; it rendered him always pleasant, mild, and agreeable to every one in conversation, though if in company the discourse turned on worldly trifles his thoughts took their flight so intensely toward God, that he was not able to listen to what was said, or he found some genteel excuse to withdraw to his closet.

It is a dangerous mistake to imagine that one can be devout merely by spending much time in prayer, and that devout persons can fall into a slothful and careless neglect of their temporal concerns. On the contrary, only solid virtue is able to do business, and to despatch it well. It taught Abraham, Isaac, and Jacob to be careful housekeepers, and excellent masters of families; it taught Moses to be a great legislator and commander, Josue to be a brave general, David a wise king, and the Maccabees invincible soldiers. In like manner St Elzear was rendered by his piety itself most faithful, prudent and dexterous in the management of temporal affairs, both domestic and public; valiant in war, active and prudent in peace, faithful in every duty and trust, and diligent in the care of his household. When he first began to keep house at Pui-Michel, he made the following regulations for his family, which he took care to see always observed.

"1) Everyone in my family shall daily hear mass, whatever business they may have. If God be well served in my house, nothing will be wanting.

2) Let no one swear, curse, or blaspheme, under pain of being severely chastised, and afterward shamefully dismissed. Can I hope that God will pour forth his heavenly blessings on my house, if it is filled with such miscreants who devote themselves to the devil? Or, can I endure stinking mouths which infect houses, and poison the souls of others?

3) Let all persons honor chastity, and let no one imagine that the least impurity in word or action shall ever go unpunished in Elzear's house. It is never to be hoped for of me.

4) Let all men and women confess their sins every week, and let no one be so unhappy as not to communicate at least on all the principal festivals; namely Christmas, Easter, Pentecost and the feasts of our Lady.

5) Let no person be idle in my house. In the morning, the first thing shall be that every one raise his heart to God with fervent prayer and oblation of himself, and of all his actions: then let all go to their business, the men abroad, the women at home. In the morning a little more time shall be allowed for meditation; but away with those who are perpetually in the church to avoid the business of

69

their employments. This they do, not because they love contemplation, but because they desire to have the work done for them. The life of the pious woman, as described by the Holy Ghost, is not only to pray well, but also to be modest and obedient, to ply her work diligently, and to take good care of the household. The ladies shall pray and read in the morning, but shall spend the afternoon at some work.

6) I will have no playing at dice, or any games of hazard. There are thousand innocent diversions, though time passes soon enough without being idly thrown away. Yet I desire not my castle to be a cloister, nor my people hermits. Let them be merry and sometimes divert themselves but never at the expense of conscience, or with danger of offending God.

7) Where peace reigns, there God dwells. Where envy, jealousy, suspicions, reports, and slanders are harbored in one family, two armies are formed, which are continually upon the watch and in ambush to surprise one another, and the master is besieged, wounded, and devoured by them both. Whoever will well serve God, he shall be dear to me; but I will never endure him who declares himself an enemy of God. Slanderers, detractors, and disorderly servants, tear one another to pieces. All such as do not fear God cannot be trusted by their master; but they will easily make a prey of his goods. Amidst such, he is in his house as in a trench, besieged on every side by enemies.

8) If any difference or quarrel happen, I will have the precept of the apostle inviolably observed, that the sun set not before it be appeased; but, in the instant that it falls out, let it be quashed, and all manner of bitterness laid in the tomb of forgetfulness. I know the impossibility of living among men, and not having something to suffer. Scarce is a man in tune with himself one whole day; and if a melancholy humor comes on him, he knows not well what he himself would have. Not to be willing to bear or pardon others, is diabolical; but to love enemies, and render good for evil, is the true touchstone of the sons of God. To such servants my house, my purse, and heart, shall be always open: I am willing to regard them as my masters.

9) Every evening all my family shall assemble to a pious conference in which they shall hear something spoken of God, the salvation of souls, and the gaining of paradise. What a shame is it, that though we are in this world only to gain heaven, we seldom seriously think of it; and scare every speak of it but at random! O life, how is it employed! O labors, how ill are they bestowed! For what follies do we sweat and toil! Discourses on heaven invite us to virtue and inspire us with a disrelish of the dangerous pleasures of

the world. By what means shall we learn to love God if we never speak of him?—Let none be absent from this conference upon pretense of attending my affairs. I have no business which so nearly toucheth my heart as the salvation of those that serve me. They have given themselves to me, and I resign all to God, master, servants, and all that is in my power.

10) I most strictly command that no officer or servant under my jurisdiction or authority injure any man in goods, honor or reputation, or oppress any poor person, or ruin any one under color of doing my business. I will not have my coffers filled by emptying those of others, or by squeezing the blood out of the veins, and the marrow out of the bones of the poor. Such blood-sucking wicked servants, to enrich their masters, damn both master and themselves. Do your imagine that a master who giveth five shillings in alms, wipeth away the theft of his servant who have torn out the entrails of the poor, whose cries for vengeance mount up to heaven? I had rather go naked to paradise, than, being clothed with gold and scarlet, be dragged with the impious rich man into hell. We shall be wealthy enough if we fear God. Any substance acquired by injustice or oppression will be like a fire hidden under the earth, which will rend, waste, and throw down or consume the whole. Let fourfold be restored if I be found to have anything which is another's; and let my dealings be public, that all who have been aggrieved on my account, may find redress. Shall a man whose treasures are in heaven, be so fond of earthly dirt? I came naked out of the womb of my mother, and shall quickly return naked into the womb of our common mother, the earth. Shall I, for a moment of life between these two tombs, hazard the salvation of my soul for eternity? If so, faith, virtue, and reason, would be wholly eclipsed, and all understanding blasted."

St. Elzear set himself the first example, in every point, which he prescribed to others. He was particularly careful that if any one let fall the least injurious or angry word against another, he should ask pardon, and make satisfaction, this humiliation being the most easy and effectual remedy of a passion which always takes its rise from pride. Delphina concurred with her husband in all his views, and was perfectly obedient to him. No coldness for so much as one moment ever interrupted the harmony or damped the affections of this holy couple. The pious countess was very sensible that the devotions of a married woman ought to be ordered in a different manner from those of a religious person; that contemplation is the sister of action, and that Martha and Mary must mutually help one another. Her time was so regulated, that she had certain hours allotted for spiritual exercises, and others for

71

household affairs and other duties. The care with which she looked into the economy of her house was a sensible proof of the interior order in which she kept her own soul. Nothing was more admirable than her attention to all her domestics, and her prudent application that peace should be observed, the fear of God and all virtues well entertained, and all brawling, tale-bearing, and other plagues of families banished. She loved her servants as her children, and she was honored by them as a mother and as a saint. In this example it appeared how truly it is said, that good and virtuous master make good servants, and that the families of saints are God's families. Alasia, sister to Delphina, lived with her, and was her faithful companion in all her pious exercises. It seemed that all that came under the roof of Elzear contracted a spirit of sincere piety; sisters and mistresses.

The gate through which the rich must enter heaven is mercy and charity to the poor. St. Elzear often visited the hospitals, especially those of lepers, whose loathsome sores he frequently kissed, cleansed, and dressed with his own hands. He every day washed the feet of twelve poor men, and often served them himself, performing the office of a carver and cup-bearer. He was the common father of all that were in distress, and provided large granaries of corn and storehouses of all other provisions for their relief. Being one day asked, why he so tenderly loved beggars, he answered with great feeling: "Because the bosom of the poor is the treasure of Jesus Christ." He used to say: "How can we ask God to bestow on us his kingdom, if we deny him a cup of water; how can we pray for his grace if we deny him what is his own? Does not he too much nor us in vouchsafing to accept anything from us?" In a time of scarcity, in 1310, his alms seemed to surpass all bounds. After his father's death he was obliged to go into the Kingdom of Arian. But the people being inclined to favor the house of Aragon against the French, and despising the meekness of the young prince, revolted, and refused to acknowledge him. Elzear opposed to their rebellion for three years no other arms than those of meekness and patience; which his friends reproachfully called indolence and cowardice. His cousin, the prince of Tarento, one day told him that his conduct hurt the common cause of his country, and said: "Allow me to take these rebels to task for you. I will hang up half a thousand, and make the rest as pliant as a glove. It is fit among the good to be a lamb, but with the wicked to play the lion. Such insolence must be curbed. Take your ease; say your prayers for me, and I will give so many blows for you, that the rabble shall give you no more trouble?" Elzear smiling, replied, "What! Would you have me begin my government with massacres and blood? I will overcome these men by good office. It is no great matter for a lion to tear lambs; but for a lamb to pull a lion in pieces is admirable. Now, by God's assistance, you will shortly see this miracle." The prince could not relish such language; the effect verified the prediction. For the citizens of Arian of their own accord became ashamed of their rebellion, and with the greatest submission and respect, invited the saint to take possession of his territory, and ever after loved and honored him as their father. Elzear discovered the true motive why he bore so patiently these insults and injuries saying: "If I receive any affront, or feel any movement of impatience begin to arise in my breast, I turn all my thoughts towards Jesus Christ crucified and say to myself: Can what I suffer bear any comparison with what Jesus Christ was pleased to undergo for me?" Thus to triumph over injuries was not want of courage, but the most heroic greatness of soul, and true Christian generosity. This was the constant conduct of our saint.

To mention one other instance: among the papers which his father left, the good count found the letters of a certain officer under his command, filled with outrageous calumnies against him, and persuading his father to disinherit him, as one fitter to be a monk than to bear arms. Delphina was moved to indignation upon reading such imprudent invectives, and said she hoped he would crush, and never foster in his breast such a scorpion, who, whilst he looked and spoke fair, could bear such deadly poison in his tail. St. Elzear told her that Christ commands us not to revenge but to forgive injuries, and to overcome the venom of hatred by charity: that therefore he would destroy and never make mention of those letters. He did so, and when this officer came to his chamber to wait upon him, he affectionately embraced him, made him a rich present, and so entirely gained his affection, that the captain offered himself afterward to be cut in a hundred pieces for his service. In like manner, on other occasions, he burnt or suppressed information that were given of injuries which others had done him, that he might spare the parties the confusion of knowing that he had received intelligence of them. In his country of Arian, he settled a rigorous administration of justice, and punished without mercy the least oppression in any of his officers. He visited malefactors that were condemned to die, and many who had persisted deaf to priests were moved by his tender exhortation to sincere compunction, and to accept their punishment in a spirit of penance. When their goods were confiscated to him, he secretly restored them to their wives and children. Writing out of Italy to St. Delphina, he said: "You desire to hear often of me. Go often to visit our amiable Lord Jesus Christ in the holy sacrament. Enter in spirit his sacred heart. You know that to be my constant dwelling. You will always find me there."

Elzear having settled his affairs in Italy, obtained leave of king Robert, the son and successor of Charles II and brother of St. Louis, bishop of Toulouse, to return into Provence for two years. He was received at Ansois with incredible joy. Not long after, Elzear being in the twenty fifth year of his age, and Delphina, after receiving the communion, pronounced publicly, at the font of the altar, in the chapel of the castle, mutual vows of perpetual chastity, which Elzear had till then kept unviolated without a vow, though Delphina had before made a secret vow. In the lives of this holy couple, the world saw pious retirement in the midst of worldly pomp, silent contemplation amidst the noise of public scenes, and in conjugal friendship a holy emulation to out view one another in piety, goodness and charity. Such happy strifes are carried on with sweet tranquility and peace, and are crowned with never-fading comfort and joy. The count had remained two years in Provence when king Robert recall him into Italy, and conferred on him the honor of knighthood, of which he had approved himself worthy by many actions of uncommon valor and address, and notable fears of arms. The saint had, according to custom, spent the night before the ceremony in the church watching in prayer; he went to confession and communicated in the morning. The king on this occasion shed tears of joy at the sight of his extraordinary devotion and piety; and the whole court admitted a prince who was at once a great soldier, a courtier, a married man, a virgin, and a saint.

King Robert chose him among all the lords of his dominions to be governor to his son Charles, duke of Calabria. The young prince was sprightly, but understood too well his high extraction, was intractable, and had contracted the contagious air of the court. The count took notice of his pupil's dangerous inclinations, but dissembled this for some time till he had won his affections, and gained sufficient credit with him. When he saw ita fit time, he made him tender remonstrances on his defects, on the necessity of a sublime virtue to support the dignity of his high rank, and on the life to come. The young prince was so penetrated with his discourses, that, leaping about his neck he said: "It is not yet too late to begin: what then must I do!" Elzear explained to him the virtues of piety, magnanimity, justice, and clemency, showing that a prince who fears God, has always a sure comfort and protection in heaven, though earth should fail him, and that he who undertakes, any business without first consulting God, deserves always to be unhappy and ruined; and is always impious. "Only assiduous devotion," said he, "can be the safeguard against the

74

dangers of vanity, flatterers, and the strong incentives of the passions. Go to confession and communion every great festival. Love the poor, , and God will multiply his favors upon your house. When you are angry, speak not a word; otherwise you undo yourself. More princes are ruined by their tongues and anger, than by the edge of the sword. You must hate flatterers as a plague; if you do not banish them, they will ruin you. Honor good men, and the prelates of the Church; this will be your principal greatness, etc. Elzear by his diligence and instructions corrected the vices of his pupil, who became a grave and virtuous prince. King Robert, going into Provence, left his son regent of Naples under the tuition of Elzear, who was chief of the council, and despatched almost all the affairs of state. Elzear entreated the duke to declare him advocate for the poor, and their agent in court. The duke heartily laughing said: "What kind of office do you beg? You will have no competitors in this ambition. I admit your request and recommend to you all the poor of this kingdom." Elzear made a low reverence, and thanked him heartily. For the discharge of this troublesome office he caused a great bag of purple velvet to be made, and with this passed through the streets, receiving in it all the requests and suits of the poor, with a cheerful countenance, full of commiseration, hearing grievances, dealing about alms, comforting the world, so that he seemed another Joseph of Egypt. He pleaded the causes of widows and orphans with wonderful eloquence, and procured them justice and charitable relief. Whilst the chief authority of the state was lodged in his hands, many offered him rich presents, which he refused, saying to those that called him on that account churlish: "It is more safe and easy to refuse all presents than to discern which might be received without danger. Neither is it easy for one who begins to take any, afterward to know where to stop, for these things are apt to create an appetite." The law of nature itself condemns as bribes all presents received by judges; they giving insensibly a bias and inclination to favor the party, as is evident by general experience. St. Elzear was so sincere a lover of truth that he was ready to die for it in the smallest points.

The emperor Henry VII invaded Naples with a great army, nor was pope Clement V able to divert him from his expedition. King Robert sent against him his brother John, and count Elzear with a great an army as he was able to raise. Two pitched battles were fought, in both which Henry was defeated, chiefly by the valor and conduct of Elzear, so that the emperor desired a peace, which was readily concluded. King Robert gave Elzear many great presents, which he accepted with one hand not to disoblige the king, but with the other distributed them all among the poor. This

75

king sent Elzear ambassador to Paris, attended with the flower of the nobility of Naples, to demand of Charles IV Mary, the daughter of the count of Valois, in marriage for the duke of Calabria. The negotiation was carried on with great success and the marriage concluded, and the good count was received at court not only with the greatest honor, but also with veneration, and as a living saint. In the meantime, the holy ambassador fell sick at Paris. He had made his will in 1317, at Toulon, by which he left his moveable goods to his wife Delphina, his real estates to his brother William of Sabran, and legacies to his relations and servants, and especially to many convents and hospitals. When the saint, three years before, made his public vow of chastity, he on the same day enrolled himself in the third order of St. Francis, into which seculars or laymen are admitted, upon condition of their wearing a part of the Franciscan habit under their clothes, and saying certain prayers every day; but these conditions are not binding under sin. St. Elzear in his sickness made a general confession, with great compunction and many tears, to the provincial of the Franciscans, and he continued to confess almost every day of his illness, though he is said never to have offended God by any mortal sin. The history of Christ's passion, which mystery had always been the favorite object of his devotion, was every day read to him, and in it he found exceeding great comfort amidst his pains. Receiving the holy viaticum he said with great joy, "This is my hope in this I desire to die."After extreme unction, and a painful agony, he happily expired on the 27th of September, in the year 1323, the twenty-eighth of his age. His death was exceedingly lamented by the kings of France and Naples, and by their whole courts. His body, according to his orders, was carried to Apt, and there interred in the church of the Franciscan Friars in that town, where it is still kept. Juridical informations were taken of his miracles by order of pope Clement VI. Urban V signed the decree of his canonization, but it was only published by Gregory XI in 1369, forty-six years after the saint's death, Delphina being still living. The king and queen of Naples would by no means suffer her to leave their court, to which she was a perfect model of piety. King Robert dying in 1343, the queen whose name was Sancia, and who was daughter to the king of Majorca, wearied with the empty greatness of the world, and loathing its vanity, put on the habit of a poor Clare in a nunnery which she had founded at Naples. In this state she lived ten years with great fervor, and would still have her dear Delphina near her, learning from her all the exercises of a spiritual life. After her death, Delphina returned into Provence, and led the life of a recluse in the castle of Ansois, in the heroic practice of penance, charity, assiduous prayer, and all other virtues. She died at Apt, near that castle, in the year 1369, the seventy-sixth of her age, on the 26th of September on which she is named in the martyrology of the Franciscan order. Her mortal remains were deposited in the same tomb with those of St. Elzear. *See the life of St. Elzear published by Surius: also Fite delli Santi del Terz. Ordine di S. Francesco. C. 14, 15, 16. 30. Suysken, t. 7, Sep. 528.*

References:

1) Marion A. Habig, O.F.M. (1979). The Franciscan Book of Saints. Franciscan Herald Press: Chicago, 722-727.

2) Hagiography Circle. Papal Canonizations before 1588 (2). St. Elzear de Sabran. Accessed 16 May 2022. http://newsaints.faithweb.com/Premodern_Canonizations2.htm

3) Reverend Alban Butler (1883). *The Lives of the Saints* as republished by Loreto Publications: Fitzwilliam, NH, 2020. Book Five, 821-831.

4) Roman Catholic Saints. St. Elzear of Sabran. Accessed 9 May 2022. https://www.roman-catholic-saints.com/saint-elzear-of-sabran.html

5) Catholic Online. Bl. Delphina. https://www.catholic.org/saints/

6) Roman Catholic Saints. Blessed Delphina of Glendeves. Accessed 16 May2022.https://delphinaroseart.com/blessed-delphina-and-saint-elzear/

7) Secular Franciscan Order USA. Accessed 16 May 2022. https://www.secularfranciscansusa.org/event/st-elzear-of-sabran-bl-delphine/2021-09-26/

St. Roch (Kingdom of Majorca [France]/Italy) (1295-1327)
Devoted himself in Italy to serve the sick during a raging pestilence
Caused many to be cured by making the Sign of the Cross over them
During the Council held in the city of Constance in 1414, the city was
delivered from the plague by imploring his intercession

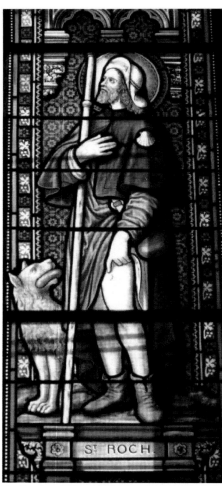

St. Roch of Montpellier at the Church of
St. Pierre-es-Liens in Dussac, France
theresadoyle-nelson.blogspot.com

Saint Roch was born in Montpellier around 1295. His father was a wealthy nobleman and possibly the governor of the town of Montpellier. His birth was in answer to his parents prayers for a child. He had a birthmark in the form of a cross that deeply marked his breast, a sign that the Blessed Virgin Mary had heard and answered his mother's prayers for her barrenness to be healed. His parents raised him in a devout manner. They all fasted twice a week as had been the custom in the early Church per the Didache c.. 60, 100 or 120 A.D.)

Both of Roch's parents died when he was 20 years old. He sold all the personal property he inherited and distribute the proceeds among the poor and then transferred the government of the city to his uncle. He then became a Third Order Franciscan and began a poor mendicant way of life. He went on pilgrimage to Rome.

In 1315, he arrived at Acquapendente near Viterbo in northern Italy and found that an

78

epidemic had broken out. Roch followed the example of Christ and offered his life in the service of his brothers and sisters in Christ. He cared for the sick both in their private homes and in the hospital — at great risk to himself. Roch served the sick without rest day and night. Reportedly, God rewarded his efforts by causing many to be cured at the mere *Sign of the Cross* which St. Roch made over them.

When the plague abated in Acquapendente, Roch continued on his journey to Rome. His miraculous healing powers were displayed in every pestilence-infested town that he passed on this way to Rome. In Rome, he also found that a pestilence had also broken out. So, in addition to visiting the holy places, Saint Roch devoted himself to the care of the sick, many of whom he miraculously cured.

When his travels brought him to the town of Piacenza (Italy), he became sick, contracting the disease in his leg. Instead of burdening anyone with his care, Roch left the house and using a staff dragged himself to a neighboring forest. There he found a dilapidated hut with a bit of straw, where he lay down. Reportedly a dog brought him bread for nourishment. His strength gradually returned.

Roch returned to Montpellier, his place of birth, where the citizens were at war. He was unrecognizable, and was accused of being a spy, arrested and imprisoned. He made no defense, wishing to conceal his true and noble identity. He entrusted himself completely to God's will. He wasted away in jail, forgotten and abandoned for five years. God sent angels to minister to him while he was held in captivity. As he felt death drawing near, he asked for a priest to administer the last sacraments. Following this, he died there on August 16, 1376.

According the Franciscan Book of Saints, when the priest entered his cell, a miraculous light filled the prison cell. Following his death inscribed on the wall, as if by angels, was his name and the prediction that the he would intercede for those afflicted by the plague. His uncle, the governor, was called to the cell. After which his mother, Roch's grandmother arrived and recognized Roch's body, due to the red, cross-shaped birthmark on his breast. They gave Roch a magnificent funeral and a church was built in his honor where he was buried. His body was moved from Montpellier to Venice in 1485, reportedly stolen by the Venetians (similar to that of

St. Mark the Evangelist which was taken to Venice from Alexandria, Egypt where St. Mark had served as the bishop). St. Roch's body is in the Chiesa di San Rocco (Church of St. Roch), Campo S. Rocco, 30125, Venice, Italy. His veneration spread throughout Europe. St. Roch was canonized by Pope Urban VIII.

St. Roch is the patron Saint of Montpellier, dogs and dog lovers. (Memorial - August 16).

The following is from *the original* Reverend Alban Butler's *Lives of Saints* (1883) republished in 2020 by Loreto Publications:[6]

> We find this eminent servant of God honored, especially in France and Italy, amongst the most illustrious saints in the fourteenth century, soon after his death, nevertheless, says F. Berthier, we have no authentic history of his life. All that we can affirm concerning him is, that he was born of a noble family at Montpellier, and making a pilgrimage of devotion to Rome, he devoted himself in Italy to serve the sick during a raging pestilence. Maldura says this happened at Placentia. Falling himself sick, and unable to assist others, and shunned and abandoned by the whole world, he made a shift to crawl rather than walk into a neighboring forest, where a dog used to lick his sores. He bore incredible pains with patience and holy joy, and God was pleased to restore him to his health. He returned into France, and in the practice of austere penance, and the most fervent piety and charity, he wore out his last years at Montpellier, where he died, as it is commonly said in 1327. Some postpone his death to the decline of the century, and think he went into Italy only in 1348, when historians mention that a pestilence made dreadful havoc in that country. Many cities have been speedily delivered from the plague by imploring his intercession, in particular that of Constance during the general council held there in 1414. His body was translated from Montpellier to Venice in 1485, where it is kept with great honor in a beautiful church; but certain portions of his relics are shown at Rome, Arles and many other places. *See Pinius the Bollandist, r. 3. Augusti, p. 380. F. Berthier, the last continuator of F. Longueva's Hist, de l Eglise de France, r. 13, 1. 37, ad an. 1327, and the life of St. Roch by Maldura, translated into French by D'Andilly. Also Pagi the Younger: Bened. XIV. etc.*

References:

1) La Comedie de Vanneau. Saint Roch: The Patron Saint of Montpellier. Accessed 9 May 2022.
https://www.lacomediedevanneau.com/saint-roch-montpellier/

2) New Advent. (60-80 A.D.). *The Didache (The Teachings of the Twelve Apostles)*. Chapter 8. Accessed 11 May 2022.
https://www.newadvent.org/fathers/0714.htm

3) Marion A. Habig, O.F.M. (1979). The Franciscan Book of Saints. Franciscan Herald Press: Chicago, 613-616.

4) Roman Catholic. Saint Roch. Accessed 27 May 2022.
https://www.roman-catholic-saints.com/saint-roch.html

5) Gretchen Filz (16Aug2017). The Story of St. Roch, Patron Saint of Dogs and Dog Lovers.
https://www.catholiccompany.com/magazine/st-roch-patron-of-dogs-6114#

6) Reverend Alban Butler (1883). *The Lives of the Saints* as republished by Loreto Publications: Fitzwilliam, New Hampshire, 2020. Book Five, Vol. VIII & IX, 199.

81

St. Bridget (Sweden) (1303–1373)

She was most zealous in serving the poor, especially the sick;
and set apart a house for their reception,
where she would often wash and kiss their feet.
Third Order Franciscan with husband;
Founded Brigittines (Order of the Most Holy Savior) following his death
Mystic

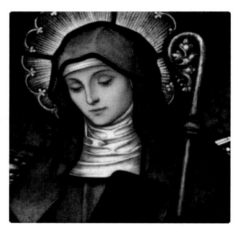

[1]**Bridget** was born in Sweden of noble and pious parents, and led a most holy life. While she was yet unborn, her mother was saved from shipwreck for her sake. At ten years of age, Bridget heard a sermon on the Passion of our Lord; and the next night she saw Jesus on the cross, covered with fresh blood, and speaking to her about His Passion. Thenceforward meditation on that subject affected her to such a degree, that she could never think of our Lord's sufferings without tears.

She was given in marriage to Ulfo prince of Nericia [a province in Sweden]; and won him, by example and persuasion, to a life of piety. She devoted herself with maternal love to the education of her children. She was most zealous in serving the poor, especially the sick; and set apart a house for their reception, where she would often wash and kiss their feet. Together with her husband, she went on pilgrimage to Compostella, to visit the tomb of the apostle St. James. On their return journey, Ulfo fell dangerously ill at Arras; but St. Dionysius, appearing to Bridget at night, foretold the restoration of her husband's health, and other future events.

Ulfo became a Cistercian monk, but died soon afterwards. Whereupon Bridget, having heard the voice of Christ calling her in a dream, embraced a more austere manner of life. Many secrets were then revealed to her by God. She founded the monastery of Vadstena under the rule of our Saviour, which was given her by our Lord himself. At his command, she went to Rome, where she kindled the

82

love of God in very many hearts. She made a pilgrimage to Jerusalem; but on her return to Rome she was attacked by fever, and suffered severely from sickness during a whole year. On the day she had foretold, she entered eternal life on July 23, 1373. Her body was translated to her monastery of Vadstena [Sweden]; and becoming illustrious for miracles, she was enrolled amongst the saints by Boniface IX.[1]

St. Bridget of Sweden the patron saint of Sweden, widows and is one of the six patron saints of Europe, together with Benedict of Nursia, Cyril and Methodius, Catherine of Siena and Edith Stein. (Memorial: October 8).

There is no sinner in the world, however much at enmity with God, who cannot recover God's grace by recourse to Mary, and by asking her assistance.

The following is from *the original* Reverend Alban Butler's *Lives of Saints* (1883) republished in 2020 by Loreto Publications:[2]

St. Birgit, more commonly called Bridget, or Birgit, was daughter of Birger, a prince of the royal blood of Sweden, legislator of Upland, and Ingeburgis, daughter to Sigridis, a lady descended from the kings of the Goths. Both the parents spent their lives in fervent exercises of piety, and had a singular devotion to the sacred passion of Christ. Birger consecrated all Fridays in a special manner to practices and penance, and never failed on that day to confess his sins, and receive Holy Eucharist, endeavoring to put himself into such a disposition as to be able to bear patiently all the crosses that might befall him till the next Friday. Ingeburgis was no less devoutly inclined, but died soon after the birth of our saint, which happened in the year 1304. Bridget was brought up by an aunt, who was a lady of singular piety. She did not begin to speak till she was three years old; and the first use she made of her tongue was to praise God: nor did she even in her childhood ever take pleasure in any discourse but what was serious. So strong and early was the grape of devotion with which God favored her, that from her cradle all her views and desires tended only to piety, and in its exercises she found her greatest delight. No symptoms ever appeared in her of anger, spite, envy, jealousy, untowardness, or disobedience. She assisted assiduously at the church office, and at sermons. At ten years of age she was most tenderly affected by a sermon which she heard on the passion of Christ; and the night following seemed to see Him hanging upon his cross, covered with wounds, and pouring forth his blood in streams in every part of his body; at the same time, she thought she heard Him say to her: "Look upon me, my daughter." "Alas," said she, "who has treated you thus?" She seemed to herself to hear him answer: "They who despised me, and are insensible to my love for them." The impression which this moving spectacle made upon her mind was never effaced; and from that time the sufferings of her redeemer became the subject of her most assiduous meditation, even when she was at work at her needle, and she could scarce ever call them to mind without shedding abundance of tears. In obedience to her father, when she was only sixteen years of age, she married Ulpho, prince of Nericia in Sweden, who was himself only eighteen. This pious couple passed the first year after their marriage in continence, and having enrolled themselves in the third order of St. Francis, lived in their own house as if they had been in a regular and austere monastery. They afterwards had eight children, four boys and four girls, who were all favored with the blessings of divine grace. Benedict and Gudma dying in their infancy, left their parents secure of their happiness; Charles and Birger died in the holy war in Palestine; Margaret and Cecily served God faithfully in the married state; and Indeburga and Catharine became nuns. The last was born in 1336, and died in 1381. She is honored among the saints on 22nd March. After the birth of these children, the parents, at the suggestion of St. Bridget, made a mutual vow of continency, and consecrated their estates more than ever to the use of the poor, whom they looked upon as their own family, and for whom they built an hospital, in which they served the sick with their own hands. Ulpho entered into the most perfect sentiments of virtue and penance, with which the example of his wife inspired him; and resigning his place in the king's council, and renouncing the court, he imitated her in all her devotion. To break all worldly ties by forsaking their country and friends, they made a painful pilgrimage to Compostella. In their return Ulpho fell sick at Arras, where he lodged with his wife and eight children, first in the street of the Lombards; but afterwards in the city, at the house of a clergyman or canon of our Lady's the cathedral, son of a nobleman named Bazentin, where , in the following century, Lewis XI lodged in 1477. He received the Viaticum and extreme unction from the hands of bishop of Arras, Andrew Ghini, a native of Florence. Bridget spared neither solicitude, pains, nor prayers for his recovery, and received assurance of it by a revelation. He was accordingly restored again to his health, and arrived in Sweden, where he died soon after, in 1344, in the odor of sanctity, in the monastery of Alvastre, of the Cistercian order, which rule, according to some, he had embraced, though others say that he was only preparing himself for that state. At least his name is inserted in the menology of that order on the 12th of February.

Bridget being by his death entirely at liberty to pursue her inclinations as to the manner of life which she desired to lead, renounced the rank of princess which she held in the world, to take upon her more perfectly the state of a penitent. Her husband's estates she divided among her children, according to the laws of justice and equity, and from that day seemed to forget what he had been in the world. She changed her habit, using no more linen except for a veil to cover her head, wearing a rough hair-shift, and, for a girdle, cords full of knots. The austerities which she practiced are incredible; on Fridays she redoubled her mortifications and other exercises, allowing herself no refection but a little bread and water. About the time of her husband's death, in 1344, she built the great monastery of Wastein, in the diocese of Lincopen, in Sweden; in which she placed sixty nuns, and, in a separate enclosure, friars, to the number of thirteen priests, in honor of the twelve apostles and St. Paul; four deacons, representing the four doctors of the church, and eight lay-brothers. She prescribed them the rule of St. Austin, with certain particular constitutions, which are said to have been dictated to her by our Savior in a vision; but this circumstances in neither mentioned by Boniface IX in the bull of her canonization, nor by Martin V in the confirmation of her order; and the popes, when they speak of this rule, mention only the approbation of the holy see, without making any inquiry about any such private revelation. The diocesan is the superior of all the monasteries of this order situated in his diocese; but no new convent can be founded but with an express license and confirmation of the pope. The chief object of the particular devotion prescribed by this rule are the passion of Christ, and the honor of His holy Mother. In this institute, as in the order of Fontevrault, the men are subject to the prioress of the nuns in temporals, but in spiritual the women are under the jurisdiction of the friars; the reason of which is, because the order being principally instituted for religious women, the men were chiefly admitted only to afford them such spiritual assistance as they want. The convents of the men and women are separated by an inviolable enclosure; but are contiguous so as to have the same church, in which the nuns keep choir above the doxal, the men underneath in the church; but they can never see one another. The number of religious persons in each double monastery is fixed as above; but most of the great or double monasteries which were situated in the

85

North, were destroyed at the change of religion, with that of Wastein, or Yatzen, which was the chief house of the order. There are two rich convents of nuns of this order at Genoa, into one of which only ladies of quality can be admitted. The greatest part of monasteries of Brigittines, or of the order of our savior, which now subsist, are single, and observe not the rule as to the number of religious, or the subjection of the friars to the nuns. There are still some double monasteries in Flanders, one at Dantzic, about ten in Germany, and some few others.

St. Bridget had spent two years in her monastery at Wastein when she undertook a pilgrimage to Rome, in order to venerate the relics of so many saints which are honored in that city, and especially to offer up her fervent prayers at the tombs of the apostles. The example of her virtue shone forth with brighter luster in that great city. The austerity of her watchings and penance, the tenderness of her devotion, her love of retirement, her fervor in visiting the churches, and in serving the sick in the hospitals, her severity towards herself, her mildness to all others, her profound humility, and her charity, appeared in all she did. Remarkable monuments of her devotion are still shown in the church of St. Paul and other places at Rome, and in its neighborhood; for the thirty last years of her life, she was accustomed to go every day to confession; and she communicated several times every week. The frequent use of the sacraments kindled every time fresh ardor in her soul. Nothing is more famous in the life of St. Bridget than the many revelations with which she was favored by God, chiefly concerning the sufferings of our blessed Savior, and revolution which were to happen in certain kingdoms. It is certain that God, who communicates Himself to His servants many ways, with infinite condescension, and distributes His gifts with infinite wisdom, treated this great saint and certain others with special marks of His goodness, conversing frequently with them in a most familiar manner, as the devout Blosius observes. Sometimes He spoke to them in visions, at other times He discovered to them hidden things by supernatural illustration of their understandings, or by representations raised in their imagination so clearly, that they could not be mistaken in them; but to distinguish the operations of the Holy Ghost, and the illusions of the enemy, requires great prudence and attention to the just criteria or rules for the discernment of spirits. Nor can any private revelations ever be of the same nature, or have the same weight and certainty with those that are public, which were made to the prophets to be by them promulgated to the church, and confirmed to men by the sanction of miracles and the authority of the church.

86

The learned divine John de Turrecremata, afterwards cardinal, by order of the council of Basel, examined the book of St. Bridget's revelations, and approved it as profitable for the instruction of the faithful; which approbation was admitted by the council as competent and sufficient. It however amounts to no more than a declaration that the doctrines contained in that book is conformable to the orthodox faith, and the revelation piously credible upon an historical probability. The learned cardinal Lambertini, afterward pope Benedict XIV, writes upon this subject as follows: "The approbation of such revelations is no more than a permission, that, after a mature examination, they may be published for the profit of the faithful. Though an assent of Catholic faith be not due to them, they deserve a human assent according to the rules of prudence by which they are probably and piously credible, as the revelations of B. Hildegardis, St. Bridget, and St. Catharine of Sienna." What is most of all praiseworthy in St. Bridget is, that in true simplicity of her heart, she always submitted her revelations to the judgment of the pastors of the church; and deeming herself unworthy even of the ordinary light of faith, she was far from every glorying in any extraordinary favors, which she never desired, and on which she never employed her mind but in order to increase her love and humility. If her revelations have rendered her name famous, it is by her heroic virtue and piety that it is venerable to the whole church. To live according to the spirit of the mysteries of religion, is something much greater and more sublime than to know hidden things, or to be favored with the most extraordinary visions. To have the science of angels without charity is to be only a tinkling cymbal; but both to have charity, and to speak the language of angels, was the happy privilege of St. Bridget. Her ardent love of Jesus Christ crucified moved her to make a painful pilgrimage to visit the holy places in Palestine, where she watered with her pious tears the chief places which Christ had sanctified by his divine steps, and purpled with His adorable blood. In her journey she visited the most renowned churches in Italy and Sicily, with a devotion that excited all who saw her to fervor. Being returned safe to Rome, she lived there a year longer, but during that interval was afflicted with grievous distempers, under which she suffered the most excruciating pains with an heroic patience and resignation. Having given her last moving instructions to her son Birger, and her daughter Catharine, who were with her, she was laid on sackcloth, received the last sacraments, and her soul, being released from its prison of clay took its flight to that kingdom after which she had always most ardently sighed, on the 23rd of July, 1373, being seventy-one years old. Her body was buried in the

Church of St. Laurence in Panis Perna, belonging to the convent of Poor Clares; but a year after her death, in July 1374, it was translated to her monastery of Wastein in Sweden, by the procurement of her son Birger and St. Catharine. She was canonized by Boniface IX in 1391, on the 7th of October, and her festival is appointed on the day following. At the petition of the clergy and nobility of Sweden the general council of Constance examined again the proofs, and unanimously declared her enrolled among the saints on the 1st of February 1415. Her canonization was again confirmed by Martin V in 1419.

The life and sufferings of our divine redeemer are the book of life, in which both souls which now begin to serve God, and those who have long exercised themselves in the most perfect practices of all heroic virtues, find the most powerful incentives and mean of spiritual improvement. The astonishing example which our most amiable and adorable savior here sets us of infinite meekness, patience, charity, and humility, if seriously considered and meditated upon, will speak a language which will reach the very bottom of our hearts, and totally reform our innermost affections and sentiments. That inordinate self-love and pride which by the contagion of sin seems almost interwoven in our very frame, will be beat down to the very ground; the poison of our passions, with which our souls are so deeply infected in all their powers, will be expelled by this sovereign antidote; and sincere compunction, patience, humility, charity, and contempt of the world will entirely possess our affections. The more a soul is advanced in the school of Christian virtues, the more feelingly she will find every circumstance in those sacred mysteries to be an unfathomed abyss of love, clemency, meekness, and humility and an inexhausted source of spiritual riches in all virtues. By this meditation she will daily learn more perfectly the spirit of our divine redeemer, and put on that blessed mind which was in Christ Jesus. In this interior conformity to Him consists the reformation and perfection of our inner man: this resemblance, this image of our divine original formed in us, entitles us to the happy portion of his promises.

References:
1) Dom Prosper Gueranger, O.S.B. (2013). The Liturgical Year: Volume XIV-Time after Pentecost Book Five. Fitzwilliam, NH: Loreto Publication.

2) Reverend Alban Butler (1883). *The Lives of the Saints* as republished by Loreto Publications: Fitzwilliam, New Hampshire, 2020. Book Six, 136-144

St. Catherine of Siena (Italy) (1347-1380) - Doctor of the Church

Her mission: to serve the poor and sick
Lay woman, 3rd Order Dominican
Stigmatic & Mystic

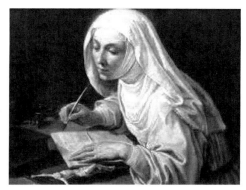

Catherine Benincasa was a lay woman, third order Dominican, virgin and doctor of the Church. She was born in 1347 in Siena, Italy to Lapa and James Benincasa. Her parents were a pious couple and her mother favored Catherine of all the children. At a young age, Catherine made a private vow of her virginity to God.

At the age of twelve her parents wanted to prepare for her a marriage engagement to which Catherine severely rejected. To distract her from her prayer life, she was assigned housework and other employments. She developed an interior prayer life able to commune with God in the interior of her soul regardless of whether at work or in solitude. Her sisters also tried to distract her with genteel dresses and worldly vanities.

Catherine liberally assisted the poor, served the sick and comforted the afflicted and prisoners. She observed several mortifications and ate sparingly. This all occurred prior to fifteen years of age.

When she was either eighteen in 1365, or twenty years old, she received the habit of the third order Dominicans. For three years she remained in a cell practicing prayer and mortifications and did not speak to anyone but God and her confessor. During a mystical vision she was told to reenter public life and to help the sick and poor.

When visiting the poor miraculously the amount of corn, oil and other necessities multiplied in her hands. She cared for a very difficult woman diagnosed with leprosy with only sweetness and humility. She cared for a woman with infectious cancer wounds with

89

great care. She obtained the conversion of both these women. She obtained the conversion of many sinners through continual tears, prayers, fasts and other austerities. When a pestilence broke out in Italy in 1374, she cared for the infected and obtained from God the cure of several.

When the Florentines were in conflict with the Holy See, which at that time was in Avignon, France, Catherine was asked to mediate the conflict. After traveling to and speaking with the chief magistrates of Florence, she traveled to Avignon where she was received by His Holiness Pope Gregory XI. Catherine encouraged Pope Gregory XI to fulfill a vow he had secretly made to return to Rome. She entreated him with several letters and eventually he did return to Rome.

She, then, resumed her activities of serving and often curing the sick, converting sinners and reconciling the most obstinate to the Church. Catherine continued to write Pope Gregory XI and exhorted him to bring peace to Italy. He, in turn, asked her again to intercede with the obstinate and disobedient Florentines. After successful negotiations and reconciliation, Catherine returned to Siena and resumed her pious practices and charitable works. She fasted once from Ash Wednesday until Ascension Thursday, receiving only the Holy Eucharist during that whole time (2-3 months).

As a mystic, she was said to have been offered to chose between two crowns, one of gold and the other of thorns. She chose the one of thorns so as to be united with and conformed to Jesus' passion. Her suffering would resume in 1378 following the death of Pope Gregory XI when the Church went into schism. Rome elected Pope Urban VI and several cardinal subsequently chose Clement VII. She wrote many letters: to Joan, queen of Sicily, the king of France, the king of Hungary, to name a few, in an attempting to unify the Church.

While still trying to reunite the Church under His Holiness Pope Urban VI, she died on April 29, 1380 in Rome at the age of thirty-three. She was burned in the church of the Minerva. Her body remains under the altar. Her skull was moved to the Dominican church in Siena. St. Catherine was canonized by His Holiness Pope Pius II in 1461. According to Butler's Lives of Saints, His Holiness Pope Urban VIII made her feast day April 30. However, it is currently (2022) celebrated on April 29th.

St. Catherine of Siena is one of the six patron saints of Europe, together with Benedict of Nursia, Cyril and Methodius, Bridget of Sweden and Edith Stein. (Memorial - April 29)

"Be who God meant you to be
and you will set the world on fire."

"Our Lord had taught her to build in her soul a private closet,
strongly vaulted with the Divine Providence, and to keep herself
always close and retired there; He assured her that by this means
she should find peace and perpetual repose in her soul,
which no storm or tribulation could disturb or interrupt."

From the Divine Office translated by Mary Ryan for the Order of St. Benedict, Inc. (1964):[2]

> Catherine, a virgin of Siena, born of devout parents, was granted the habit of St. Dominic worn by the Sisters of Penance. Her abstinence was most strict and her whole life was one of marvelous austerity. When she was staying at Pisa on the Lord's day, refreshed by the Bread of heaven and rapt in ecstasy, she saw the crucified Lord coming with a great light and from the marks of His wounds, five rays coming down to the same places in her body. Aware of the mystery, she implored the Lord that the wounds would not be visible, and the color of the rays immediately changed from that of blood to brightness, in the form of pure light touching her hands and feet and heart. But such was the pain she suffered, even though the signs of the bleeding wounds could not be seen, that she believed she would soon have died if God had not lessened it. Her learning was infused, not acquired. She went to Pope Gregory XI at Avignon and showed him that she knew by divine means of the vow he had made to return to the City, a vow known to God alone, and she was the cause of the Pope's going to occupy in person his See in Rome. In about the thirty-third year of her age, she went to her Bridegroom, and Pius II enrolled her among the holy virgins.

The following is from *the original* Reverend Alban Butler's *Lives of Saints* (1883) republished in 2020 by Loreto Publications:[3]

> Title: St. Catharine of Sienna - Virgin and Doctor of the Church.
>   St. Catharine was born at Sienna, in 1347. Her father,

91

James Benincasa, by trade a dyer, was a virtuous man; and though blessed with temporal prosperity, always chiefly solicitous to leave to his children a solid inheritance of virtue, by his example, and by deeply instilling into them lessons of piety. Her mother, Lapa, had a particular affection for this daughter above her other children; and the accomplishments of mind and body with which she was adorned made her the darling and delight of all that knew her, and procured her the name of Euphrosyna. She was favored by God with extraordinary graces as soon as she was capable of knowing Him. She withdrew very young to a solitude a little out of the town, to imitate the lives of the fathers of the desert. Returning after some time to her father's house, she continued to be guided by the same spirit. In her childhood she consecrated her virginity to God by a private vow. Her love of mortification and prayer, and her sentiments of virtue, were such as are not usually found in so tender an age. But God was pleased to put her resolution to a great trial, At twelve years of age, her parents thought of engaging her in a married state. Catharine found them deaf to her entreaties that she might live single; and therefore redoubled her prayers, watching, and austerities, knowing her protection must be from God alone. Her parents, regarding her inclination to solitude as unsuitable to the life for which they designed her, endeavored to divert her from it, and began to thwart her devotions, depriving her in this view of the little chamber or cell they had tell then allowed her. They loaded her with the most distracting employments, and laid on her all the drudgery of the house, as if she had been a person hired into the family for that purpose. The hardest labor, humiliations, contempt, and the insults of her sisters, were to the saint a subject of joy; and such was her ardent love of crosses, that she embraced them in all shapes with a holy eagerness, and received all railleries with an admirable sweetness and heroic patience. If any thing grieved her, it was the loss of her dear solitude. But the Holy Ghost, that interior faithful master, to whom she listened, taught her to make herself another solitude in her heart; where, amidst all her occupations, she considered herself always as alone with God; to whose presence she kept herself no less attentive than if she had no exterior employment to distract her. In that admirable Treatise of God's Providence, which she wrote, she saith, "That our Lord had taught her to build in her soul a private closet, strongly vaulted with the divine providence, and to keep herself always close and retired there; he assured her that by this means she should find peace and perpetual repose in her soul, which no storm or tribulation could disturb or interrupt." Her sisters and other friends persuaded her to join with them in the diversions of the wold, alleging, that virtue is not an enemy to neatness in dress, or to cheerfulness; under which soft names they endeavored to recommend the dangerous liberties of worldly pastimes and vanities. Catharine was accordingly prevailed upon by her sister to dress in a manner something more genteel; but she soon repented of her compliance, and wept for it during the remainder of her life, as the greatest infidelity she had ever been guilty of to her heavenly spouse. The death of her eldest sister, Bonaventura, soon after confirmed her in those sentiments. Her father, edified at her patience and virtue, at length approved and seconded her devotion, and all her pious desires. She liberally assisted the poor, served the sick, and comforted the afflicted and prisoners. Her chief subsistence was on boiled herbs, without either sauce or bread. Which last she seldom tasted. She wore a very rough haircloth, and a large iron girdle armed with sharp points, lay on the ground, and watched much. Humility, obedience, and a denial of her own will, even in her penitential austerities, gave them their true value. She began this course of life when under fifteen years of age. She was moreover visited with many painful distempers, which she underwent with incredible patience; she had also suffered much from the use of hot baths prescribed her by physicians. Amidst her pains, it was her constant prayer that they might serve for the expiation of her offences, and the purifying of her heart... She long desired, and in 1365, but eighteenth years of her age, (but two years later, according to some writers,) she received the habit of the third order of St. Dominic, in a nunnery contiguous to the Dominican's convent. From that time her cell became her paradise, prayer her element, and her mortifications had no longer any restraint. For three years she never spoke to any one but to God and her confessor. Her days and nights were employed in the delightful exercises of contemplation; the fruits whereof were supernatural lights, a most ardent love of God, and zeal for the conversion of sinners. The old serpent, seeing her angelical life, set all his engines at work to assault her virtue. He first filled her imagination with the most filthy representations, and assailed her heart with the basest and most humbling temptations. Afterwards, he spread in her soul such a cloud and darkness that it was the severest trial imaginable. She saw herself a hundred times on the brink of the precipice, but was always supported by an invisible hand. Her arms were fervent prayer, humility, resignation, and confidence in God. By these she persevered victorious, and was at last delivered from those trials which had only served to purify her heart. Our savior visiting her after this bitter conflict, she said to him: "Where wast Thou, my divine spouse, while I lay in such an abandoned, frightful

93

condition." "I was with thee," He seemed to reply. "What!" said she, "amidst the filthy abominations with which my soul was infested!" He answered: "They were displeasing and most painful to thee. This conflict therefore was thy merit, and the victory over them was owing to My presence." Her ghostly enemy also solicited her to pride, omitting neither violence not stratagem to seduce her into this vice; but invincible humility was a buckler to cover her from all his fiery darts. God recompensed her charity to the poor by many miracles, often multiplying provisions in her hands, and enabling her to carry loads of corn, oil, and other necessaries to the poor, which her natural strength could not otherwise have borne. The greatest miracle seemed her patience in bearing the murmurs, and even the reproaches, of these ungrateful and importunate people. Catharine dressed and served an old woman named Tocca, infected to that degree with a leprosy, that the magistrates had ordered her to be removed out of the city, and separated from all others. This poor wretch nevertheless made no other return to the tender charity of the saint, but continual bitter complaints and reproaches; which, instead of wearing out her constancy, only moved the saint to show her still greater marks of sweetness and humility. Another, whose infectious cancer the saint for a long time sucked and dressed, published against her the most infamous calumnies; in which she was seconded by a sister of the convent. Catharine bore in silence the violent persecution they brought upon her, and continued her affectionate services till, by her patience and prayers, she had obtained of God the conversion of both these enemies, which was followed by a retraction of their slander.

The ardent charity of this holy virgin made her indefatigable in laboring for the conversion of sinners, offering for that end continual tears, prayers, fasts, and other austerities, and thinking nothing difficult or above her strength. All her discourses, actions, and her very silence powerfully induced men to the love of virtue, so that no one, according to pope Pius II, even approached her who went not away better. Nannes, a powerful turbulent citizen, being brought to our saint to be reclaimed, all she could say to him to bring him to a right sense of his duty was of no effect; upon which she made a sudden pause in her discourse, to offer up her prayers for him: they were heard that very instant, and an entire change was wrought in the man, to which his tears and other tokens bore evidence. He accordingly reconciled himself to all his enemies, and embraced a most penitential life. When he afterwards fell into many temporal calamities, the saint rejoiced at his spiritual advantage under them, saying, God purged his heart from the poison with which it was infected by its inveterate attachment to creatures. Nannes gave to the saint a stately house which he possessed within two miles of the city. This, by the pope's authority, she converted into a nunnery. We omit the miraculous conversion of James Tholomei and his sisters, of Nicholas Tuldo, and many others; particularly of two famous assassins going to die with blasphemies in their mouths, and in transports of rage and despair, who were suddenly converted in their last moments, on the saints, praying for them, confessed their crimes to a priest with great signs of repentance, and appeared thoroughly resigned to the punishment about to be inflicted on them. A pestilence laying waste the country in 1374, Catharine devoted herself to serve the infected, and obtained of God te cure of several amongst others, of two holy Dominicans, Raymund of Capua , and Bartholomew of Sienna. The most hardened sinners could not withstand the force of her exhortations to a change of life. Thousands flocked from places at a distance in the country to hear or only to see her, and were brought over by her words or example to the true dispositions of sincere repentance. She undertook a journey to Monte Pulciano to consecrate to God two of her nieces, who there took the religious veil of Saint Dominic: and another journey to Pisa, by order of her superiors, at the earnest suit of the citizens. She there restored health to many in body, but to a far greater number in soul, Raymund of Capua and two other Dominicans were commissioned by pope Gregory XI, then residing at Avignon, to hear the confessions at Sienna, of those who were induced by the saint to enter upon a change of life; these priests were occupied, day and night, in hearing the confessions of many who had never confessed before; besides those of other who had acquitted themselves but superficially of that duty. While she was at Pisa, in 1375, the people of Florence and Perugia, with a great part of Tuscany, and even of the Ecclesiastical State, entered into a league against the holy see. The news of this disturbance was delivered to Catharine by Raymund of Capua, and her heart was pierced with the most bitter sorrow on account of those evils, which she had foretold three years before they came to their height. The two furious factions of the Guelphs and Ghibellines, who had so disturbed and divided the state of Florence, then a powerful commonwealth, united at last against the pope, to strip the holy see of the lands it possessed in Italy. The disturbance was begun in June, 1373, and a numerous army was set on foot: the word Libertas, written on the banner of the league, was signal. Perugia, Bologna, Viterbo, Ancona, and other strongholds, soon declared for them. The inhabitants of Arezzo, Lucca, Sienna, and other places, were kept within the bounds of duty by the prayers, letters, and exhortations of St. Catharine, and generously contemned the threats of the Florentines. Pope Gregory XI, residing at Avignon, wrote to the city of Florence, but without success. He therefore sent the cardinal Robert of Geneva, his legate, with an army, and laid the diocese of Florence under an interdict. Internal divisions, murders, and all other domestic miseries amongst the Florentines, joined with the conspiracy of the neighboring states, concurred to open their eyes, and made them sue for pardon. The magistrates sent to Sienna to beg St. Catharine would become their mediatrix. She could not resist their pressing entreaties. Before she arrived at Florence, she was met by the priors or chiefs of the magistrates; and the city left the management of the whole affair to her discretion, with a promise that she should be followed to Avignon by their ambassadors, who should sign and ratify the conditions of reconciliation between the parties at variance, and confirm every thing she had done. The saint arrived at Avignon on the 18th of June, 1376, and was received by the pope and cardinal with great marks of distinction. His holiness, after a conference with her, in admiration of her prudence and sanctity, said to her: "I desire nothing but peace, I put the affair entirely into your hands; only I recommend to you the honor of the church." But the Florentines sought not peace sincerely, and they continued to carry on secret intrigues to draw all of Italy from its obedience to the holy see. Their ambassadors arrived very late at Avignon, and spoke with so great insolence, that they showed peace was far from being the subject of their errand. God suffered the conclusion of this work to be deferred in punishment of the sins of the Florentines, by which means St. Catharine sanctified herself still more by suffering longer amidst a seditious people.

The saint had another point no less at heart in her journey to Avignon. Pope John XXII, a Frenchman, born at Cahors, bishop, first of Frejus, then of Avignon, lastly of Porto, being made pope in 1314, fixed his residence at Avignon, where John's successors, Benedict XII, Clement VI, Innocent VI, and Urban V, also resided. The then pope Gregory XI had made a secret vow to return to Rome; but not finding this design agreeable to his court, he consulted the holy virgin on this subject, who answered; "Fulfil what you have promised to God." The pope, surprised she should know by revelation what he had never discovered to any person on earth, was immediately determined to carry his good design into execution. The saint soon after left Avignon. We have several letters written by her to him, to press him to hasten his return; and he shortly after followed her, leaving Avignon on the 13th of September, in 1376. He overtook the saint at Genoa, where she made a short stay. At Sienna, she continued her former way of life, serving and often curing the sick, converting the most obstinate sinners, and reconciling the most inveterate enemies, more still by her prayers than by her words. Such was her knowledge of heavenly things, that certain Italian doctors, out of envy, and with the intent to expose her ignorance, being come to hold a conference with her, departed in confusion and admiration at her interior lights. The same had happened at Avignon, some time before, where three prelates, envying her credit with the pope, put to her the most intricate questions on an interior life, and many other subjects; but admiring her answers to all their difficulties, confessed to the pope they had never seen a soul so enlightened, and so profoundly humble as Catharine. She had many disciples: among others, Stephen, son of Conrad, a senator of Sienna. This nobleman was reduced by enemies to the last extremity. Seeing himself on the brink of ruin, he addressed himself to the saint, who, having first made a thorough convert of him from the world and its vanities, by her prayers miraculously, on a sudden, pacified all his persecutors, and calmed their fury. Stephen, from that time, looked upon as dust all that he had formerly most passionately loved and pursued; and he testified of himself, that by her presence, and more by her zealous discourses, he always found the divine love vehemently kindled in his breast, and his contempt of all earthly things increased. He became the most fervent among her disciples, made a collection of all her words as oracles, would be her secretary to write her letters, and her companion in her journeys to Avignon, Florence, and Rome; and at length, by her advice, professed himself a Carthusian monk. He assisted at her death, and wrote her life at the request of several princes; having been witness of her great miracles and virtues, and having experienced often in himself her spirit of prophecy, her knowledge of the consciences of others, and her extraordinary light in spiritual things.

St. Catharine wrote to pope Gregory XI, at Rome, strongly exhorting him to contribute by all means possible to the general peace of Italy. His holiness commissioned her to go to Florence still divided and obstinate in its disobedience. She lived some time in that factious place, amidst daily murders and confiscations, in frequent dangers of her own life many ways; in which she always showed herself most undaunted, even when swords were drawn against her. At length she overcame that obstinate people, and brought them to submission, obedience, and peace, though not under Gregory XI, as Baillet mistakes, but his successor, Urban VI, as her contemporary historian informs us. This memorable reconciliation was effected in 1378; after which Catharine hastened

97

to her solitary abode at Sienna, where her occupation, and, we may say, her very nourishment, was holy prayer; in which intercourse with the almighty, he discovered to her very wonderful mysteries, and bestowed on her a spirit which delivered the trust of salvation in a manner that astonished her hearers. Some of her discourses were collected, and composed the treatise *On Providence*, under her name. Her whole life seemed one continual miracle; but what the servants of God admired most in her, was the perpetual strict union of her soul with God. For, though obliged often to converse with different persons on so many different affairs, and transact business of the greatest moment, she was always occupied on God, and absorbed in him. For many years she had accustomed herself to so rigorous an abstinence, that the blessed Eucharist might be said to be almost the only nourishment which supported her. Once she fasted from Ash Wednesday till Ascension day, receiving only the blessed Eucharist during that whole time. Many treated her as a hypocrite, and invented all manner of calumnies against her; but she rejoiced at humiliations, and gloried in the cross of Christ as much as she dreaded and abhorred praise and applause. In a vision, our Savior is said one day to have presented her with two crowns, one of gold and the other of thorns, bidding her choose which of the two she pleased. She answered: "I desire, O Lord to live here always conformed to your passion, and to find pain and suffering my repose and delight." Then eagerly taking up the crown of thorns, she forcibly pressed it upon her head. The earnest desire and love of humiliations and crosses was nourished in her soul by assiduous meditation on the sufferings of our divine redeemer. What, above all things, pierced her heart was scandal, chiefly that of the unhappy great schism which followed the death of Gregory XI in 1378, when Urban VI was chosen at Rome, and acknowledged there by all the cardinals, though his election was in the beginning overawed by the Roman people, who demanded an Italian pope. Urban's harsh and austere temper alienated from him the affections of the cardinals, several of whom withdrew; and having declared the late election null, chose Clement VII, with whom they retired out of Italy, and resided at Avignon. Our saint, not content to spend herself in floods of tears, weeping before God for these evils of his church, wrote the strongest and most pathetic letters to those cardinals who had first acknowledged Urban, and afterward elected another; pressing them to return to their lawful pastor, and acknowledge Urban's title. She wrote also to several countries and princes in his favor, and to Urban himself, exhorting him to bear up cheerfully under the troubles he found himself involved in, and to abate somewhat of a temper that had made him so many enemies, and mollify that rigidness of disposition which had driven the world from him, and still kept a very considerable part of Christendom from acknowledging him. The pope listened to her, sent for her to Rome, followed her directions, and designed to send her, with St. Catharine of Sweden, to Joan, queen of Sicily, who had sided with Clement. Our saint grieved to see this occasion of martyrdom snatched from her when the journey was laid aside on account of the dangers that were foreseen to attend it. She wrote however to queen Joan: likewise two letters full of holy fire to the king of France, also to the king of Hungary, and others, to exhort them to renounce the schism.

We pass over the ecstasies and other wonderful favors this virgin received from heaven, and the innumerable miracles God wrought by her means. She has left us, besides the example of her life, six treatises in form of a dialogue, a discourse on the Annunciation of the Blessed Virgin, and three hundred and sixty-four letters, which show that she had a superior genius, and wrote perfectly well. While she was laboring to extend the obedience of the true pope, Urban VI, her infirmities and pains increasing, she died at Rome on the 29th of April, in 1380, being thirty-three years old. She was buried in the church of the Minerva, where her body is still kept under an altar. Her skull is in the Dominicans' church at Sienna, in which city are shown her house, her instruments of penance, and other relics. She was canonized by pope Pius II in 1461. Urban VIII transferred her festival to the 30th of this month.

When we read the lives of the saints, and consider the wonderful graces with which God enriched them, we admire their happiness in being so highly favored by him, and say to ourselves that their labors and sufferings bore no proportion to the sweetness of heavenly peace and love with which their souls were replenished, and the spiritual joy and consolation which were a present superabundant recompense and support. But is was in the victory over their passion, in the fervor of their charity, and in the perfection of their humility, patience, and meekness, that their virtue and their happiness chiefly consisted. Nor are we to imagine that God raised them to these sublime graces without their assiduous application to the practice both of exterior and interior mortification, especially of the latter. Self-denial prepared them for this state of perfect virtue, and supported them in it. What pity is it to hear persons talk of sublime virtue and to see them pretend to aspire after it, without having studied in earnest to die to themselves. Without this condition, all their fine discourses are mere speculation, and their endeavors fruitless. *(From her life by Raymund of Capua, her confessor, afterwards general of the*

99

Dominicans; also by Stephen, prior of the Carthusians, near Pavia, who had intimately known the saint, and from other contemporary authors. Likewise Diva Catharine Senesis Vita per Joan, Pinum, Tolosanum. Bononise, 4to. 1505. See her history judiciously and elegantly compiled by F. Touron, t.2, a writer justly extolled in the Journal de Scavants, and honored with great encomiums by pope Benedict XIV. Her life by her confessor, containing things omitted in other editions, is printed in Italian at Florence, in 1477, 4to., in a Gothic character; yet this is a translation from the Latin: also another printed at Sienna, in 1524, 4to. See also Papebroke's Remarks, Apr. T. 3, p. 851. A.D. 1380)

References:

1) Catholic Online. St. Catherine of Siena. https://www.catholic.org/saints/saint.php?saint_id=9 (Accessed 10Dec2021)

2) The Hours of the Divine Office in English and Latin (1964). Volume Two: Passion Sunday to end of July. The Proper of the Saints translated by Mary Ryan for the Order of St. Benedict, Inc. Collegeville, MN: The Liturgical Press, 1761-1762

3) Reverend Alban Butler (1883). *The Lives of the Saints* as republished by Loreto Publications: Fitzwilliam, New Hampshire, 2020. Book Three, Vol. IV & V - April and May, 292-301. (*Reprinted with permission*)

St. Frances of Rome (Italy) (1384-1440)

Dedicated to the care of the sick, dying and starving in Rome[5]
Grain and wine miraculously replenished after all given away
Founded Oblates of Mary (Collatines) dedicated to pray for the Holy
Father and care for the sick and poor in Rome — Mystic

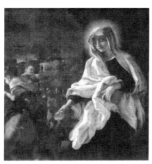

St. Francis of Rome
aesaintoftheday.blogspot.com

Saint Frances of Rome (mother, widow, mystic, Third Order Franciscan, Benedictine Oblate) was born in 1384 to Paul de Buxo and Jacobella Rofredeschi. Both parents were from wealthy families of noble Roman descent 1384. She desired to become a nun, however, her parents had other ideas and reportedly forced her into an arranged marriage at the age of twelve with Lorenzo Ponziani, a young nobleman. They had a good marriage and with him she bore three children.

Lorenzo and Frances lived in the Ponziani palace in the Trastevere section of Rome around the corner from the little church of San Francesco a Ripa. This church had been given by Brother Jacoba (the Roman lady Giacoma di Settesoli) to St. Francis in 1212. At this time there was an adjoining friary. Here Frances Ponziani was received as a Third Order Franciscan. Father Bartholomew Bondi, OFM, became her spiritual director.

Frances became seriously ill and Lorenzo, desiring for her cure, called to their home a man who practiced magic, whom Frances drove from their house. Reportedly St. Alexis appeared to her and cured her.

Frances was conscious of the presence and inspiration of her guardian angel. If she fell into any fault, he would give her a little nudge.

In 1401, at the age of 17, Frances gave birth of their first child, a son whom she named John Baptist. Soon thereafter, her mother-in-law died, leaving Frances to run the household which she did in a competent and Christian manner.

Frances found great companionship in the wife of her husband's brother, who also wished to live a life of service and prayer. Together, Frances and Vannozza, with their husbands' permission, would care for the poor, especially in hospitals.

101

As Frances family size increased to three, giving birth first to two sons and then a daughter, she focused her energies and attentions on caring for her family and household.

In 1402, the Black Plague swept Italy, devastating Rome. Frances' second son died. Frances used all her money and then sold her possessions to buy whatever the sick needed. Her husband initially objected. However when he went to look at the empty granary and found it miraculously filled with forty measures of wheat, he allowed her to continue her charity work.

A similar event occurred after Frances gave away all the wine held in the cask in their cellar. Her father-in-law found this empty and chastised her. Together she went with him to the cellar, turned open the spigot and the best wine any of them had ever tasted flowed. Her father-in-law reportedly stated, "Oh, my dear child, dispose henceforward of everything I possess, and multiply without end those alms that have gained you such favor in God's sight!"[2]

In 1410, when Frances was 26 years old, Rome was invaded. Lorenzo was wounded fighting with the papal troops. Frances nursed him back to health and he returned to the war. Their eldest son, John Baptist, was taken hostage and was only returned after peace was restored. Quickly following this civil war, the Black Plague devastated Rome taking the lives of her second son and daughter.

The peasants, who worked on the now war torn and wasted Ponziani farm, went to Frances asking for food. Frances dedicated herself to the care of the sick, starving and dying.[5] She reportedly opened a section of her home as a hospital. She organized a group of Roman women to assist her work. She also was stricken by the plague but suddenly recovered and resumed her charity work.

Another mystical experience was the encounter of her second son following his death. He brought her an archangel to take the place of her guardian angel. "The archangel's light was visible to her so that she could read by it. When she committed a slight fault, the archangel would hide himself and his light would not shine until she had made an act of contrition."[2]

In 1425, the group of Roman women, about a half dozen were clothed as oblates of St. Benedict which apparently did not cancel Frances' membership in the Franciscan Third Order. They called themselves the Oblates of Mary and were dedicated to God and the service of the poor.

102

Frances turned over the household care to her remaining son's wife and dedicated her energies to charity work in the city. Frances and Vanozza walked on pilgrimage over 100 miles from Rome to Assisi, the town of St. Francis and St. Clare. "Near Assisi St. Francis himself appeared to them, and provided the hungry and thirsty pilgrims with fresh juicy pears by striking a wild pear tree with his stick."[2]

In 1433, when Frances was 49 years old, Lorenzo died. After his death, Frances lived in community with the Oblates of Mary. They served the poorest of the poor in Rome. They prayed for the Holy Father and peace in Rome which was again in turmoil.

In 1944, at the age of 56, after returning to the convent from caring for her sick son, Frances became ill. She died seven days later on March 9, 1440. A few months after her burial, her tomb was open and her body was found incorrupt and emanating a pleasant fragrance. When it was again opened in 1638, only Frances' bones remained. Her tomb is located in Rome beneath the high altar in the crypt of the church now named in her honor: Santa Francesca Romana.

St. Frances of Rome was canonized by Pope Paul V in 1608. Patron of the Benedictine Oblates. (Memorial March 9)

A married woman must, when called upon,
quit her devotions to God at the altar,
to find Him in her household affairs."

God hath given, and God hath taken away. I rejoice
in those losses, because they are God's Will. Whatever He sends
I shall continually bless and praise His Name for."

The following is from *the original* Reverend Alban Butler's *Lives of Saints* (1883) republished in 2020 by Loreto Publications:[3]

Title: St. Frances, Widow, Foundress of the Collatines.
St. Frances was born at Rome in 1384. Her parents, Paul de Buxo and Jacobella Rofredeschi, were both of illustrious families. She imbibed early sentiments of piety, and such was her love of purity from her tender age, that she would not suffer her own father to touch even her hands, unless covered. She had always an aversion to the amusements of children, and loved

103

solitude and prayer. At eleven years of age she desired to enter a monastery, but, in obedience to her parents, was married to a rich young Roman nobleman, name Laurence Ponzani, in 1396. A grievous sickness showed how disagreeable this kind of life was to her inclination. She joined with it her former spirit; kept herself as retired as she could, shunning feasting and public meetings. All her delight was in prayer, meditation, and visiting churches. Above all, her obedience and condescension to her husband was inimitable, which engaged such a return of affection, that for forty years which they lived together, there never happened the least disagreement; and their whole life was a constant strife and emulation to prevent each other in mutual complaisance and respect. While she was at her prayers or other exercises, if called away by her husband, or the meanest person of her family, she laid all aside to obey without delay, saying: "A married woman must, when called upon, quit her devotions to God at the altar, to find Him in her household affairs." God was pleased to show her the merit of this her obedience; for the authors of her life relate, that being called away four times in beginning the same verse of a psalm in our Lady's office, returning the fifth time, she found that verse written in golden letters. She treated her domestics not as servants, but as brothers and sisters, and future heirs in heaven; and studied by all means in her power to induce them seriously to labor for their salvation. Her mortifications were extraordinary, especially when, some years before her husband's death, she was permitted by him to inflict on her body what hardships she pleased. She from that time abstained from wine, fish, and dainty meats, with a total abstinence from flesh, unless in her greatest sicknesses. Her ordinary diet was hard and moldy bread. She would procure secretly, out of the pouches of the beggars, their dry crusts in exchange for better bread. When she fared the best, she only added to bread a few unsavory herbs without oil, and drank nothing but water, making use of a human skull for her cup. She ate but once a day and by long abstinence had lost all relish of what she took. Her garments were of coarse serge, and she never wore linen, not even in sickness. Her discipline was armed with rowels and sharp points. She wore continually a hair shirt, and a girdle of horse-hair. An iron girdle had so galled her flesh, that her confessor obliged her to lay it aside. If she inadvertently chanced to offend God in the least, she severely that instant punished the part that had offended; as the tongue, by sharply biting it, etc. Her example was of such edification, that many Roman ladies having renounced a life of idleness, pomp, and softness, joined her in pious exercises, and put themselves under the direction of the Benedictine monks of the congregation of Monte Oliveto, without leaving the world, making vows, or wearing any particular habit. St. Frances prayed only for children that they might be citizens of heaven, and when she was blessed with them, it was her whole care to make them saints.

It pleased God, for her sanctification, to make trial of her virtue by many afflictions. During the troubles which ensured upon the invasion of Rome by Ladislas, king of Naples, and the great schism under pope John XXIII at the time of opening the council of Constance, in 1413, her husband, with his brother-in-law Paulucci, was banished Rome, his estates confiscated, his house pulled down, and his eldest son, John Baptist, detained a hostage. Her soul remained calm amidst all those storms: she said with Job: "God hath given, and God hath taken away. I rejoice in those losses, because they are God's will. Whatever he sends I shall continually bless and praise his name for." The schism being extinguished by the council of Constance, and tranquility restored at Rome, her husband recovered his dignity and estate. Some time after, moved by the great favors St. Frances received from heaven, and by her eminent virtue, he gave her full leave to live as she pleased; and he himself chose to serve God in a state of continency. He permitted her in his own lifetime to found a monastery of nuns, called Oblates, for the reception of such of her own sex as were disposed to embrace a religious life. The foundation of this house was in 1425. She gave them the rule of St. Benedict, adding some particular constitutions of her own, and put them under the direction of the congregation of the Olivetans. The house being too small for the numbers that fled to this sanctuary from the corruption of the world, she would gladly have removed her community to a larger house; but not finding one suitable, she enlarged it, in 1433, from which year the founding of the order is dated. It was approved by pope Eugenius IV in 1437. They are called Collatines, perhaps from the quarter of Rome in which they are situated; and Oblates, because they call their profession oblation, and use in it the word offero, not profiteor. St. Frances could not yet join her new family; but as soon as she had settled her domestic affairs, after the death of her husband, she went barefoot with a cord about her neck, to the monastery which she had founded and there, prostrate on the ground, before the religious, her spiritual children, begged to be admitted. She accordingly took the habit on St. Benedict's day, [July 11], in 1437. She always sought the meanest employments in the house, being fully persuaded she was of all the most contemptible before God; and she labored to appear as mean in the eyes of the world as she was in her own. She continued the same humiliations, and the same universal poverty though soon after chosen superioress of her congregation. Almighty God bestowed on her humility, extraordinary graces, and supernatural favors, as frequent visions, raptures, and the gift of prophesy. She enjoyed the familiar conversation of her angel guardian, as her life and the process of her canonization attest. She was extremely affected by meditating on our Savior's passion, which she had always present to her mind. At mass she was so absorbed in God as to seem immoveable, especially after holy communion: she often fell into ecstasies of love and devotion. She was particularly devout to St. John the Evangelist, and above all to our Lady, under whose singular protection she put her order. Going out to see her son John Baptist, who was dangerously sick, she fell so ill herself that she could not return to her monastery at night. After having foretold her death, and received the sacraments, she expired on the 9th of March, in the year 1440, and of her age the fifty-sixth. God attested her sanctity by miracles: she was honored among the saints immediately after her death, and solemnly canonized by Paul V in 1608. Her shrine in Rome is most magnificent and rich; and her festival is kept as a holy day in the city, with great solemnity. The Oblates make no solemn vows, only a promise of obedience to the mother-president, enjoy pensions, inherit estates, and go abroad with leave. Their abbey in Rome is filled with ladies of the first rank.

In a religious life, in which a regular distribution of holy employments and duties takes up the whole day, and leaves no interstices of time for idleness, sloth, or the world, hours pass in these exercises with the rapidity of moments, and moments by fervor of the desires bear the value of years. There is not an instant in which a soul is not employed for God, and studies not with her whole heart to please Him. Every step, every thought and desire, is a sacrifice of fidelity, obedience, and love offered to Him. Even meals, recreation, and rest, are sanctified by this intention; and from the religious vows and habitual purpose of the soul of consecrating herself entirely to God in time and eternity, every action, as St. Thomas teaches, renews and contains the fervor and merits of this entire consecration, of which it is a part. In a secular life, a person by regularity in the employment of his time, and fervor in devoting himself to God in all his actions and designs, may in some degree enjoy the same happiness and advantage. This St. Frances perfectly practised, even before she renounced the world. She lived forty years with her husband without ever giving him the least occasion of offence; and by the fervor with which she conversed of heaven, she seemed already to have quitted the earth, and to have made paradise her ordinary dwelling. *(Abridged from her life by her confessor Canon. Mattiotti; and that by Magdalen Dell'Anguillara, superioress of the Oblates, or Collatines. Helyot, Hist, des Ordr. Mon. T. 6, p. 208. A.D. 1440.)*

References:

1) Franciscan Media. (9Mar2021). Saint Frances of Rome. Accessed 14 May 2022. https://www.franciscanmedia.org/saint-of-the-day/saint-frances-of-rome

2) Marion Habig. OFM. St. Frances of Rome. Accessed 14 May 2022. https://www.roman-catholic-saints.com/st-frances-of-rome.html

3) Hagiography Circle. 9 March. Saint Frances [Francesca] of Rome. Accessed 14 May 2022. http://newsaints.faithweb.com/martyrology/March/09.htm

4) Reverend Alban Butler (1883). *The Lives of the Saints* as republished by Loreto Publications: Fitzwilliam, New Hampshire, 2020. Book Two, Vol. II & III - February and March, 344-348. (*Reprinted with permission*)

5) Marion A. Habig, O.F.M. (1979). *The Franciscan Book of Saints.* Franciscan Herald Press: Chicago, 174-177.

St. Didacus (Spain) (d. 1463)

He was entrusted with the care of the sick in the convent of Ava Caeli.
With such loving charity did he acquit himself of this duty,
that the sick wanted for nothing even during a famine in the city;
...for his great faith and his gift of healing;
for by signing the cross upon the sick with oil from a
lamp burning before an image of the Mother of God, to whom
he had the greatest devotion, he miraculously cured many of them.

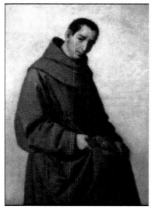

St. Didacus
Source: scborromeo.org

Didacus, (lay Franciscan brother) was born around 1400 in San Nicolas in the diocese of Seville, in Andalusia (Spain). As a young man, he led the life of a hermit under the guidance of a devout hermit priest. He returned to his parents after some time and subsequently took the habit of the Observantine Friar Minors (St. Francis's of Arrizafa) becoming a lay brothers who served in manual labor and the humble offices of the convent (as opposed to serving in the choir).

After his profession, Brother Didacus was sent to the Canary Islands with a priest, where he was instrumental in converting many to Christianity. There he served for several years. Though only a brother, he was selected as the first guardian or warden of the convent. Returning to Spain, he served in various convents in Seville.

In 1450, when over three thousand eight hundred religious persons of the order of St. Francis assembled in Rome to celebrate the canonization of St. Bernardine, he accompanied F. Alfonsus de Castro in his journey. His companion suffered a serious illness and Didacus cared for him with such fervor of spirit and ardent charity that it was easy to see how much God aided and favored him. He cared for many of the order who were sick in Rome, during the thirteen weeks that he stayed there.

He returned to Seville and lived thirteen more years at the convent of Saussaye and in the Castille, in the convent of Alcala of Henares. He fell ill in 1463 from what began as an abscess in his arm. With his brethren surrounding his bed, he asked for the cord the

108

friars wore, which he placed around his neck. He then held a wooden cross in his hands and tearfully begged pardon from those surrounding his bed. With his brethren praying for him, he then gazed upon the crucifix praying the words of the hymn on the cross, *"O faithful wood, O precious nails! You have borne an exceedingly sweet burden, for you have been deemed worthy to bear the Lord and King of heaven."* St. Didacus died on November 12, 1463, around the age of 63. His burial was delayed due to the voluminous number of pilgrims who came to honor his remains. His body was incorrupt and exuded a pleasant odor. He was eventually buried in the Franciscan church at Alcala de Henares.

St. Didacus performed many miracles during his lifetime. Following his death, many miracles continued to occur at his tomb. A miracle of note which lead to his formal canonization was the cure of Don Carlos, son of king Philip II, who, at the age of seventeen, had fallen at the palace of Alcala sustaining a head wound judged by the surgeons to be mortal. King Philip II had the shrine of Didacus brought to the room of the dying prince, which was done with great devotion and holy pomp and thereupon the prince's wound was immediately healed.[2]

King Philip requested that Didacus be canonized which was done by His Holiness Pope Sixtus V (1585-1590) in 1588, twenty-five years after Didacus' death. His Holiness Blessed Pope Innocent XI (1676-1689)[4] ordered his office in the Roman Breviary be celebrated to November 13. St. Didacus is a special patron saint of the Franciscans who are brothers.[3] The Spanish Mission in San Diego, California (Mission Basilica San Diego de Alcala) founded by the Franciscan St. Junipero Serra, O.F.M. (1713-1784) was named for St. Didacus. (Memorial - November 13).

From the Divine Office translated by Mary Ryan for the Order of St. Benedict, Inc. (1964):

> Didacus was a Spaniard from the town of San Nicholas del Puerto in the diocese of Seville. From his early youth he served his apprenticeship in the life of holiness under the guidance of a good priest. Then, in order to unite himself more closely with God, he was professed as a lay brother, in the convent of Arizafa under the rule of St. Francis of Assisi. There he submitted eagerly to the yoke of humble obedience and regular observance, devoting himself

109

primarily to contemplation. And God's light was so wonderfully poured out on him that although he was unlettered, he used to speak of heavenly things in a remarkable way which was clearly due to divine inspiration. At a mission in the Canary islands he endured many hardships, burning with the desire for martyrdom, and brought many unbelievers by his word and example to faith in Christ. He was sent to care for the sick at the convent of Ara Coeli in Rome, and carried out this work in a wonderful spirit of charity, the grace of healing shining out from him. Finally at Alcala he departed this life in a most holy way in the year 1463. Famous for miracles, he was numbered among the Saints by Sixtus V.[1]

The following is from the *original* Reverend Alban Butler's Lives of Saints (1883) republished in 2020 by Loreto Publications:[2]

Title: St. Didacus, Confessor

Didacus or Diego (that is, in Spanish, James) was a native of the little town of St. Nicholas, in the diocese of Seville, in Andalusia, of mean condition, but from his childhood fervent in the love of God, and the practice of all virtues. Near that town a holy priest led an eremitical life, and Didacus in his youth obtained his consent to live with him. Though very young he imitated the austerities and devotions of his master and they cultivated together a little garden; and also employed themselves in making wooden spoons, trenches, and such like mean utensils. After having lived thus a recluse for some years, he was obliged to return to his parents; but desiring most ardently to walk in the footsteps of his divine redeemer, he soon after betook himself to a convent of the Observantine Friar Minors, called St. Francis's of Arrizafa, and there took the habit among the lay-brothers who belong not to the choir, but serve the convent in humble offices, and are much employed in manual labor. After his profession he was sent with a priest of his order into the Canary Islands, where he did wonders in instructing and converting many idolaters, and though only a lay-brother, was appointed by his superiors the first guardian or warden of a convent which was erected in one of those islands called Forteventura. By the mortification of his flesh and of his own will, and assiduous prayer, he offered himself a continual sacrifice to our Lord, and by this long martyrdom prepared himself to shed his blood for the faith among the barbarians, if such had been the will of God. After some time, he was recalled into Spain, and lived in divers convents about Seville with great fervor, simplicity, austerity, and recollection; he seemed so much absorbed in God as

110

scare to be able to speak but to him, or of him; and the humility, ardor, and lively sentiments with which he always discoursed of heavenly things, discovered how much he was dead to himself and replenished with the divine Spirit.

In the year 1450, a great jubilee was celebrated at Rome; and St. Bernadine of Sienna being canonized at the same time, three thousand eight hundred religious persons of the of the order of St. Francis were assembled there, in their great convent, called Aracaeli. Didacus went thither with F. Alfonsus de Castro. In this journey our saint attended his companion during a dangerous illness with such fervor of spirit, and such an ardent charity, that it was easy to see how much God aided and favored him, and how wonderfully he was animated with his spirit in all the pains he took night and day for his love. This appeared still more in the charity and devotion with which he waited on many other of his order that were sick at Rome, during thirteen weeks that he stayed there. From Rome the servant of God returned back to Seville, and lived thirteen years longer in the convent, first of Saussaye, and chiefly of Alcala of Henares, in Castile, shining in all kinds of virtue, going forward every day in perfection, and moving wonderfully all who conversed with him to aspire to the same. Not content punctually to keep the rule of his holy father St. Francis, he endeavored with all his strength to draw in himself the most perfect portraiture of his heavenly life. His admirable humility, by which he put himself under the feet of everyone, was a great source of the constant peace of mind which he enjoyed; for, so perfect was the mastery which he had gained over his passions, and his soul was so much raised above all earthly things, that nobody ever saw him troubled, heard from his mouth an angry or unbeseeming word, or discerned anything in his conduct which did not seem to breathe an air of perfect virtue. Having no other will but that of our Lord, in whose cross he gloried, he accepted everything with equal cheerfulness from his hand, and equally praised him in adversity and prosperity. He treated his body very rigorously: his habit was always mean, and his attire and whole exterior deportment was an image of the interior mortification of his soul. With the perfect spirit and practice of penance he joined her good sister, continual prayer, and the elevation of his soul to God. In contemplation his body was sometimes seen raised from the ground, while his soul was ravished and absorbed in God. The passion of our divine Redeemer was the ordinary object on which his thoughts and affections were employed; he often meditated upon it with a crucifix in his hand, and with frequent raptures. When he passed from the contemplation of the bloody sacrifice in which the same

111

sacred victim continues daily to be offered on our altars, his love and fervor were redoubled. A God in the Holy Eucharist made the spiritual food of our souls, was the object of his admiration, and the nourishment of his love; and the oftener he received this God of love in his breast, the more were the flames of his love increased. His tender devotion to the Son extended to the mother, whom he honored as his advocate.

In 1463, he was taken ill at Alcala, where he had spent the last years of his life. His distemper began by an imposthume in his arm. During this illness his preparation for his last hour was most fervent and edifying. In his agony he called for a cord (such as the friars wear) and put it about his neck, and holding a cross of wood in his hands, with tears in his eyes he begged pardon of all his religious brethren that were assembled about his bed in prayer. Then fixing his eyes on the crucifix he repeated with great tenderness the words of the hymn on the cross: *Dulce lignum, dulces clavos, etc.*, and calmly expired on the 12th of November, in 1462. Several miracles were performed by him in his lifetime; and many more through his intercession after his death. Don Carlos, son of king Philip II, having by a fall at the palace of Alcala, hurt his head so grievously that they wound was judge mortal by the surgeons; and miracles being then frequently wrought at the tomb of St. Didacus, the king caused his shrine to be brought into the chamber of the dying prince, which was done with great devotion and holy pomp; and thereupon the prince's wound was immediately healed. Philip II, out of gratitude, solicited the saint's canonization, which was performed by Sixtus V in 1588. Innocent XI appointed his office in the Roman Breviary, and ordered his feast to be transferred to the 13th of November, though in his order it continues to be observed on the 12th. See on this saint, Mark of Lisbon in the chronicle of his order; and the history of the life, miracles and canonization, compiled by Peter Gelasinius, apostolic prothonotary, and Francis Pegna, the celebrated auditor of the Rota, by order of his holiness. See also Sedulius's Historia Seraphica.[2]

References:

1) The Hours of the Divine Office in English and Latin (1964). Volume Two: Passion Sunday to end of July. The Proper of the Saints translated by Mary Ryan for the Order of St. Benedict, Inc. Collegeville, MN: The Liturgical Press, 1806-1807

2) Reverend Alban Butler (1883). The Lives of the Saints as republished by Loreto Publications: Fitzwilliam, New Hampshire, 2020. Book Six, Volume X & XI - October and November, 728-731.

3) Marion A. Habig, O.F.M. (1979). The Franciscan Book of Saints. Franciscan Herald Press: Chicago, 833-835.

St. John of God (Portugal/Spain) (1495-1550)
Patron Saint of Nurses and Nurses' Associations
declared by Pope Pius XI in 1930.[1][2]
His followers formed the Brothers Hospitallers of St. John of God,
a world-wide Catholic religious institute
dedicated to the care of the poor,
sick and those suffering from mental disorders[3]

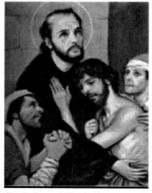

St. John of God, Patron of Nurses   Hospitallers.org

St. John of God is one of two saints who were declared patrons of nurses and nursing associations by Pope Pius XI in 1930. He was born on March 8, 1495, in Portugal, to poor devout Christian parents. He left home and worked as a shepherd in Castile for the count of Oropeusa. At age 22, to avoid marriage to the shepherd's daughter, he enlisted in the Roman Emperor's army where he lived a dissolute life. He left the army in 1535, and went to Andalusia in 1536. He repented of his past sins and began exercises of prayer and mortification. With some companions he planned to go to Africa to help the slaves and perhaps suffer martyrdom. En route he was waylaid to help a gentleman and his family in Gibraltar who was condemned to banishment by King John III who had confiscated their estate. He journeyed with them to Ceuta supporting them by what he made from day-labor.

He returned to Gibraltar and worked as a peddler selling little pictures and books of devotion. In 1538, at age forty-three, he opened a shop in Granada selling his increasing stock. Here he heard a sermon preached by St. John D'Avila, Doctor of the Church, on the soldier St. Sebastian's day, which caused him great anguish in regards to his past sins. He exhibited so much anguish and remorse and was physically self destructive that he was placed in a "madhouse."

There St. John D'Avila came to visit him and convinced him to be more moderate in his mortifications. John of God remained in the hospital until 1539 when he was released on St. Ursula's day. He focused on doing something for the poor. He went on pilgrimage to our Lady of Guadaloupa asking her intercession. He began selling

114

wood to feed the poor. He soon rented a house of harbor for poor sick persons. Thus in 1540, he began the foundation which would become a world wide ministry. He cared for the sick day and night while the townspeople brought him all the necessaries for his little hospital. The archbishop of Granada, seeing the great charitable work, was also a benefactor. The bishop of Tuy bestowed upon him the name, John of God, and gave him a habit. The marquis of Tarisa tested his charity by disguising himself and asking for alms. When he observe that John gave all he had, the marquis returned this money along with 150 crowns of gold and daily sent bread, sheep and hens to the hospital. When the hospital caught fire, St. John of God walked through the fire to carry out on his back the patients. He was seen to stand in the fire and was not burned.

Additionally, he assisted many person exposed to misfortune in their own homes. He provided doweries for young maidens who otherwise would not be able to marry and he helped remove others for desolate living. He fell sick after ten years of hard service in the hospital. The cause of his illness was severe fatigue after attempting to rescue, in full habit, a person in danger of being drown in a flood. The lady Anne Osorio found him confined in his bed with a basket under his head for a pillow, covered by an old coat for a blanket. She notified the Archbishop and had him removed to her home. She with her own hands and her maids fed him broths and read to this the history of the passion of our Lord.

The archbishop ordered him to give the city his dying benediction. The archbishop heard his confession, gave him viaticum and extreme unction, promised to pay his debts and provide for the poor. St. John of God died on March 8, 1550. He was buried by the archbishop. His followers formed the Brothers Hospitallers of St. John of God, a world-wide Catholic religious institute. The rules were drawn up in 1556, six years after his death. Religious vows were introduced in 1570. His order of charity to serve the sick was approved by pope St. Pius V (1566-1572).[4]

St. John of God was beatified by His Holiness Pope Urban VIII (1623-1644)[3] in 1630 and canonized by Pope Alexander VIII (1689-1691)[3] in 1690. His relics were moved into the church of his brethren in 1664. St. John of God is the patron saint of nurses and nurses associations, hospitals, hospital workers, the sick and dying. (Memorial - March 8).[1]

"Labor without intermission to do all the good works in your power, while time is allowed you."
"In the twilight of life, God will not judge us on our earthly possessions and human success, but rather, on how much we have loved."

"Lord, Thy thorns are my roses, and Thy sufferings my paradise."

The following is from the *original* Reverend Alban Butler's Lives of Saints (1883) republished in 2020 by Loreto Publications:[5]

Title: St. John of God, Confessor "Founder of the Order of Charity.
St. John, surnamed of God, was born in Portugal, in 1495. His parents were of the lowest rank in the country, but devout and charitable. John spent a considerable part of his youth in service, under the mayoral or chief shepherd of the count of Oropeusa in Castile, and in great innocence and virtue. In 1522, he listed himself in a company raised by the count, and served in the wars between the French and Spaniards; as he did afterward in Hungary, against the Turks, while the emperor Charles V was king of Spain. By the licentiousness of his companions, he by degrees lost his fear of offending God, and laid aside the greatest part of his practices of devotion. The troop which he belonged to being disbanded, he went into Andalusia in 1536, where he entered the service of a rich lady near Seville, in quality of shepherd. Being now about forty years of age, stung with remorse for his past misconduct, he began to entertain very serious thoughts of a change of life, and doing penance for his sins. He accordingly employed the greatest part of his time, both by day and night, in the exercises of prayer and mortification; bewailing almost continually his ingratitude towards God, and deliberating how he could dedicate himself in the most perfect manner to His service. His compassion for the distressed moved him to take a resolution of leaving his place, and passing into Africa, that he might comfort and succor the poor slaves there, not without hopes of meeting with the crown of martyrdom. At Gibraltar he met with a Portuguese gentleman condemned to banishment, and whose estate had also been confiscated by king John III. He was then in the hand of the king's officers, together with his wife and children, and on his way to Ceuta in Barbary, the place of his exile. John, out of charity and compassion, served him

without any wages. At Ceuta, the gentleman falling sick with grief and the change of air, was soon reduced to such straits as to be obliged to dispose of the small remains of his shattered fortune for the family's support. John, not content to sell what little stock he was master of to relieve them, went to day-labor at the public works, to earn all he could for their subsistence. The apostasy of one of his companions alarmed him; and his confessor telling him that his going in quest of martyrdom was an illusion, he determined to return to Spain. Coming back to Gibraltar, his piety suggested to him to turn peddler, and sell little pictures and books of devotion, which might furnish him with opportunities of exhorting his customers to virtue. His stock increasing considerably he settled in Granada, where he opened a shop, in 1538, being then forty-three years of age.

The great preacher and servant of God, John D'Avila, surnamed the Apostle of Andalusia, preached that year at Granada, on St. Sebastian's day, which is there kept as a great festival. John, having heard his sermon, was so affected that it, that, melting into tears, he filled the whole church with his cries and lamentations; detesting his past life, beating his breast, and calling aloud for mercy. Not content with this, he ran about the streets like a distracted person, tearing his hair, and behaving in such a manner that he was followed everywhere by the rabble with sticks and stones, and came home all besmeared with direct and blood. He then gave away all he had in the world, and having thus reduced himself to absolute poverty, that he might die to himself, and crucify all the sentiments of the old man, he began again to counterfeit the madman, running about the streets as before, till some had the charity to take him to the venerable John D'Avila, covered with dirt and blood. The holy man, full of the Spirit of God, soon discovered in John the motions of extraordinary graces, spoke to him in private, heard his general confession, and gave him proper advice, and promised his assistance ever after. John, out of a desire of the greatest humiliations, returned soon after to his apparent madness and extravagances. He was, thereupon, taken up and put into a madhouse, on supposition of his being disordered in his senses, where the severest methods were used to bring him to himself, all which he underwent in the spirit of penance, and by way of atonement for the sins of his past life. D'Avila, being informed of his conduct, came to visit him, and found him reduced almost to the grave by weakness, and his body covered with wounds and sores; but his soul was still vigorous, and thirsting with the greatest ardor after new sufferings and humiliations. D'Avila however told him, that having now been sufficiently exercised in

117

that so singular a method of penance and humiliation, he advised him to employ himself for the time to come in something more conducive to his own and the public good. His exhortation had its desired effects; and he grew instantly calm and sedate, to the great astonishment of his keepers. He continued, however, sometime longer in the hospital, serving the sick, but left the hospital entirely on St. Ursula's day, in 1539. This his extraordinary conduct is an object of the fervor of his conversion, his desire for humiliation, and a holy hatred of himself and his past criminal life. By it he learned in a short time perfectly to die to himself and the world; which prepared his soul for the graces which God afterwards bestowed on him. He then thought of executing his design of doing something for the relief of the poor; and, after a pilgrimage to our Lady's in Guadaloupa, to recommend himself and his undertaking to her intercession, in a place celebrated for devotion to her, he began by selling wood in the marketplace, to feed some poor by the means of his labor. Soon after he hired a house to harbor poor sick persons in, whom he served and provided for with an ardor, prudence, economy, and vigilance, that surprised the whole city. This was the foundation of the order of charity, in 1540, which by the benediction of heaven, has since been spread all over Christendom. John was occupied all day in serving his patients: in the night he went out to carry in new objects of charity, rather then to seek out provisions for them; for people, of their own accord, brought him in all necessaries for his little hospital. The archbishop of Granada, taking notice of so excellent an establishment, admiring the incomparable order observed in it, both for the spiritual and temporal care of the poor, furnished considerable sums to increase it, and favored it with his protection. This excited all persons to vie with each other in contributing to it. Indeed, the charity, patience and modesty of St. John, and his wonderful care and foresight, engaged everyone to admire and favor the institute. The bishop of Tuy, president of the royal court of judicature in Granada, having invited the holy man to dinner, put several questions to him, to all which he answered in such a manner, as gave the bishop the highest esteem of his person. It was this prelate that gave him the name of John of God, and prescribed him a kind of habit, though St. John never thought of founding a religious order: for the rules which bear his name were only drawn up in 1556, six years after his death; and religious vows were not introduced among his brethren before the year 1570.

To make trial of the saint's disinterestedness, the marquis of Tarisa came to him in disguise to beg an alms, on pretense of a necessary lawsuit, and he received from his hands twenty-five ducats, which was all he had. The marquis was so much edified by his charity, that, besides returning the sum, he bestowed on him one hundred and fifty crowns of gold, and sent to his hospital every day, during his stay at Granada, one hundred and fifty loaves, four sheep, and six pullets. But the holy man gave a still more illustrious proof of his charity when the hospital was on fire; for he carried out most of the sick on his own back: and though he passed and repassed though the flames, and stayed in the midst of them a considerable time, he received no hurt. But his charity was not confined to his own hospital: he looked upon it as his own misfortune if the necessities of any distressed person in the whole country had remained unrelieved. He therefore made strict inquiry into the wants of the poor over the whole province, relieved many in their own houses, employed in a proper manner those that were able to work, and with wonderful sagacity laid himself out every way to comfort and assist all the afflicted members of Christ. He was particularly active and vigilant in settling and providing for young maiden in distress, to prevent the danger to which they were often exposed, of taking bad courses. He also reclaimed many who were already engaged in vice: for which purpose he sought out public sinners, and holding a crucifix in his hand, with many tears exhorted them to repentance. Though his life seemed to be taken up in continual action, he accompanied it with perpetual prayer and incredible corporal austerities. And his tears of devotion, his frequent raptures, and his eminent spirit of contemplation, gave a luster to his other virtues. But his sincere humility appeared most admirable in all his actions, even amid the honors which he received at the court of Valladolid, whither business called him. The king and princes seemed to vie with each other who should show him the greatest courtesy, or put the largest alms in his hands; whose charitable contributions he employed with great prudence in Valladolid itself, and the adjacent country. Only perfect virtue could stand the test of honors, amid which he appeared the most humble. Humiliation seemed to be his delight; these he courted and sought, and always underwent them with great alacrity. One day when a woman called him hypocrite, and loaded him with invectives, he gave her privately a piece of money, and desired her to repeat all she had said in the marketplace.

Worn out at last by ten years' hard service in his hospital, he fell sick. The immediate occasion of his distemper seemed to be excess of fatigue in saving wood and other such things for the poor in a great flood, in which, seeing a person in danger of being drowned, he swam in his long clothes to endeavor to rescue him, not without imminent hazard of his own life: but he could not see

119

his Christian brother perish without endeavoring at all hazards to succor him. He at first concealed his sickness, that he might not be obliged to diminish his labors and extraordinary austerities; but in the mean time he carefully revised the inventories of all things belonging to his hospital, and inspected all the accounts. He also reviewed all the excellent regulations which he had made for its administration, the distribution of time, and the exercise of piety to be observed in it. Upon a complaint that he harbored idle strollers and bad women, the archbishop sent for him, and laid open the charge against him. The man of God threw himself prostrate at his feet, and said: "The Son of God came for sinners, and we are obliged to promote their conversion, to exhort them, and to sigh and pray for them. I am unfaithful to my vocation because I neglect this; and I confess that I know no other bad person in my hospital but myself; who, as I am obliged to own with extreme confusion, am a most base sinner, altogether unworthy to each the bread of the poor." This he spoke with so much feeling and humility that all present were much moved, and the archbishop dismissed him with respect, leaving all things to his discretion. His illness increasing, the news of it was spread abroad. The lady Anne Osorio was no sooner informed of his condition, but she came in her coach to the hospital to see him. The servant of God lay in his habit in his little cell, covered with a piece of an old coat instead of a blanket, and having under his head, not indeed a stone, as was his custom, but a basket, in which he used to beg alms in the city for his hospital. The poor and sick stood weeping round him. The lady, moved with compassion, dispatched secretly a message to the archbishop, who sent immediately an order to St. John to obey her as he would do himself, during his illness. By virtue of this authority she obliged him to leave his hospital. He named Anthony Martin superior in his place, and gave moving instructions to his brethren, recommending to them, in particular, obedience and charity. In going out he visited the blessed sacrament, and poured forth his heart before it with extraordinary fervor; remaining there absorbed in his devotions so long, that the lady Anne Ossorio caused him to be taken up and carried into her coach, in which she conveyed him to her own house. She herself prepared with the help of her maids, and gave him with her own hands, his broths and other things, and often read to him the history of the passion of our Redeemer. He complained that while our Savior, in his agony, drank gall, they gave him, a miserable sinner, broths. The whole city was in tears; all the nobility visited him; the magistrates came to beg he would give his benediction to their city. He answered, that his sins rendered him the scandal and reproach of their country; but

120

recommended to them his brethren, the poor, and his religious that served them. At last, by order of the archbishop he gave the city his dying benediction. His exhortations to all were most pathetic. His prayer consisted of most humble sentiments of compunction and inflamed aspirations of divine love. The archbishop said mass in his chamber, heard his confession, gave him the viaticum and extreme unction, and promised to pay all his debts, and to provide for all his poor. The saint expired on his knees, before the altar, on the 8th of March in 1550, being exactly fifty-five year old. He was buried by the archbishop at the head of all the clergy, both secular and regular, accompanied by all the court, noblesse, and city, with the utmost pomp. He was honored by many miracles, beatified by Urban VIII in 1630, and canonized by Alexander VIII in 1690. His relics were translated into the church of his brethren in 1664. His order of charity to serve the sick was approved by pope Pius V. The Spaniards have their own genera: but the religious in France and Italy obey a general who resides at Rome. They follow the rule of St. Austin.

One sermon perfectly converted one who had been long enslaved to the world and his passion, and made him a saint. How comes it that so many sermons and pious books produce so little fruits in our soul? It is altogether owing to our sloth and wilful hardness of heart, that we receive God's omnipotent word in vain, and to our most grievous condemnation. The heavenly seed can take no root in hearts which receive it with indifference and insensibility, or it is trodden upon and destroyed by the dissipation and tumult of our disorderly affections, or it is choked by the briers and thorns of earthly concerns. To profit by it, we must listen to it with awe and respect, in the silence of all creatures, in interior solitude and peace, and must carefully nourish it in our hearts. The holy law of God is comprised in the precept of divine love; a precept so sweet, a virtue so glorious and so happy, as to carry along with it its present incomparable reward. St. John, from the moment of his conversion, by the penitential austerities which he performed, was his own greatest persecutor; but it was chiefly by heroic works of charity that he endeavored to offer to God the most acceptable sacrifice of compunction, gratitude, and love. What encouragement has Christ given us in every practice of this virtue, by declaring, that whatever we do to others he esteems as done to himself! To animate ourselves to fervor, we may often call to mind what St. John frequently repeated to his disciples, "Labor without intermission to do all the good works in your power, while time is allowed you." His spirit of penance, love, and fervor he inflamed by meditating assiduously on the sufferings of Christ, of which he often used to say: "Lord, thy thorns are my roses, and thy sufferings my paradise."[2] *From his life, written by Francis de Castro, twenty-five years after his death, abridged by Baillet, p. 92, and F. Helyot, Hist, des Ordes Relig. T. 4, p. 131. AD 1550.*

References:

1) "patrons of nurses". Patrons of the Faith. CatholicSaints.Info. 21 January 2022. Web. 28 May 2022. <https://catholicsaints.info/patrons-of-nurses/>

2) The Monks of Solesmes (1960). The Human Body: Papal Teachings, Boston: Daughters of St. Paul, 189.

3) Catholic Online. Accessed 28 May 2022.
https://www.catholic.org/saints/saint.php?saint_id=68

4) The List of Popes (1911). In the Catholic Encyclopedia. New York: Robert Appleton Company. Retrieved May 28, 2022 from New Advent: http://www.newadvent.org/cathen/12272b.htm.

5) Reverend Alban Butler (1883). March 8, St. John of God in The Lives of the Saints as republished by Loreto Publications: Fitzwilliam, New Hampshire, 2020. Book Two, Volume II & III - October and November, 330-340.

St. Camillus de Lellis (Italy) (1550-1614)

Patron Saint of Nurses and Nurses' Association
declared by Pope Pius XI in 1930.[1][2]
Established an order known initially as "Servants of the Sick," then
"Order of the Ministers of the Infirm" or now simply the "Camillians."
Cared for the sick both in hospital and home.
Priest

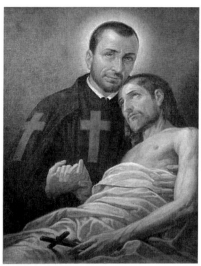

St. Camillus de Lellis
Source: littleportionhermitage.org

Camillus de Lellis was born on May 25, in the holy year 1550 (on the day dedicated to St. Urban, Pope and Martyr), in Bacchianico, Abruzzi, Kingdom of Naples, Italy To Camilla Compellio of Laureto and Giovanni de Lellis. His mother was a noble lady who was nearly 60 years old when Camillus was born. She died when he was young. His brother Giuseppe, born many years prior, had died as a child. His father was a military officer who was intimate friends of King Ferdinand and served in the rank of captain, under the Emperor Charles V in almost all the enterprises which were undertaken in Italy in his time.

Two unique events occurred in conjunction with his birth. A few days before his birth, his mother *dreamed that she had given birth to a son with a cross on his breast, who was followed by several children all decorated in the same way*...if she had lived she would *"see her son with many religious followers of his holy example, and full of his fervent zeal, all armed with the venerable sign of the cross, robbing the devil of multitudes of souls, and this chiefly at the time of their agony, when he always uses all his strength to assault them with greater fury."*

His mother's labor pains began while attending the Holy Sacrifice of the Mass which compelled her to return home. In unbearable pain, *"she was unable to give birth to the child on the place prepared for her; but almost beside herself, she rushed*

123

impetuously to the stable, and throwing herself down on the hay, she there immediately brought forth with the greatest ease: so that we may say, that Camillus would not consent to be born in a palace, or on a bed more luxurious than that in which his Lord willed to be born."

As a young man, he served as a soldier fighting against the Turks first for the Venetians and then for the Kingdom City State of Naples in the Neapolitan troops until 1574. As a young man he was addicted to cards and gaming to the point where he lost even what was necessary. For his subsistence, he was obliged to work for the Capuchin friars driving two donkeys and also working on a building. Through their influence he was converted in 1575 and never again resumed his gaming and gambling life. He attempted to enter the Capuchin friars and then the Grey Friairs. Due to a leg injury which resulted in a oozing sore, he was not admitted. He went to Rome for medical treatment. He moved into San Giacomo (St. James) Hospital for the incurable where he worked for four years. He was especially attentive to the sick who were dying, both their temporal and spiritual needs. To better serve them he prepared himself to receive holy orders. He was ordained to the priesthood in 1584 by Thomas Goldwell, bishop of Asaph. As a priest he moved from the hospital to serve at the chapel of Our Lady's ad miracula.

Within the year, at age 32, he founded the Congregation of the Servants of the Sick (the Camillians or Fathers of a Good Death), caring for the sick first in the hospital of the Holy Spirit in Rome and then in hospitals and homes that they established in several countries. In addition to the evangelical vows of poverty, chastity and obedience, the Camillians added a fourth vow of perpetually serving the sick. Camillus honored the sick as living images of Christ[3] and he taught his companions to do the same.

One of his companions, Sanzio Cicatelli, reported that, *"the three fervent laborers* (Camillus, Bernardino and Curzi) *began to attend the hospital of St. Spirito everyday, where they served the sick with the most fervent charity... They gave them their food, they made their beds, they cleansed their tongues, they exhorted them to patience and the devout receiving of the sacraments, they suggested pious ejaculations, they recommended their souls, and, in fine, they performed acts of charity so intense, that it would be absurd to expect anything of the kind from even the most active of ordinary*

124

servants. Whoever saw them acting with such tenderness, easily perceived that persons of that stamp did not look at the sick simply as men, but by a living faith and ardent charity served them as though they saw in them the very person of Jesus Christ, wounded and fainting, so that they occasioned great wonder and edification."[45]

Camillus viewed sickness as a time in which a Christian stands in need of the greatest constancy and fortitude and yet is the weakest. In Butler's Lives of Saints, it describes how Camillus exhorted his fellow companions to care for the sick, especially in their last hour. He exhorted them to provide every type of spiritual nourishment for the sick and dying: to suggest to them short acts of compunction and other virtues, to read to them, pray for them, teach them suitable ejaculations. He encouraged the sick to settle their temporal affairs so they might focus on their soul, disposing themselves to receive the last sacraments: extreme unction (the Sacrament of the Anointing of the Sick), viaticum (the Holy Eucharist as "food for the journey") and an apostolic pardon. He instructed the dying to unite their death with that of the Savior. He instituted prayers for all those in agony or who were near their death. In addition, concerned that many hospitals were allowing people to be buried alive, he ordered his religious to continue the prayers for souls for a quarter of an hour after the patient seemed to have drawn their last breath. He also instructed that their face was not to be immediately covered thereby stiffling their breathing.

In 1588 when a plague broke out upon ships anchored near Naples, the Servants of the Sick (Camillians), boarded the ships and cared for the sailors. Two died, the Order's first martyrs of charity. The Camillians cared for the sick also when a pestilence broke out in Rome. When others would not do so, the Camillians cared for those sick with contagious disease even risking their own lives.

In the last year of his life Camillus moved from Genoa to Rome. Admitted to the infirmary, Camillus de Lellis died 14 July 1614. When the infirmarian asked him whether he would take a little jelly, he answered, "Wait a quarter of an hour, and I shall be refreshed." And in exactly a quarter of an hour he died. "During his whole sickness he was so absorbed in God, and so often breathed forth the most tender affections of love, thankfulness, and devotion, that it did not appear to be a man that was praying, but an angel

125

already enjoying the beatific vision. And, lastly, when he received the Holy Viaticum, his face appeared to shine, and his eyes were fixed on the Blessed Sacrament, as though he saw there the most holy Humanity of our Saviour. All these circumstances prove that at the time God favored him with some heavenly vision."

St Camillus was initially buried near the high altar in St. Mary Magdalen's church in Rome, the Mother House of the Order of St. Camillus. After miracles were authentically proved, his remained were placed under the altar. He was beatified in 1742 and canonized in 1746 both by His Holiness Pope Benedict XIV (1740-1758). The symbol of the "red cross" originated with St. Camillus. (Memorial: July 14; July 18 in USA)[6]

"Think well, speak well, do well. These three things, through the mercy of God, will make a man go to heaven."

"The minister of the sick must be a man
who approaches his brother,
who needs to open his heart to the hope of a better tomorrow,
who must be understood and supported in this effort of openness to
the goals of the time that ends,
but also on those of eternity, which never ends."[7]

The following is from the *original* Reverend Alban Butler's Lives of Saints (1883) republished in 2020 by Loreto Publications:[8]

He was born in 1550 at Bacchianico in Abruzzo, in the kingdom of Naples. He lost his mother in his infancy, and six years after his father, who was a gentleman, and had been an officer, first in the Neapolitan and afterwards in the French troops in Italy. Camillus having learned only to read and write, entered himself young in the army, and served first in the Venetian, and afterwards in the Neapolitan troops, till, in 1574, his company was disbanded. He had contracted so violent a passion for cards and gaming, that he sometimes lost even necessaries. All playing at lawful games for exorbitant sums, and absolutely all games of hazard for considerable sums are forbidden by the law of nature, by the imperial or civil law, by the severest laws of all Christian or civilized nations, and by the canons of the Church. No contract is justifiable in which neither reason nor proportion is observed. Nor

126

can it be consistent with the natural law of justice for a man to stake any sum on blind chance, or to expose, without a reasonable equivalent or necessity, so much of his own or antagonist's money, that the loss would notably distress himself or any other person. Also many other sins are inseparable from a spirit of gaming, which springs from avarice, is so hardened as to rejoice in the loss of others, and is the source and immediate occasion of many other vices. The best remedy for this vice is, that those who are infected with it be obliged, or at least exhorted, to give whatever they have won to the poor.

Camillus was insensible of the evils attending gaming, till necessity compelled him to open his eyes; for he at length, was reduced to such straits, that for a subsistence he was obliged to drive two asses, and to work at a building which belonged to the Capuchin friars. The divine mercy had not abandoned him through all his wanderings, but had often visited him with strong interior calls to penance. A moving exhortation which the guardian of the Capuchins one day made him, completed his conversion. Ruminating on it as he rode from him upon his business, he at length alighted, fell on his knees, and vehemently striking his breast, with many tears and loud groans deplored his past unthinking sinful life, and cried to heaven for mercy. This happened in February in the year 1575, the twenty-fifth of his age; and from that time to his last breath he never interrupted his penitential course. He made an essay of a novitiate both among the Capuchins and the Grey Friars, but could not be admitted to his religious profession among either on account of a running sore in one of his legs, which was judged incurable. Therefore leaving his own country he went to Rome, and there served the sick in St. James's hospital of incurables four years with great fervor. He wore a knotty hair shirt, and a rough brass girdle next to his skin; watched night and day about the sick, especially those that were dying, with the most scrupulous attention. He was most zealous to suggest to them devout acts of virtue and to procure them every spiritual help. Fervent humble prayer was the assiduous exercise of his soul, and he received the holy communion every Sunday and holiday, making use of St. Philip Neri for his confessarius. The provisors or administrators having been witnesses to his charity, prudence and piety, after some time appointed him director of the hospital.

Camillus grieving to see the sloth of hired servants in attending the sick, formed a project of associating certain pious persons for that office who should be desirous to devote themselves to it out of a motive of fervent charity. He found proper persons so disposed, but met with great obstacles in the execution of his design. With a view of rendering himself more useful in spiritually assisting the sick, he took a resolution to prepare himself to receive holy orders. For this purpose he went through a course of studies with incredible alacrity and ardor, and received all his orders from Thomas Goldwell, bishop of St. Asaph's, suffragan to cardinal Savelli, the bishop viceregent in Rome, under pope Gregory XIII. A certain gentleman of Rome named Firmo Calmo, gave the saint six hundred Roman sequines of gold (about two hundred and fifty pounds sterling), which he put out for an annuity of thirty-six sequines a year during his life; this amounting to a competent patrimony for the title of his ordination, required by the council of Trent and the laws of the diocese. The same pious gentleman, besides frequent great benefactions during his life, bequeathed his whole estate real and personal on Camillus's hospital at his death. The saint was ordained a priest at Whitsuntide in 1584, and being nominated to serve a little chapel called our Lady's ad miracula, he quitted the direction of the hospital. Before the close of the same year he laid the foundation of his congregation for serving the sick, giving to those who were admitted into it a long black garment with a black cloth for their habit. The saint prescribed them certain short rules, and they went every day to the great hospital of the Holy Ghost, where they served the sick with much affection, piety, and diligence, that it was visible to all who saw them, that they considered Christ himself as lying sick or wounded in his members.

They made the beds of the patients, paid them every office of charity, and by their short pathetic exhortations disposed them for the last sacraments, and a happy death. The founder had powerful adversaries and great difficulties to struggles with; but by confidence in God he conquered them all. In 1585 his friends hired him a large house and the success of his undertaking encouraged him to extend further his pious views; for he ordained that the members of his congregation should bind themselves by the obligation of their institute, to serve persons infected with the plague, prisoners, and those who lie dying in private houses.

Sickness is often the most severe and grievous of all trials; whence the devil made it his last assault in tempting Job. It is a time in which a Christian stands in need of the greatest constancy and fortitude yet through the weakness of nature, is generally the least able to keep his heart united with God, and usually never stands more in need of spiritual comfort and assistance. The state of sickness is always a visitation of God, who by it knocks at the door of our heart, and puts us in mind of death; it is the touchstone of patience, and the school or rather the harvest of penance, resignation, divine love, and every virtue. Yet by a most fatal abuse is this mercy often lost and perverted by sloth, impatience, sensuality, and forwardness. Those who in time of health were backward in exercising fervent acts of faith, hope and charity, contrition, etc., in sickness are still more indisposed for practices which they are unacquainted; and to their grievous misfortune sometimes pastors cannot sufficiently attend them, or have not a suitable address which will give them the key of their hearts, or teach them the art of insinuating into the souls of penitents the heroic sentiment and an interior relish of those essential virtues.

This consideration moved Camillus to make it the chief end of his new establishment, to afford or procure the sick all spiritual succor, discreetly to suggest to them short pathetic acts of compunction and other virtues, to read by them, and to pray for them. For this end he furnished his priests with proper books of devotion, especially on penance and on the sufferings of Christ; and he taught them to have always at hand the most suitable ejaculations extracted from the psalms and other devotions. But dying persons were the principal object of our saint's pious zeal and charity. A man's last moments are the most precious of his whole life; and are of infinite importance; as on them depends his eternal lot. Then the devil useth his utmost efforts to ruin a soul, and cometh down, having great wrath, knowing that he hath but a short time. The saint therefore redoubled his earnestness to afford every spiritual help to persons who seemed in danger of death. He put them early in mind to settle their temporal concerns, that their thoughts might be afterward employed entirely on the affair of their soul. He advised those friends not to approach them too much, whose sight or immoderate grief could only disturb or afflict them. He disposed them to receive the last sacraments by the most perfect acts of compunction, resignation, faith, hope, and divine love; and he taught them to make death a voluntary sacrifice of themselves to the divine will, and in satisfaction for sin; of which it is the punishment. He instructed them to conjure their blessed redeemer by the bitter anguish which His heart felt in the garden and on the cross, and by His prayer with a loud voice and tears, in which he deserved to be heard for his reverence, that He would show them mercy, and give them the grace to offer upon their death in union with His most precious death, and to receive their soul as he with His last breath recommended His own divine soul into the hands of His heavenly Father, and with it those of all his elect to the end of the world. He instituted prayers for all persons in their agony, or who were near their death.

129

Everyone was charmed at so perfect a project of charity, and all admired that such noble views and so great an undertaking should have been reserved to an obscure illiterate person. Pope Sixtus V confirmed this congregation in 1586, and ordered that it should be governed by a triennial superior. Camillus was the first, and Roger, and Englishman, was one of his first companions. The church of St. Mary Magdalen was bestowed on him for the use of his congregation. In 1588 he was invited to Naples, and with twelve companions founded there a new house. Certain galleys having the plague on board were forbid to enter the harbor. Wherefore these pious Servants of the Sick (for that was the name they took) went on board and attended them; on which occasion two of their number died of the pestilence, and were the first martyrs of charity in this holy institute. St. Camillus showed a like charity in Rome when a pestilential fever swept off great numbers, and again when that city was visited by a violent famine. In 1591 Gregory XV erected his congregation into a religious order, with all the privileges of the mendicant order, and under the obligation of the four vows of poverty, chastity, obedience and perpetually serving the sick, even those infected with the plague; he forbade these religious men to pass to any other order except that of the Carthusians. Pope Clement VIII in 1592 and 1600 again confirmed this order with additional privileges. Indeed the very end of this institution engaged all men to favor it; especially those who considered how many thousands die, even in the midst of priests, without sufficient help in preparing themselves for that dreadful hour which decides their eternity; what superficial confessions, what neglect in acts of contrition, charity, restitution, and other essential duties, are often to be feared; which grievous evils might be frequently remedied by the assiduity of well qualified ministers.

Among many abuses and dangerous evils which the seal of St. Camillus prevented, his attention to every circumstance relating to the care of dying persons soon made him discover that in hospitals many are buried alive, of which Cicatello relates several examples, particularly of one buried in a vault, who was found walking about in it when the next corpse was brought to be there interred. Hence the saint ordered his religious to continue the prayers for souls yet in their agony for a quarter of an hour after they seem to have drawn their last breath, and not to suffer their faces to be covered so soon as is usual, by which means those that are not dead are stifled. This precaution is most necessary in cases of drowning, apoplexies, and such accidents and distempers which arise from mere obstructions or some sudden revolution of humors, St. Camillus showed still a far greater solicitude to provide all

130

comforts and assistance for the souls of those that are sick, suggesting frequent short pathetic aspirations, showing them a crucifix, examining their past confessions and present dispositions, and making them exhortations with such unction and fervor that his voice seemed like a shrill trumpet, and pierced the hearts of all who heard him. He encouraged his disciples to these duties with words of fire. He did not love to hear anything spoken unless divine charity made part of the subject; and if he had a sermon in which it was not mentioned, he would call the discourse a gold ring without a stone.

He was himself afflicted with many corporal infirmities, as a sore in his leg for forty-six years; a rupture for thirty-eight years which he got by-serving the sick; two callous sore in the sole of one of his feet, which gave him great pain; violent nephritic colics, and for a long time before he died, a loss of appetite. Under this complication of diseases he would not suffer anyone to wait on him, but sent all his brethren to serve poor sick persons. When he was not able to stand he would creep out of his bed, even in the night, by the sides of the beds, and crawl from one patient to another to exhort them to acts of virtue, and see if they wanted anything. He slept very little, spending great part of the night in prayer and in serving the sick. He used often to repeat with St. Francis: "So great is the happiness which I hope for, that all pain and suffering is a pleasure." His friars are not obliged to recite the Church office unless they are in holy orders; but confess and communicate every Sunday and great holidays, have every day one hour's meditation, hear mass, and say the litany, beads, and other devotions. The holy founder was most scrupulously exact in every word and ceremony of holy mass, and of the divine office. He despised himself to a degree that astonished all who knew him. He laid down the generalship in 1607, that he might be more at leisure to serve the poor. He founded religious houses at Bologna, Milan, Genoa, Glorence, Ferrara, Messina, Palermo, Mantua, Viterbo, Bocchiano, Theate, Burgonono, Sinuessa, and other places, he had sent several of his friars into Hungary, and to all other places which in his time were afflicted with the plague. When Nola was visited with that calamity in 1600, the bishop constituted Camillus his vicar general, and it is incredible what succors the sick received from him and his companions, of whom five died of that distemper. God testified his approbation of the saint's zeal by the spirit of prophecy and the gift of miracles, on several occasions, and by many heavenly communications and favors.

He assisted in the fifth general chapter of his order in Rome in 1613, and after it, with the new general, visited the houses in Lombardy, giving them his last exhortations, which were everywhere received with tears. At Genoa he was extremely ill, but being a little better, duke Doria Tursi sent him in his rich galley to Civita Vecchia, whence he was conveyed in a litter to Rome. He recovered so as to be able to finish the visitation of his hospitals, but soon relapsed, and his life was despaired of by the physicians. Hearing this, he said; "I rejoice in what hath been told me: 'We shall go into the house of the Lord'" He received the Viaticum from the hands of cardinal Ginnasio, protector of his order, and said with many tears; "O Lord, I confess, I am the most wretched of sinners, most undeserving of they favor; but save me by thy infinite goodness. My hope is placed in they divine mercy through thy precious blood." Though he had lived in the greatest purity of conscience ever since his conversion, he had been accustomed to go every day to confession with great compunction and many tears. When he received the extreme unction he made a moving exhortation to his religious brethren, and having foretold that he should die that evening, he expired on the 14th of July, 1614, being sixty-five years one month and twenty days old. He was buried near the high altar in St. Mary Magdalen's church; but upon the miracles which were authentically approved, his remains were taken up and laid under the altar; they were enshrined after he was beatified in 1742, and in 1746 he was solemnly canonized by Benedict XIV. *(See the life of Camillus by Cicatello his disciples , and the acts of his canonization with those of Sts. Fidelis of Sigmaringa, Peter Regalati, Joseph of Leonissa, and St. Catharine de Ricci, printed at Rome in 1749, p. 10, 65, and 529, and Bullar. Rome. T. 16, p. 88. Heylor, Hist, des Ordres Relig. T. 4, p. 263.)*[8]

References:

1) "patrons of nurses". Patrons of the Faith. CatholicSaints.Info. 21 January 2022. Web. 28 May 2022. <https://catholicsaints.info/patrons-of-nurses/>

2) The Monks of Solesmes (1960). The Human Body: Papal Teachings, Boston: Daughters of St. Paul, 189.

3) "Saint Camillus of Lellis". CatholicSaints.Info. 1 December 2021. Web. 10 December 2021. <https://catholicsaints.info/saint-camillus-of-lellis/>

4) M. Mueller, O.S.CAM. (1926). St. Camillus of Lellis: Founder of the Clerks Regular Servants of the Sick. Translated from Italian by F.W. Faber. Accessed 10Dec2021 https://archive.org/details/LifeOfSt.CamillusOfLellis. Milwaukee: The Servants of the Sick, 49.

5) Fr. Sanzio Ciccatelli (1615). Life of St. Camillus of Lellis. Accessed 10 December 2021. https://archive.org/details/LifeOfSt.CamillusOfLellis

6) Catholic News Agency. St. Camillus de Lellis. Accessed 18 April 2022. https://www.catholicnewsagency.com/saint/st-camillus-704

7) Phrase of St. Camillus in article Father Enrico Rebuschini: angel of suffering. Ministers of the Sick Camillian Religious. Accessed 4 April 2022. www.camilliani.org/padre-enrico-rebuschini-angelo-dei-sofferenti/

8) Reverend Alban Butler (1883). July 14, St. Camillus de Lellis in The Lives of the Saints as republished by Loreto Publications: Fitzwilliam, New Hampshire, 2020. Book Four, Volume VI & VII- June and July, 558-566

9) The List of Popes. (1911). In The Catholic Encyclopedia. New York: Robert Appleton Company. Retrieved May 28, 2022 from New Advent: http://www.newadvent.org/cathen/12272b.htm

St. Michael Kozaki (Mie, Japan) (1551-1597)
Worked as a nurse in a Franciscan hospital in Japan
Married layman and father, hospital nurse
Holy Martyrs of Nagasaki of 1597 / First martyrs of the Far East

St. Michael Kozaki was born in 1551 in Ise, Mie, Japan. He was a married lay man and the father of St. Thomas Kozaki. He was a bow maker and carpenter. When the Franciscans started their missionary work in Japan, he was already Christian and he joined as a secular Franciscan. He worked with them as a catechist, and as a nurse in their hospital. He helped to build convents and churches in Kyoto and Osaka. On February 5, 1597, he was crucified at Tateyama (Hill of Wheat) in Nagasaki, Japan along with his son St. Thomas, Kozaki, St. Peter Baptist, St. Paul Miki and companions.[1] St. Michael Kozaki was 46 years old. His son, an altar server, was about 15 years old. St. Michael Kozaki was beatified on September 14, 1627 by Pope Urban VIII (1623-1644)[4] and canonized on June 8, 1862 by Pope Pius IX (1846-1878).[2][4] (Feast Day - February 6)

From the letters of Saint Peter Baptist of January 4 and February 2, 1597 (Archivio Ibero-Americano 6 [1916] 16-17)[3]

> We forfeit our lives for the preaching of the Gospel
> Of the friars here six were arrested and kept in prison for several days. With them were three Japanese of the Society of Jesus – one of them professed – and also other Christian faithful. There are twenty of us all together. We are now traveling in this rather cold month of the winter. They are conducting us with cavalry and a strong guard. On some days more than two hundred men were assigned to keep us under guard. In spite of this we have great consolation, and we continue to rejoice in the Lord because according to the sentence pronounced against us we are to be crucified for having preached the law of God contrary to the king's command. The rest were condemned because they are Christians.
> Those who wish to die for Christ now have a golden opportunity. I think that the faithful of this region would have been greatly consoled if religious of our Order had been here, but they may rest assured that as long as this king rules, men in our habit will not live long in Japan because he will quickly send them to eternal life. May he get us there.
> The sentence pronounced against us was written on a sign and carried before us. The sign read that we were condemned to

death because we preached the law of Nauan (i.e., the law of Christ) contrary to the command of Taycosama, and would be crucified when we reached Nagasaki. For this we were very happy and consoled in the Lord since we had forfeited our lives to preach his law.

There are six friars here and eighteen Japanese, all condemned to death; some because they are preachers, other because they are Christians. From the Society of Jesus there is a brother, a catechist and a third, a layman. They took us out of the prison and put us on carts. Each had a part of an ear cut off and thus they conducted us through the streets of Miyako with very many people and soldiers following. Then we were again remanded to prison. On the following day, our hands were tied securely behind our backs, as they took us to Osaka while mounted soldiers urged us on.

On still another day they brought us out of prison again, mounted us on horses and conducted us through the streets of the city. We were also taken to Sakai where they did the same thing. On each occasion there was a public proclamation by the town crier. We knew we had been condemned to death but only while in Osaka were we informed that our execution was to take place in Nagasaki.

For the love of God let your charity commend us to God that the sacrifice of our lives may be acceptable in his sight. From what I have heard here I think we will be crucified this coming Friday because it was on a Friday that they cut off a part of each one's ear at Miyako, an event we accepted as a gift from God. We all ask you then with great fervor to pray for us for the love of God.

Dearest brothers, help us with your prayers that our death may be acceptable to the majesty of God in heaven where, God willing, we hope to go. We will remember you. We have not forgotten your love here. I have loved you and still love you with all my heart. I wish you the peace and love of our Lord Jesus Christ. Farewell, dearest brothers, because there is no longer any time to speak to you. Until we meet in heaven. Remember me.

The list of the "Martyrs of Nagasaki (5-11-1957) from the Proper Offices of Franciscan saints and blesseds in the LOH[3]

Franciscan Friars:
San Pedro Bautista Blázquez, superior of the mission (1542-1597)
San Felipe de Jesus or de las Casas (1571-1597)
San Francisco Blanco (1567-1597)
San Francisco or La Parrilla de San Miguel (1543-1597)

135

San Gonzalo García (1562-1597)
San Martín Aguirre of the Ascension (1567-1597)

Secular Franciscans:
Nagasaki San Antonio (13 years old)
St. Bonaventure of Miyako
St. Cosmas Takeya
Miyako San Francisco Fahelante
Miyako San Francisco Medical
San Gabriel Ize
San Joaquin Sakakibara Osaka
San Juan Kinuyo Miyako
San Leon Kasasumara
San Luis Ibaraki (12 years old)
St. Matthias of Miyako
St. Michael Kozaki, father of St. Thomas Kozaki (nurse)
San Pablo Ibaraki, Ibaraki uncle of St. Louis
St. Paul Suzuki
Miyako San Pedro Sukejiro
Thomas Idauki Miyako or Ize
St. Thomas Kozaki (14 years), son of St. Michael Kozaki

Jesuits:
Saint Paul Miki, professed priest
San Juan de Goto, catechist
San Diego Kisai, catechist"[3]

References:

1) Catholic Online. "St. Michael Kozaki." Accessed 29 January 2022.
https://www.catholic.org/saints/saint.php?saint_id=5114

2) "Saint Michael Kozaki." CatholicSaints.Info. 13 August 2016. Web. 23
November 2021. <https://catholicsaints.info/saint-michael-kozaki/>

3) Secular Franciscans KC. Accessed 28 May 2022.
https://secularfranciscanskc.blogspot.com/2010/02/

4) The List of Popes. (1911). In The Catholic Encyclopedia. New York:
Robert Appleton Company. Retrieved May 28, 2022 from New Advent:
http://www.newadvent.org/cathen/12272b.htm

St. Aloysius (Luigi) Gonzaga (Italy) (1568-1591)

*During the 1591 epidemic, requested to interrupt theological studies and
assist in hospital erected by the fathers of Jesuit Society in Rome[1]
Catechized and exhorted the poor patients, washed their feet, made their
beds, changed their clothes, performed, with wonderful assiduity and
tenderness, the most painful and loathsome offices of the hospital.[1]
Went among the plague victims to heal and help them,
working alongside St. Camillus de Lellis.[2]
Begged alms for the sick and
physically carried those he found in the streets to a hospital
where he washed and fed them and prepared them for the sacraments[3]*

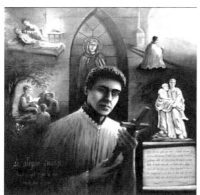

St. Aloysius Gonzaga
ignatiusloyola.org

Aloysius (Lewis/Luigi) Gonzaga was born on March 9, 1568 in the castle of Castiglione, in the town of Castiglione delle Stiviere, in the province of Mantua, in Lombardy, Italy located in the diocese of Brescia. His parents were Ferdinand Gonzaga, prince of the holy empire and marquis of Castiglione and Martha Tana Santena, daughter of Tanus Santena, lord of Cherry in Piemont. Aloysius was the eldest of three children having a younger brother Ralph, and a sister Isabel who died in Spain when he was thirteen. Aloysius was a very pious youth. His mother had prayed for a son who would love and serve God entirely. Throughout his youth he spent many hours in prayer and meditation. He suffered some illnesses in his youth from which he recovered.

At the age of eight, Aloysius and his younger brother Ralph, were set to the court of Francis of Medicis to learn Latin and Tuscan languages and other behaviors suitable to their station in life. After two years they were placed in the court of duke William Gonzaga, governor of Montserrat. In both locations, Aloysius continued to practice his acts of piety and prayer. At the age of 11 years and 8 months he decided to resign, to his brother, his title of the marquisate at Castiglione, even though the emperor had already invested him in this position. Again Aloysius fell sick suffering from

137

"retention of urine." During this time he read Surius's *Lives of Saints*. During his prayer he receive mystical experiences and ecstasies.

At age 12 he received his First Holy Communion from St. Charles Borromeo, who was on a preaching mission. From that time on, he had a great devotion to the Holy Eucharist and the Holy Sacrifice of the Mass which would bring tears to his eyes. The next year in 1581, Aloysius and Ralph were made pages to the James, the son of King Phillip II. During his time at court in Spain, Aloysius read Lewis of Granada's excellent book *On Mental Prayer* and continued his pious practices when he was not attending James. He remained in Spain two years and then returned to Italy in July 1584 on board the galleys of the famous John Andrew Doria, of the Battle of La Ponto.

Aloysius had a great desire to enter the Society of Jesus (Jesuits) which his father opposed. He attempted to subvert Aloysius' desires assigning him to various secular tasks. Eventually Aloysius' persistence prevailed and his father acquiesced giving his blessing. Aloysius then renounced his titles and inheritance giving these to his younger brother Ralph (Rodolfo) and left for Rome. In Rome, he met Pope Sixtus V and then entered the novitiate of the Jesuits on November 25, 1585 at St. Andrews at the age of 17. Aloysius was humble and obedient throughout his novitiate. He never spoke of himself nor did he make excuses when people found fault with his actions, even when they misjudged him. He suffered an illness and was sent to Naples for six month to recover. He, then, returned to Rome and on November 20, 1587, he made his religious vows and soon after received minor orders. He had studied logic while a page in the Spanish court and philosophy during his nine months stay in Milan. He therefore studied divinity under Gabriel Vasquez and others. His studies were interrupted to settle an estate inheritance disagreement between his brother, now the Marquis, and his cousin which occurred when his uncle Horatio Gonzaga died without children. He also made family peace when Ralph married secretly failing to notify his uncle Alphonsus Gonzaga, lord of Castle Godfrey, whose heir he was to be. After settling the family issues, Aloysius was sent to Milan on March 22, 1590 for theological studies. After receiving a revelation notifying him that he would soon die, his superiors moved him back to Rome in

November to finish his theological studies.

In 1591 when a contagious pestilence infected many in Rome, the Jesuits set up a new hospital to care for the sick. Aloysius asked in earnest to be allowed to care for the sick. Granted permission, Aloysius catechized and exhorted the poor patients, made their beds, changed their clothes, and performed, with wonderful assiduity and tenderness, the most painful and loathsome offices of the hospital.[1] He also went among the plague victims to heal and help them, working alongside St. Camillus de Lellis.[2] He begged alms for the sick and physically carried those he found in the streets to a hospital where he washed and fed them and prepared them for the sacraments.[3] So many of the Jesuit fathers had died contracting this contagious disease that Aloysius was forbidden to return to the hospital. He did receive permission, however, to work at Our Lady of Consolation (Consolata) hospital which did not treat anyone with contagious diseases. Aloysius contracted the plague when he cared for a man there. Aloysius fell sick and took to bed on March 3, 1951 with a severe fever lasting seven days. Thinking that he might die, Aloysius received viaticum and extreme unction. He recovered, to his dismay, though he strongly desired to be with God. His confessor, the famous Cardinal Bellarmine informed him that it was not an unusual grace to desire death, not out of impatience, but to be united to God.[1] His fever continued for three month causing excessive weakness. The physicians gave him and another brother bitter medicine which he drank slowly as a mortification, not revealing or showing signs of its bitterness.

He continued to have mystical experiences and ecstasies during which it was revealed to him that he would die on the octave day of Corpus Christi. Though he appeared to be improving, at his request, he was given viaticum and extreme unction on the Octave day. Around midnight, between June 20th and June 21st, 1591, Aloysius Gonzaga died. He was 23 years old and had lived with the Jesuits 5 years and 7 months. He was buried in the Jesuit Church of the Annunciation in Rome. His relics were moved to a chapel built in his honor, by the marquis Scipio Lancelotti, in the same Church. His body is now kept in the Church of St. Ignatius in Rome.[3]

Butler's Lives of Saints reported that St. Aloysius Gonzaga was beatified by His Holiness Pope Gregory XV in 1621. However, the Vatican Dicastery for the Causes of Saints[2] and Hagiography

Circle[4] records that his beatification occurred 16 years earlier on October 19, 1605 by Pope Paul V. He was canonized by Pope Benedict XIII on December 31, 1726 at the Vatican Basilica.

Three years after his canonization, Pope Benedict XIII declared him the protector of students. His Holiness Pope Pius XI designated him as the patron of Catholic youth in 1926. Pope St. John Paul II in 1991, consecrated him as the patron of AIDS patients. (Memorial - June 21).

St. Aloysius or Lewis GOnzaga, Confessor (June 21), from the *original* Rev. Alban Butler's (1883) *Lives of Saints:*[1]

Aloysius Gonzaga was son of Ferdinand Gonzaga, prince of the holy empire, and marquis of Castiglione, removed in the third degree of kindred from the duke of Mantua. His mother was Martha Tana Santena, daughter of Tanus Santena, lord of Cherry, in Piemont. She was lady of honor to Isabel, the wife of Phillip II of Spain, in whose court the marquis Gonzaga also lived in great favor. When she understood this nobleman had asked her in marriage both of the king and queen, and of her friends in Italy, being a lady of remarkable piety, she spent her time in fasting and prayer; in order to learn the will of heaven, and to draw down upon herself the divine blessing. The marriage was solemnized in the most devout manner, the parties at the same time performing their devotions for the jubilee. When they left the court and returned to Italy, the marquis was declared chamberlain to his majesty, and general of part of the army in Lombardy, with a grant of several estates. The marchioness made it her earnest petition to God that He would bless her with a son, who should devote himself entirely to His love and service. Our saint was born in the castle of Castiglione, in the diocese of Brescia, on the 9th of March, 1568. William, duke, of Mantua, stood godfather, and gave him the name of Aloysius. The holy name of Jesus and Mary, with the sign of the cross and part of the catechism, were the first words which his devout mother taught him as soon as he was able to speak; and from her example and repeated instructions the deepest sentiments of religion, and the fear of God were impressed upon his tender soul. Even in his infancy he showed an extraordinary tenderness for the poor; and such was his devotion that he frequently hid himself in corners, where after long search he was always found at his prayers, in which so amiable was his piety, and so heavenly did his recollection appear, that he seemed to resemble an angel clothed with a human body. His father designing to train him up to the army, in order to give him an inclination to that state, furnished him with little guns, and other weapons, took him to Casal to show him a muster of three thousand Italian foot, and was much delighted to see him carry a little pike, and walk before the ranks. The child stayed there some months, during which time he learned from the officers certain unbecoming words, the meaning of which he did not understand, not being then seven years old. But his tutor hearing him use bad words, chid him for it, and from that time he could never bear the company of any persons who in his hearing ever profaned the holy name of God. This offence, though excusable by his want of age and knowledge, was to him during his whole life a subject of perpetual humiliation, and he never ceased to bewail and accuse himself of it with extreme confusion and compunction. Entering the seventh year of his age he began to conceive greater sentiments of piety, and from that time he used to date his conversion to God. At that age, being come back to Castiglione, he began to recite every day the office of our Lady, the seven penitential psalms, and other prayers, which he always said on his knees, and without a cushion a custom which he observed all his life. Cardinal Bellarmine, three other confessors, and all who were best acquainted with his interior, declared after his death their firm persuasion, that he had never offended God mortally in his whole life. He was sick of an ague at Castiglione eighteen months; yet never omitted his task of daily prayers, though he sometimes desired some of his servants to recite them with him.

When he was recovered, being now eight years old, his father placed him and his younger brother Ralph, in the polite court of his good friend Francis of Medicis, grand duke of Tuscany, that they might learn the Latin and Tuscan languages, and other exercises suitable to their rank. At Florence the saint made such progress in the science of the saints that he afterwards used to call that city the mother of his piety. His devotion to the Blessed Virgin was much inflamed by reading a little book of Gaspar Loartes on the mysteries of the Rosary. He at the same time conceived a great esteem for the virtue of holy chastity; and he received of God so perfect a gift of the same, that in his whole life he never felt the least temptation either in mind or body against purity, as Jerome Platus and cardinal Bellarmine assure us from his own mouth. He cultivated this extraordinary grace by assiduous prayer, universal mortification, and the most watchful flight of all occasions; being well apprized that this virtue is so infinitely tender, that it fades and dies if blown upon by the least vapor: and that it is a bright and clear mirror which is tarnished with the least breath, and even by the sight. He never looked at any women, kept his eyes strictly

141

guarded, and generally cast down; would never stay with his mother alone in her chamber, and if she sent any message to him by some lady in her company, he received it, and gave his answer in a few words, with his eyes shut, and his chamber door only half open; and when bantered on that score, he ascribed such behavior to his bashfulness. It was owing to his virginal modesty, that he did not know by their faces many ladies among his own relations, with whom he had frequently conversed, and that he was afraid and ashamed to let a footman see so much as his foot uncovered. But humility, which is the mother of all virtues, was in our saint the guardian of his purity. He never spoke to his servants by way of command, but with such modesty that they were ashamed not to obey. He would only say to them: "Pray dispatch this or that: You may do this" or, "If it be no trouble you may do this or that." No novice could practice a more exact and ready obedience than Aloysius set an example of towards all his superiors, especially Francis Tuccius, whom his father had appointed tutor to his sons, and governor of his family at Florence.

      The two young princes had stayed there a little more than two years, when their father removed them to Mantua, and placed them in the court of the duke William Gonzaga, who had made him governor of Montserrat. Aloysius left Florence in November 1579, when he was eleven years and eight months old. He, at that time, took a resolution to resign to his brother Ralph his title to the marquisate at Castiglione, though he had already received the investiture from the emperor. And the ambitious or covetous man is not more greedy of honors or riches than this young prince from a better principle appeared desirous to see himself totally disengaged from the ties of the world, by entirely renouncing its false pleasures, which begin with uneasiness, and terminate in remorse, and are no better than real pains covered over with a bewitching varnish. He knew the true delights which virtue brings, which are solid without alloy, and capable of filling the capacity of man's heart, and these he thirsted after. In the meantime, he fell sick of an obstinate retention of urine, of which distemper he cured himself only by the rigorous rules of abstinence which he observed. He took the opportunity of this indisposition to rid himself more than ever of company and business, seldom going abroad, and spending most of his time in reading Surius's *Lives of the Saints* and other books of piety and devotion. It being the custom in Italy and other hot climates to pass the summer months in the country, the marquis sent for his sons from Mantua to Castiglione in that season. Aloysius pursued the same exercises, and the same manner of life in the town, at court, and in the country. The servants, who watched him in his chamber, saw him employed in prayer many hours together, sometimes prostrate on the ground before a crucifix, or standing up absorbed in God so as to appear in an ecstasy. When he went downstairs, they took notice that at every standing place he said a Hail Mary. It was in this retirement that his mind was exceedingly enlightened by God, and without the help of any instructor he received an extraordinary gift of mental prayer, to which his great purity of heart and sincere humility disposed his soul. He sometimes passed whole days in contemplating, with inexpressible sweetness and devotion, the admirable dispensation of divine providence in the great mysteries of our redemption, especially the infinite goodness and love of God, His mercy, and other attributes. In this exercise he was not able to contain the spiritual joy of his soul in considering the greatness and goodness of his God, not to moderate his tears. Falling at last on a little book of father Canisius, which treated Meditation, and on certain letters of the Jesuit missionaries in the Indies, he felt a strong inclination to enter the Society of Jesus [Jesuits], and was inflamed with an ardent zeal for the salvation of souls.

He began even then to frequent the schools of Christian doctrine and to encourage other boys, especially among the poor, in learning their catechism, and often instructed them himself. So excellently did he then discourse of God as astonished grown persons of learning and abilities. It happened that in 1580 St. Charles Borromeo came to Brescia in quality of apostolic visitor, and preached there on the feast of Mary Magdalen. No importunities of the marquis or other princes could prevail upon the great saint to visit them at their country seats, or to take up his lodgings anywhere but with the clergy of the churches where he came. Wherefore Aloysius, being only twelve years old, went to Brescia to receive his blessing. It is incredible how much the good cardinal was taken with the piety and generous sentiments of the young prince. But finding that he had never yet received the holy communion, he exhorted him to prepare himself for that divine sacrament, and to receive it very frequently; prescribing him rules for his devout preparation, and with regard to many other practices of piety; all which the holy youth constantly observed, remembering ever after with wonderful joy the happiness of having seen so great a saint. He from that time conceived so tender a devotion to the blessed Eucharist, that in hearing mass, after the consecration, he often melted into tears, in profound sentiments of love and adoration; and he frequently received wonderful favors in communicating; and this holy sacrament became his greatest comfort and joy. The marquis after this carried his whole family to

143

Casal, the residence of his government of Montferrat. There the saint made the convents of the Capuchins and Barnabites the usual places of his resort. He fasted three days a week. Fridays at least on bread and water, boiled together for his whole dinner; his collation was a little piece of dry bread. On other days his meals were so slender that his life seemed almost a miracle. He secretly thrust a board into his bed to rest on in the night, and rose at midnight to pray even in the coldest season of winter, which is very sharp under the Alps. He spent an hour after rising, and two hours before going to bed in private prayer.

In 1581, his father attended the empress Mary of Austria, wife to Maximilian II and sister to Philip II of Spain, in her journey from Bohemia to Spain, and took with him his three children; a daughter named Isabel who died in Spain, and his to sons, who were both made by king Philip pages to his son James, elder brother of Philip III. Aloysius was then thirteen years and a half old. He continue his studies but never neglected his long meditations and devotions, which he often performed by stealth in secret corners. Though he every day waited on the infant of Spain, James, to pay his duty to the empress, he never once looked on the face of the princess, or took notice of her person; and so great was his guard over all his senses, and so universal his spirit of mortification, that it was a proverb at court, that the young marquis of Castiglione seemed not to be made of flesh and blood. While he remained in Spain he found great pleasure and benefit in reading Lewis of Granada's excellent book *On Mental Prayer*.

He prescribed himself a daily task of an hour's meditation, which he often prolonged to three, four, or five hours. He at length determined to enter the Society of Jesus [Jesuits], in order to devote himself to the instructing and conducting souls to God; and he was confirmed in this resolution by his confessor, who was one of that order. When he disclosed it to his parents, his mother rejoiced exceedingly; but his father, in excessive grief and rage, said he would have him scourged naked. "O that it would please God," replied modestly the holy youth, "to grant me so great a favor as to suffer that for His love." What heightened the father's indignation, was a suspicion that this was a contrivance on account of his custom of gaming, by which he had lately lost six hundred crowns in one evening; a vice which his son bitterly deplored, not so much, as he used to say, for the loss of the money, as for the injury done to God. However, the consent of the marquis was at length extorted through the mediation of friends. The infant or prince of Spain dying a fever, Aloysius was at liberty, and after two years' stay in Spain, returned to Italy in July, 1584, on board the

144

galley of te famous John Andrew Doria, whom his Catholic majesty had lately appointed admiral. He brother traveled in rich apparel, but the saint in a suit of black Flanders serge. In his journey he either conversed on holy things, or entertained himself secretly in his heart with God. As soon as he came to an inn he sought some private little chamber, and fell to prayer on his knees. In visiting religious houses he went first to the church, and prayed some time before the blessed sacrament. When he had arrived at Castiglione he had new assaults to bear, from the eloquence and authority of a cardinal, many bishops, and eminent men, employed by the duke of Mantua and his own uncles; yet he remained firm, and brought over some of these ambassadors to his side, so that they pleaded in his favor. But his father flew back from his consent, loaded his son with opprobrious language, and employed him in many distracting secular commissions. The saint had recourse to God by prostrating himself before a crucifix, and redoubling his severities, till the marquis no longer able to oppose his design, cordially embraced him, and recommended him to Claudius Aquaviva, general of the society, who appointed Rome for the place of his novitiate. The father repented again of his consent, and detained his son nine months at Milan, during which time he used the most tender entreaties, and every other method to bring him from his purpose. He again removed him to Mantua, and thence to Castiglione; but finding his resolution invincible, left him at liberty, saying to him: "Dear son, your choice is a deep wound in my heart. I ever loved you, as you always deserved. In you I had founded the hopes of my family, but, you tell me God calls you another way. Go, therefore, in His name, whither you please, and may His blessing everywhere attend you." Aloysius having thanked him, withdrew, that he might not increase his grief by his presence, and betook himself to his prayers. His cession of the marquisate to his brother Ralph, with the reserve of two thousand crowns in ready money, and four hundred crowns a year for life, was ratified by the emperor, and the writings were delivered at Mantua, in November, 1585. The excessive grief and tears of his subjects and vassals at his departure, only drew from him these words, "That he sought nothing but the salvation of his soul, and exhorting them all to the same." Arriving at Rome, he visited the churches and chief places of devotion, then kissed the feet of pope Sixtus V, and entered his novitiate at St. Andrews's on the 25th of November, 1585, not being completely eighteen years old. Being conducted to his cell, he entered it as a celestial paradise, in which he was to have no other employment than that of praising God without interruption; and exulting in his heart, he repeated with the prophet: This is my

145

rest forever: here will I dwell for I have chosen it.

The saint in his noviceship condemned himself as guilty of sloth if he did not in every religious duty surpass in fervor all his companions; he respected them all, and he behaved himself towards them as if he had been the last person in the family, and indeed such he always reputed himself. He loved and rejoiced most in the meanest and most contemptible employments. His mortifications, though great, were not so severe as he had practiced in the world, because limited by obedience, which gave a merit to all his actions. He used to say that a religious state in this resembles a ship, in which they sail as fast who sit idle, as they who sweat at the oar in rowing. Yet such was the general mortification of his senses, that he seemed totally inattentive to exterior things, only inasmuch as they regarded God. He never took notice of the difference of villas where he had been, the order of the refectory in which, he every day ate, or the rich ornaments of the chapels and altars where he prayed. He seemed entirely inattentive to the taste of what he ate, only he endeavored to avoid whatever seemed savory. He never listened to reports or to discourse about worldly matters; spoke very little, and never about himself, thinking himself justly deserving to be forgotten by the whole world, and to be made no account of in everything.

He was a capital enemy to any artifice or dissimulation, which he called the bane and canker of Christian simplicity. Nothing gave him so much mortification as the least marks of honor or distinction. It was his delight to carry a wallet through the streets of Rome begging from door to door, to serve the poor and the hospitals, or to sweep the kitchen, and carry away the filth; in which actions he usually had before his eyes Christ humbled for us. On holidays he used to catechize the children of poor laborers. He changed his new gilt breviary for an old one, and often did so in his habit and other things. His whole life seemed a continued prayer, and he called holy meditation the short way to Christian perfection. He found in that exercise the greatest spiritual delights, and remained in it on his knees, as if he were motionless, in a posture of wonderful recollection and respect. It is not possible to describe the sweet raptures and abundant tears which often accompanied his devotion, especially in presence of the blessed Eucharist, and after communicating. He spent the three first days after communion in thanksgiving for that inestimable favor; and the three following in languishing aspirations and desires to receive on the Sunday his savior, his God, his physician, his king, and his spouse: on the eve of his communion his mind was wholly taken up with the dignity and infinite importance and advantages of that great action, nor

146

could he speak of anything else. Such was the first of his words whenever he spoke on that mystery of love, that it inflamed all who heard him. He made every day at least four regular visits to pray before the blessed sacrament. The passion of Christ was also a most tender object of his devotion. From his infancy he had chosen the Blessed Virgin for his special patroness and advocate. He had a singular devotion to the holy angels, especially his angel guardian. In the beginning of his noviceship he was tried by an extreme spiritual dryness and interior desolation of soul, which served perfectly to purify his heart, and was succeeded by the greatest heavenly consolations. He bore the pious death of his father with unshaken constancy, because he considered it and all other events purely in the view of the divine will and providence. It happened six weeks after Aloysius had taken the habit. From the day on which his son had left him to enter the society, the marquis had entirely devoted himself to the practice of perfect virtue and penance.

Humility and obedience were the young novice's favorite virtues, and by them he gained a perfect mastery over himself. To appear poor, little and contemptible, was his delight, and he rejoiced to see the last and worst portion in anything fall to his share. He was never known guilty of the least transgression of the rule of silence or any other, and feared to arrive one moment too late at any duty. He would not, without the leave of his master, speak one word even to his kinsman, cardinal Roborei; nor would he ever stay with him so long as to fail one minute in any rule. It happened that the pious and learned Jerome Platus, while he was his master of novices, thinking his perpetual application to prayer and study prejudicial to his health, ordered him to spend, in conversing with others after dinner, not only the hour allotted for all, but also the half hour longer which is allowed to those who dined at the second table. Father minister not knowing this order punished him for it, and obliged him publicly to confess his fault, which he underwent without offering any excuse. The minister learning afterwards how the matter was, admired very much his silence, but for his greater merit enjoined him another penalty for not telling him the order of his master. The saint bore in silence and joy the imputation and chastisement of the faults of any others, because this afforded him an opportunity of exercising patience, meekness, and humility. By a habit of continual application of his mind to God, attention at prayer seemed so easy and natural to him, that he told his superior, who put to him that questions, that if all the involuntary distractions at his devotions during six months were joined together, they would not amount to the space of one Hail

147

Mary. His health decaying, he was forbid to meditate or pray, except at regular times. This he found the hardest task of his whole life; so great a struggle did it cost him to resist the impulse with which his heart was carried towards God. For the recovery of his health he was sent to Naples, where he stayed half a year, and then returning to Rome. In that city, after completing his novitiate of two years, he made his religious vows on the 20th of November, 1587, and soon after received minor orders.

Aloysius had finished his logic while a page in the Spanish court, and his course of natural philosophy during his nine months' stay at Milan. After this he commenced student in divinity under Gabriel Vasquez, and other celebrated professors. But a family contest obliged him to interrupt his studies. His uncle, Horatio Gonzaga, died without issue, and bequeathed by will his estate of Sulphurino to the duke of Mantua. Ralph, the saint's brother, pleaded that the donation was invalid, the estate being a fief of the empire, which inalienably devolves on the next heir in blood, and he obtained a rescript of the emperor Maximilian in his favor. But the duke refused to acquiesce in this sentence; and the archduke Ferdinand and several other princes had in vain attempted to reconcile the two cousins. At length St. Aloysius was sent for to be the mediator of peace. He had then just finished his second year of divinity, and was at the Jesuits' villa at Frescati during the vacation, when father Robert Bellarmine brought him an order from the general to repair to Mantua about this affair. A discreet lay brother was appointed to be his companion, to whom a charge was given to take care of his health, with an order to Aloysius to obey him as to that particular. Most edifying were the examples of his profound humility, mortification, love of poverty, and devotion, and incredible the fruits of his zeal, both on the road, and at Mantua, Castiglione, and other places where he went. Though both parties were exceedingly exasperated, no sooner did this angel of peace appear, than they were perfectly reconciled. The duke, though before much incensed, was entirely disarmed by the sight and moving discourse of the saint; he readily pardoned and yielded up the estate to the marquis, who as easily consented to bury in oblivion all that had passed, and the two cousins made a sincere and strict alliance and friendship together. Many others who were at variance, or at law, were in the same manner made friends by the means of the saints, friendly interposing. No enmity seemed able to withstand the spirit of meekness and charity which his words and whole deportment breathed. Great numbers were by him converted from sinful habits, and many brought to a profession of perfect virtue. His brother Ralph had fallen in love with a young gentlewoman, much inferior to him in birth, and had secretly married her before private witnesses, but durst not publish his marriage for fear of offending his uncle, Alphonsus Gonzaga, lord of Castle Godfrey, whose heir he was to be. The saint represented to him that by such a conduct, notwithstanding his precautions, he offended God by the scandal he gave to his subjects and others, who looked upon his behavior as criminal. He, moreover, undertook to satisfy his uncle, mother, and other friends, and thus engaged him publicly to declare his marriage, and the uncle and others, through the saint's mediation, took no offence at the alliance. Aloysius having happily restored peace among all his relations, and settled them in the practice of true virtue, by the direction of his superiors went to Milan on the 22nd of March, 1590, there to pursue his theological studies. These he accompanied with his usual exercises of devotion, and all virtues, especially humility, to nourish and improve which in his heart, he embraced every kind of humiliation. He often begged to serve in the kitchen and refectory, and it was his delight to draw water for the cook, wash the dishes, cover the table, or sweep the scullery. While he was at Milan, one day in his morning prayer he was favored with a revelation, that he had only a short time to live. And by this heavenly visitation he found his mind wonderfully changed, and more than ever weaned from all transitory things. This favor he afterwards disclosed at Rome, in great simplicity, to F. Vincent Bruno and others. The general would not suffer him to finish his studies at Milan, but recalled him to Rome in November the same year, to perform there the fourth or last year of his theological courses. The saint chose a dark and very small chamber over the staircase in the garret, with one window in the roof; not had he in it any other furniture than a poor bed, a wooden chair, and a little stool to lay his books upon. He appeared even in the schools and cloisters quite absorbed in God, and often at table, or with his companions at recreation time after dinner, he fell into ecstasies, and appeared unable to contain the excessive heavenly joy with which his soul overflowed. He frequently spoke in raptures on the happiness of dying, the more speedily to enjoy God.

In 1591 an epidemical distemper swept off great multitudes in Rome. In this public distress the fathers of the society [Jesuits] erected a new hospital, in which the general himself, with other assistants, served the sick. Aloysius obtained by earnest entreaties to be one of this number. He catechized and exhorted the poor patients, washed their feet, made their beds, changed their clothes, and performed, with wonderful assiduity and tenderness, the most painful and loathsome offices of the hospital. The

149

distemper being pestilential and contagious, several of these fathers died martyrs of charity, and Aloysius fell sick. It was on the 3rd of March, 1591, that he took to his bed: at which time he was overwhelmed with excessive joy as the thought that he was called to go to his God. This joy gave him afterwards a scruple whether it was not immoderate. But his confessor, who was the famous cardinal Bellarmine, comforted him, saying, that it is not an unusual grace to desire death, not out of impatience, but to be united to God. The pestilential fever in seven days became so violent, that the saint received the viaticum and extreme unction. However, he recovered; but from the relics of this distemper succeeded a hectic fever, which in three months reduced him to an excessive weakness. He studied to add continual mortifications to the pains of his disease, and rose in the night to pray before a crucifix, till being caught by the infirmarian, he was forbid doing so for the future; which direction he punctually obeyed. The physicians having ordered him and another sick brother to take a very bitter draught, the other drank it at once with the ordinary helps to qualify the bitterness of the taste; but Aloysius sipped it slowly, and as it were drop by drop, that he might have the longer and fuller taste of what was mortifying; nor did he give the least sign of perceiving any disagreeable taste. After speaking with father Bellarmine on the happiness of speedily enjoying God, he fell into a rapture through excess of inward delights, and it continued almost the whole night, which seemed to him in the morning to have been but one moment, as he told F. Bellarmine. It seems to have been in this ecstasy that he learned he should die on the octave day of Corpus Christi, which he often clearly foretold. In thanksgiving for his death being so near, he desired one to recite with him the Te Deum; with which request the other complied. To another he cried out, his heart exulting with joy; "My father, we go rejoicing! We go rejoicing!" He said every evening the seven penitential psalms with another person, in great compunction. On the octave day, he seemed better, and the rector had thought of sending him to Frescati. But he repeated still that he should die before next morning, and he received the viaticum and extreme unction. At night he was thought to be in no immediate danger, and was left with two brothers to watch by him. These, about midnight, perceived on a sudden, by a wanness and violent sweat with which he was seized, that he was falling into his agony. His most usual aspirations during his illness were the ardent languishings of a soul aspiring to God, extracted from the psalms. After saying; "Lord, into Thy hands I commend my spirit," he frequently repeated the holy name of Jesus with which sacred word he expired a little after midnight between the 20th and 21st days of June, the octave of Corpus Christi that year, 1591, being twenty-three years, three months, and eleven days old, of which he had lived five years and almost seven months in the society. He was buried in the church of the Annunciation, belonging to the Jesuits of the Roman college. A rich chapel being afterwards built in that church under his name, by the marquis Scipio Lancelotti, his relics were translated into it. St. Aloysius was beatified by Gregory XV in 1621, and canonized by Benedict XIII, in 1726. Ceparius gives a history of many miracles wrought through the intercession and by the relics of this saint, several being cures of noblemen and eminent prelates. A much more ample history of his miracles may be read in Janning the Bollandist, in an appendix to the life of St. Aloysius.

When we see a young prince, the darling of this family and country, sacrifice nobility, sovereignty, riches, and pleasures, the more easily to secure the treasure of divine love, and of eternal happiness, how ought we to condemn our own sloth, who live as if heaven were to cost us nothing!

(From his life, written in the most authentic manner by F. Ceparius, his master of novices. See also other memoirs collected by Tanning the Bellandist, Junij, t. 4. p847, ad p. 1169, and his life in French by F. Orleans. A.D. 1591).

References:

1) Reverend Alban Butler (1883). *The Lives of the Saints*. Book Four, Vol VI-VII, June and July. Re-published by Loreto Publications: Fitzwilliam, New Hampshire, 2020, 243-255

2) Dicastero delle Cause dei Santi. Luigi Gonzaga (1568-1591). Accessed 23 June 2022. http://www.causesanti.va/it/santi-e-beati/luigi-gonzaga.html

3) Tom Rochford, SJ. Saint Aloysius Gonzaga. Accessed 23 June 2022. https://www.jesuits.global/saint-blessed/saint-aloysius-gonzaga/

4) Hagiography Circle. Beatifications before 1662. Accessed 23 June 2022. http://newsaints.faithweb.com/Premodern_Beatifications.htm

St. Pedro de San Jose de Betancur (Canary Islands/Guatemala) (1626-1667)

Known as "St. Francis of the Americas"
Opened a hospital for the convalescent poor,
Opened a shelter for the homeless and a school for the poor
Rang bell on streets of city calling rich to repentance & begging alms
Founded Bethlehemites (Order of the Brethren of Bethlehem)

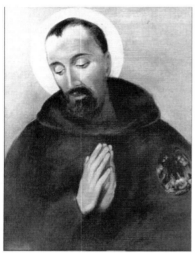

Bl. Pedro de San Jose de Betancur
hermanosdebelenlalaguna.es

St. Pedro de Betancur (Third Order Franciscans, Bethlehemite) was born on March 21, 1626, on Tenerife in the Canary Islands. He was poor and worked as a shepherd to the age of 24. He then planned to journey to Guatemala where he had a relative working in government service. Unfortunately he ran out of money in Havana, Cuba so remained there for about a year.

In 1651, he arrived in Guatemala. He was destitute and found himself in a breadline run by the Franciscans.

Pedro enrolled in a Jesuit College hoping to study for the priesthood. He was unsuccessful in his studies and withdrew from school in 1655.

At this time he became a Third Order Franciscan and took the name Pedro de San Jose. Within three years, he opened a hospital for the convalescent poor, a shelter for the homeless and a school for the poor. The hospital of Our Lady of Bethlehem was reportedly the first convalescent hospital in the world and cared for the sick poor who were expelled from hospitals. He served immigrants, the enslaved, abandoned children and anyone that needed him. He also established an inn for priests and several small chapels in poor areas.

So as not to neglect the rich, he walked through the streets of rich neighborhoods ringing a bell begging for alms and calling the wealthy to repentance. Soon other men came to share in his work and formed a community which, after Pedro's death, was given

152

Papal approval as the Bethlehemite Congregation. A woman's community was also founded after his death inspired by his life of prayer and compassion for the sick, poor and destitute..

Pedro de San Jose is credited with introducing the Christmas *posadas* procession, in which people representing Mary and Joseph seek a night's lodging from their neighbors. This custom spread to Mexico and other Central American countries.

Pedro died in April 25, 1667 in the City of Santiago de los Caballeros in Guatemala, at age 41 from pneumonia. His remains rest in the Church of San Francisco el Grande in Antigua, Guatemala.

Pedro de San Jose Betancur was beatified on June 22, 1980 at Saint Peter's Basilica in the Vatican City and canonized at the Southern Hippodrome in Guatemala City by Pope St. John Paul II on July 30, 2002. He is the first and only saint from the Canary Islands, Guatemala and Central America. He is often referred to as the *"Saint Francis of the Americas"* due to his work with the marginalized and poor. (Memorial April 25).

References:

1) Franciscan Media. (26Apr2021). Saint Pedro de San Jose Betancur. https://www.franciscanmedia.org/saint-of-the-day/saint-pedro-de-san-jose-b etancur. Accessed 14 May 2022.

2) Our Lady of Mercy, Sunderland, Diocese of Hexham & Newcastle. St. Pedro de San Jose Betancur. Accessed 14 May 2022. https://sunderlandcatholic.com/news/st-pedro-de-san-jose-betancur-april-25

3) Hagiography. 2002. Accessed 14 May 2022. http://newsaints.faithweb.com/2002.htm

4) Congregazione delle Cause dei Santi. Accessed 28 May 2022. http://www.causesanti.va/it/celebrazioni.html

St. Jeanne (Jane) Antide Thouret (France/Italy) (1765-1826)

Cared for the sick, wounded and poor
during the chaos of the French Revolution
Founded congregation of the
Sisters of Charity of St. Jeanne Antide (SCSJA)
In 1810 placed in charge of the Hospital of the Incurables,
the largest hospital in Naples
The sisters often visited poor and sick in their homes

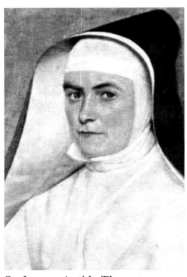

St. Jeanne Antide Thouret.
https://daughters-of-charity.com/feast-of-st-jeanne-antide-thouret/

St. Jeanne (Jane/Joan) Antide Thouret was born on November 27, 1765 in the little village of Sancey-le-Long, Doubs, in eastern France near the Swiss border to a poor farming family. She was the fourth child and the first daughter born to her parents. Her mother died when she was 16 years old and she assumed the management of the household.

When she was 22 years old, she joined the Daughters of Charity in Paris in 1787 and worked caring for the sick in various hospitals. However 6 years later, in 1793, when the French Revolution was at its height, all religious congregations were banned. She refused the government's order to return to secular life, and when she tried to escape the authorities, she was badly beaten.[1] She was forced to leave and returned home and cared for the sick, wounded and the poor --- all of which grew numerous during the chaos of the French Revolution. She taught children and opened a small school for girls, helped hide priests and gathered Christians in prayer.

In 1795 she joined the Solitaires, an itinerant religious community established by Father Antoine-Sylvestre Receveur. They traveled across Switzerland and parts of the Kingdom of Bavaria (Germany) caring for the sick. In 1797 she left this community now in Wiesent and alone, without money, papers or knowing German, traveled to Switzerland.

154

In 1799 she returned to Besancon and opened a school, dispensary and soup kitchen for the poor in the Diocese of Besancon. There she founded a new congregation, the Sisters of Charity of St. Jeanne Antide (SCSJA). The challenges in establishing and maintaining the community are described below from the Rome, Italy website of the Sister of Saint Jeanne Antide Thouret. In addition to the three vows that all religious take, poverty, chastity and obedience, SCSJA also take a fourth vow of Service to the Poor.

In 1810 she was called to Naples where she was in charge of the Hospital of the Incurable, the largest hospital in the city. The sisters often visited poor and sick in their homes. She died from a cerebral hemorrhage on the evening of August 24, 1826 in Naples, Italy.

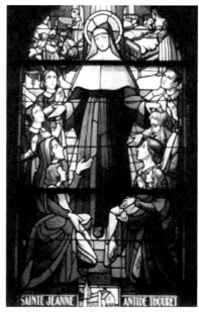

St. Jeanne-Antide-Stained glass of the church of Malbuisson (France). https://www.suoredellacarita.org/en/jeanne-antide-thouret-life/

St. Jeanne Antide Thouret was declared venerable with the decree of heroic virtue promulgated on July 9, 1922, beatified on May 23, 1926, which is celebrated as her feast day, and canonized on January 14, 1934 all by Pope Pius XI.[2] Today approximately 2,500 Sisters of Charity of St. Jeanne Antide serve in 27 different countries. (Memorial - May 23)[3]

"I'm a daughter of the Church, you be also with me"
(April 11, 1820 circular).

"Remember to consider only Christ in the person of the poor. Serve them always as you would serve Christ himself."[4]

When God calls, and is listened to, He gives all that is necessary.

155

From the Sisters of Charity of Saint Jeanne Antide Thouret (Suore Della Carita di Santa Giovanna Antide Thouret), Via santa Maria in Cosmedin, 5-ROMA, (0039) 06 57 17 081[6]

"**1765 - The first Daughter** - The Thourets had already three sons when Jeanne Antide is born the 27th November 1765 at Sancey, a village in Franche-Comte. She is baptized the same day and receives the name of her God-mother.

1781 Mother of Her Family When She is Sixteen - Her mother dies when she is sixteen years old and she becomes mother of her numerous family, dealing with an auntie who does not agree with the father's decision of entrusting this responsibility to his daughter. In the relative calm at the end of the Ancient Regime, when the surging ideas of the revolution were creeping already in the countryside. Jeanne Antide knows the hard work of the village people with the charge of a family. She succeeds in everything she does. But against the wishes of her family, who wanted a suitable man for her, she chooses to leave everything, with a departure she thinks it will be forever, to follow a mysterious call to serve Christ and the poor.

1787 Small Sister in Formation at Langres in the Region of Paris — 1787 marks the first beginning. She is 22 and a new life begins for her. She is not anymore the respected mistress of the house, but a humble little sister receiving everything from the community and those who are in charge. At Langres as in Paris, with the Daughters of Charity she learns to serve the sick poor as a spouse of Christ.

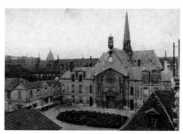

The hospital Laennec-service place of Jeanne-Antide in Paris. Source: https://www.suoredellacarita.org/en /jeanne-antide-thouret-life/

The itinerary for the formation of the young religious seems to unfold without unexpected events. This is true if we do not consider the illness, the grief for her father's death, the revolution and its confusion, the disorder inside the convents, the religious persecution. Nonetheless, nothing makes Jeanne Antide stray from her project, not even, in 1793, the forced return to her village.

1793 Educator and Nurse in the Parish of Sancey — Since her return to Sancey, Jeanne Antide is urged to help the children for whom there was no school, the sick who lacked doctors, the Christians without priests and the priests who were hidden. After all, she makes a gift of her talents and competence. Loved by

156

everybody, she has everything to succeed. However she still dreams of solitude, poverty, prayer! The project of living a religious life still dwells in her and makes her join the ideal of life presented by Father Receveur. Therefore she leaves for Switzerland following the Solitaries who will be soon persecuted, hunted, transformed from migrants into fugitives traveling towards Germany.

1795 European Citizen — In this aimless flight with the Solitaries, among the many dangers of the journey, threatened by the Imperial army as well as the Austrian army, among poverties, epidemics, and daily problems inside the community Jeanne Antide loses neither her head nor her love for God and for the poor sick entrusted to her and for whom she gives herself completely; at Neustschtadt, in Bavaria [Kingdom of Bavaria which after 1871 united with Kingdom of Saxony, and Prussia to form Germany], she sees her younger sister and many others die. She does everything with competence and wisdom yet... she cannot bear anymore not being able to express her love for the sick as she wishes: God is calling her once again somewhere else, but where?...

1797 Along on the Way of Exile — A new interruption! In 1797, she leaves Wiesent near Ratisbona [Kingdom of Bavaria] where the Solitaries are established, alone, with no money, without papers, not knowing German, without a steering compass beside her abandonment and her trust in God. She reaches Einsiedein, in Switzerland, and then closer to France, which she had promised to God not to see anymore. It is here that she receives from the Church the beautiful and difficult mission of going back to Besancon [France] to contribute in re-establishing the Diocese at human and Christian level, after the disasters of the Revolution.

1798 Prisoner Waiting for the Hour of God — At Landeron (Switzerland), busy educating children and taking care of a sick priest, Jeanne Antide had found again a calmer life. But she has to pack again and go where she did not choose. How to prepare herself for the uncertain and dangerous future that she could foresee? She does not have to search long. The Terror wakes up again. Having been in exile, Jeanne Antide must hide for almost a year at La Grange, a silent and prayerful prisoner in a tiny room offered by a friend at the risk of life.

157

1799 Foundress under Obedience — Finally she is in Besancon with no other certainty than the mission entrusted to her and her abandonment to Providence! When she opens the first school the 11ᵗʰ April 1799, the calm has not yet been re-established, Foundress under obedience of a

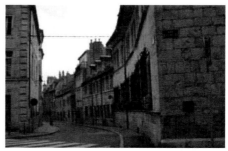

The rue des Martelots, place of the first community. Source: Ibid

Congregation that claims to belong to Saint Vincent de Paul from whom she draws the first elements of her Rule of Life. In ten years time, Jeanne Antide works, struggles, forms young sisters, takes care of the sick, establishes services, cooperates with the local authorities in taking charge of the poor and supports the Church. Recognized at a civil level by the Prefects, then by Napoleon himself, her foundation acquires a fame that expands to the neighbor countries, in Savoy, in Switzerland, and in Naples, the great city rich of its properties, of its history, still wounded by the passage of the French army.

1810 A Woman with a Universal Love — Jeanne Antide accepts the Neapolitan adventure suggested by Madam Letitia, mother of Napoleon, with trust; she and her sisters prepare themselves as best as possible. A European citizen, in Naples, Jeanne Antide sows goodness, care, education, wonder for this new way of living among the world. But she is always at the mercy of adversities,

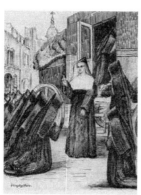

poverty, jealousy. And her restlessness about the communities left in France, where a wind of division is blowing, grows. The beautiful trunk of the tree rooted in Besancon does not recognize her anymore. She is tried by the division, at the same time, in 1819, the Church recognizes and approves her Rule of Life, one of the first presenting an apostolic feminine religious life.

1823 Daughter of the Church — Will a trip to Paris to meet the authorities who refuse her, obtain a reconciliation among the two parties? It's a failure. Jeanne Antide keeps standing in the heart of the storm, with the constant pain of not having been able to rebuild the bonds with the communities in Franche-Comte opening them to the universal Church.

Jeanne-Antide on leaving to Naples. Source: Ibid

1825 A Christian at the Foot of the Cross — Passing through Savoy, at Saint-Paul en Chablais, Jeanne Antide re-takes the way to Naples. At each moment her prayer, nourished by a suffering lived with the Lord on the cross, overcomes the horizon of space and time and allows her to keep loving till death the rebel communities and to maintain the hope in spite of the definitive separation.

1826 Saint for the Church and the Poor — Entrusting everything to the One who called her, filled with his love which supported her many trials, Jeanne Antide, sick, dies in Naples, the 24ᵗʰ August 1826, for the grief of the whole Neapolitan people. Woman of transition, to whom everything seemed to succeed, Jeanne Antide won great struggles through her sufferings and the grace received, through her love for God and for the poor, love for the Church and her Congregation. The Church proclaimed her holiness the 14ᵗʰ January 1934."

Jeanne-Antide Thouret: Spiritual Profile by Father Luigi Mezzadri:[5]

God Alone - The Church - The Poor

Jeanne-Antide was a women with a strong character. Since her youth she was accustomed to take up responsibility first at home and then in the choices of her life. As a novice and young sister, she never wavered from the fundamental orientation of her life and was never accommodating in her religious life. In the dramatic choices of the Revolution she had a strong sense of the Church; she faced openly the representatives of the Revolution in her hometown. While being in exile with the Solitaires of Fr. Receveur, she knew how to detach herself and to face a tough journey in a foreign country supported only by her faith and her determination.

Since the origin of her community she had to make difficult choices, from which she never intended to run away. Throughout her life she showed intelligence, broad vision, a strong sensitivity, but also a mature maternal sense. In other words, she was an upright and resolute woman. On this human foundation a sense of humility, surely not innate, was grafted. Her humility was the results of a constant asceticism and a fine sense of contemplation and solitude, which found the appropriate expression only in the service of the poor.

The Poles of Her Spirituality

The First pole is "God Alone," which implies a deep interior detachment from things, and a continued reference to God and His glory. Because of this basic foundation she commits her life in total consecration to the Lord: *"when God calls and is*

159

listened to, He gives all that is necessary" (letter of February 23, 1813). In one of her letters of 1826 she concludes by saying that she *"would have crossed the seas would go at the end of the world, if she believed that God wanted it for his glory."*

In second place there is "the Church." Mother Thouret repeated: *"I'm a daughter of the Church, you be also with me,"* as she wrote in the circular of April 11, 1820; for her attachment to the Church she deserved to be called *Filia Petri*. The authority of the Pope was strongly opposed by the limited and myopic horizons of gallicanism and by the short-sighted Diocesan particularity.

The third pole of her spirituality is constituted by "the poor;" she was a true daughter of St. Vincent, whom she considered as initiator, founder, father, patron Saint, model and protector of the Institute. Besides the many concepts which reflect St. Vincent's thoughts, she also acquired the same tenderness for the poor, recommending respect, compassion, generosity, patience, charity.

There were many difficulties within the Institute especially in relation with Abbe Bacoffe, who claimed the role of superior. In the mentality of the time it was unacceptable for a female community to be led by a woman. Among other things, Abbe Bacoffe forbade her from having contacts with Archbishop Claude Lecoz (1802-1815), who despite the fact of being a constitutional Bishop, was the rightful pastor of the Church of Besancon and therefore the direct superior of the Sisters of Mother Thouret.

In 1810 the sisters were called to the Kingdom of Naples, by Madame Letizia, the mother of the emperor. During her stay in Italy sister Thouret asked for the Pontifical approval of the Constitutions, which she herself had composed and had been approved by the Archbishop of Besancon. The minor changes demanded by the Pontifical approval provoked in the new Archbishop Gabriel Courtois de Pressigny (1817-1823), a rather wayward bishop with feelings of gallicanism, a complete refusal. Indeed, he forbade the sisters of his diocese to receive the foundress who had visited France to prevent division of the Institute. The split was, however, inevitable. Mother Thouret returned to Naples where she lived painfully the last three years of her life. She died on August 24, 1826. She was beatified on May 23, 1926 and canonized on January 14, 1934. The two branches of the Institute were united in 1954.

Putting her own steps on the footsteps of St. Vincent led the saint to Christ. From here a series that has come down to use was born."[5]

160

References:

1) Catholic News Agency. "St. Jane Antide Thouret." Accessed 29January 2022. https://www.catholicnewsagency.com/saint/st-jane-antide-thouret-477

2) Hagiography Circle: An Online Resource on Contemporary Hagiography. 1826. Accessed 19 April 2022.
http://newsaints.faithweb.com/year/1826.htm

3) Sister Elyse Staab, D.C. "Saint Jeanne Antide Thouret." Daughters of Charity of St. Vincent de Paul. Accessed 29 January 2022.
https://daughters-of-charity.com/feast-of-st-jeanne-antide-thouret/

4) McClarey, Donald R. (2019). "Saint of the Day Quote - St. Jane Antide Thouret." Accessed 29 January 2022.
https://the-american-catholic.com/2019/08/24/saint-of-the-day-quote-saint-jane-antide-thouret/

5) Father Luigi Mezzadri, C.M. "Jeanne-Antide Thouret: Spiritual Profile." Sisters of Charity of Saint Jeanne Antide Thouret. Accessed 29Jan2022.
https://www.suoredellacarita.org/en/jeanne-antide-thouret-spiritual-profile/

6) Sisters of Charity of Saint Jeanne Antide Thouret. Accessed 28 May 2022. https://www.suoredellacarita.org/en/jeanne-antide-thouret-life/

St. Vincenza Gerosa (Italy) (1784-1847)

Practiced charitable works especially nursing the sick.
Founded a hospital.
Founded the Sisters of Charity of Lovere with St. Bartolomea Capitanio

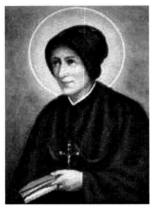

St. Vincenza Gerosa
Source: catholic.org

Caterina Gerosa was born October 29, 1784 to a well-off Italian family in Lovere, Bergamo, Italy. When she was seventeen, her father died, and she saw her uncles push her mother out of the family home. During this time of interior suffering, she began to practice charitable works, especially nursing the sick.

Caterina Gerosa lost her family in rapid succession and was left alone to manage the family business. She used her family's money to provide charitable activities to the community. Caterina became involved with her parish Church, organizing the women's oratory at meetings and retreats, and established a practical school to teach poor girls the domestic work of the community to improve their station of life. In one of these meetings, Caterina met 16 year old Bartolomea Capitanio. Bartolomea had suffered under an alcoholic father before being sent to a convent school. She had since made a perpetual vow of chastity and begun a school for poor girls. Together they embarked on a new mission to start a hospital to care for those who could not afford medical care.

After doing so, they decided to expand their mission to establish a special religious institution with the goals of providing assistance to the sick, free education for girls, Christian orphanages, and programs designed to promote goodness of youth. To accomplish this mission, they together founded the Sisters of Charity of Saints Bartolomea Capitanio and Vincenza Gerosa (SCCG) in 1824. Together they consecrated themselves to God in a simple ceremony on November 21, 1832, in the presence of Fr. Rusticiano and Fr. Angelo Bosio at the altar of the parish church of St. George at Casa Gaia. Thus began the Congregation of the Sisters of Charity of Lovere. Bartolomea Capitanio was 26 and Caterina was 48.

They were God's merciful witnesses in the area of nursing

and education. Bartolomea composed a rule based "on the rules and example left to us by our Redeemer." Only six months later, Bartolomea fell gravely ill of tuberculosis and died on July 26, 1833. Vincenza assumed the work of building and spreading the charism of the order. Caterina was elected Mother Superior and went on to serve as Sister Vincenza, taking her name after St. Vincent. She introduced charitable service in prisons and went on to build hospitals for the needy.[1]

The Order of the Sisters of Charity of Lovere was approved by His Holiness Pope Gregory XVI in 1840 and quickly spread throughout Italy and later to India and other countries. Vincenza oversaw the order until her death in 1847. The Order is known today as "The Institute of the Sisters of Charity of Saints Bartolomea Capitanio and Vincenza Gerosa (SCCG) and also the Sisters of Maria Bambina.

Vincenza died on June 29 1847 after a long illness and was succeeded by Sister Crocifissa Rivellini. She was declared venerable with the promulgation of the decree on heroic virtue on July 24, 1927 and beatified on May 7, 1933 both by His Holiness Pope Pius XI. She was canonized on May 18, 1950[3] by Venerable Pope Pius XII. (Memorial - June 28).

He who has not learned what the crucifix means knows nothing, and he who knows His crucifix has nothing more to learn.

References:

1) Sisters of Charity of Saints Bartolomea Capitanio and Vincenza Gerosa (Sccg). Accessed 29 January 2022. https://newsventure.org/en/Sisters_of_Charity_of_Saints_Bartolomea_Capitanio_and_Vincenza_Gerosa_(SCCG)-4026648824

2) Dicastero delle Cause dei Santi. Vincenza Gerosa (1784-1847). http://www.causesanti.va/it/santi-e-beati/vincenza-gerosa.html. Accessed 17 June 2022.

3) Hagiography Circle: 1847. Accessed 17 June 2022. http://newsaints.faithweb.com/year/1847.htm

St. Marianne Cope, O.S.F. (Germany/USA) (1838-1918)

Opened two of the first Catholic Hospitals in Central New York:
St. Elizabeth in Utica and St. Joseph's Hospital in Syracuse
Answering the request of King Kalakaua of Hawaii, Sister Marianne and
several sisters traveled to Molaki to care for lepers with Fr. Damian.
Operated a school and hospital and cared for Fr. Damian after he
contracted leprosy.[1]

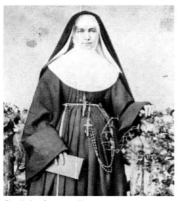

St. Marianne Cope
Source: mercyhour.org

Maria Anna Barbara Koob was born on January 23, 1838 in Heppenheim, Grand Duchy of Hesse [Germany]. Just a year after her birth, Barbara Koob immigrated to the United States of America (USA) at which time the family name was changed to Cope. Her family settled in Utica, New York where she attended the parish school until 8th grade. When her father became an invalid, Barbara Cope worked in a factory to assist the family financially. She first learned about medical care from the Sisters of St. Francis of Syracuse who came into her home to care for her ailing father.[2] Her father died in 1862 when she was 24 years old. This along with her siblings' maturity, permitted her to leave the factory to purse religious life.

Barbara entered the Sisters of St. Francis of Syracuse, New York taking the name Sister Marianne. The first sisters of St. Francis were all nurses or teachers for the first 50 years or so. Sister Marianne was both. Speaking German, she initially became a teacher and later a principal at a school for immigrant children in New York.

She, then, helped direct the opening of the first two Catholic hospitals in central New York. She arrange for students from the Geneva Medical College in New York to work at the hospital, but also stipulated that patients should be able to refuse treatment by them. It was one of the first times in history that the rights of a patient to refuse treatment was recognized.

By 1883 Sister Marianne Cope became the Superior General of her congregation. She answered the request of Hawaiian King Kalakaua, who had invited more than fifty religious institutes, to

164

care for the victims of leprosy. Sister Marianne and six Franciscan sisters traveled to the Hawaiian Island in 1883 first operating a hospital and school for the leper community on Oahu and subsequently on Molokai. It was at the hospital on the island of Oahu, where victims of leprosy were sent for triage. The most severe patients were then sent to the island of Molokai.

Sister Marianne Cope also cared for St. Father Damian who ministered among the lepers after he contracted leprosy and died in 1889. Mother Marianne miraculously never suffered from Leprosy. She died at age 80 on Molokai on August 9, 1918. She was buried on Molokai.

Her remained were returned to the Syracuse, New York mother house, St. Anthony Convent chapel, 1024 Court Street in Syracuse, New York in 2005 and then enshrined in the Honolulu cathedral in 2014. Mother Marianne Cope was beatified on May 14, 2005 and canonized on October 21 2012 by Pope Benedict XVI. (Memorial - January 23).[3]

"Let us make the very best use of the precious moments
and do all in our power for His dear sake
and for His greater honor and glory."

Saint Marianne Cope's biography for the Sisters of St. Francis of the Neumann Communities' Museum:[4]

Marianne Cope was a Professed Member of the Sisters of St. Francis and is Recognized as an Extraordinary Woman of the 1800's and Early 1900's. Her Call to Act as a Servant of God and the Franciscan Spirit she Embraced, provided a Foundation of Values that Gave her the Courage and Compassion to Accept Difficult Challenges with Diplomacy and Grace.

As a leader in her community, Mother Marianne was instrumental in opening two of the first Catholic Hospitals in Central New York: St. Elizabeth in Utica and St. Joseph's Hospital in Syracuse. Recognizing the need for basic health care in a city of immigrants, she and a small group of women defied convention by purchasing a saloon in Syracuse, New York and transforming it into a hospital to serve the needs of a diverse community. Here they welcomed everyone and provided the same quality of care regardless of race, ethnicity, religion, or economic means. They pioneered rules of patient's rights and cleanliness practices not seen before in the United States. And this was just the beginning.

165

Throughout upstate New York, Mother Marianne and her growing community educated and provided healthcare to children and adults with dignity and compassion for all.

In 1883, Mother Marianne and a group of six other Sisters of St. Francis bravely journeyed across the United States by train and took a ship to the Sandwich Islands (now Hawaii) to care for individuals believed to have leprosy (now known as Hansen's disease). They initially served at the Branch hospital at Kaka'ako on the island of Oahu to provide care for those exiled from their families. The king and queen then asked that the sisters open a home to care for the healthy children of patients and Marianne named it the Kapiolani Home in honor of the queen.

Mother Marianne traveled to Maui in 1884 where she was asked to manage Malulani Hospital, the island's first general hospital, as well as St. Anthony School. In 1888, she and the sisters moved to Kalaupapa to care for those with Hansen's disease who had been exiled to the remote peninsula on the island of Molokai. There she cared for Father Damien in his last months and attended temporarily to the boy's home that he had established there until the Sacred Heart Fathers sent a permanent replacement.

Mother Marianne not only provided healthcare to the girls in her care at Bishop Home in Kalaupapa, she offered healing for mind, body and spirit by creating a community that supported individual creativity, dignity and respect. A community of family was established enhanced by gardens, music, art, games and laughter. The grave sites of thousands of people who died from Hansen's disease cover the peninsula on Molokai. It is heartening to know that the sisters provided them with some measure of peace and comfort during their time there.

References:

1) "Saint Marianne Cope". CatholicSaints.Info. 21 September 2021. Web. 9 April 2022. <https://catholicsaints.info/saint-marianne-cope/>

2) Kristin Barrett-Anderson (9 June 2022). Personal Communication. Saint Marianne Cope Shrine and Museum, Syracuse, New York.

3) https://www.simplycatholic.com/st-marianne-cope-a-saint-for-outcasts-and-lepers/ (accessed 16Oct2021).

4) Sisters of St. Francis of the Neumann Communities Museum. Saint Marianne Cope (1938-1918) Biography. Accessed 28 May 2022. https://www.saintmarianne.org/her-story.html

St. Bernadette of Lourdes (France) (1844-1879), Incorrupt

Served as an "intern au pair" at the Hospice de Lourdes
run by the Sisters of Charity of Nevers
As a novice, cared for the sick, was head of the infirmary,
sacristan and most often was the patient herself[1]
It was noted that her sympathetic manner made her a favorite with sick
people. Her very presence brought comfort.
Mystic receiving 18 apparitions of the Blessed Virgin Mary at Lourdes

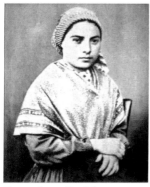

Bernadette Soubirous
Source: giveninstitute.com

Bernadette Soubirous was born on January 7, 1844 in Lourdes, Hautes-Pyrenees, France to Francois Soubirous and Louise Casterot. Bernadette was baptized on January 9–her parent's first wedding anniversary by Father Dominique Forgue in the parish church in Lourdes. As an infant, Bernadette was sent to the neighboring mountain hamlet of Bartres to be nursed by Marie Lagues who had lost an infant. Bernadette referred to Marie as her "foster mother." Bernadette was eldest of nine children and was followed by six brothers and two sisters, only three of whom lived beyond the age of ten. Her brother Justin died in 1865 at the age of 9 and four others died as infants. Her father was a miller and operated a mill that had been in his wife's family. Her childhood was initially comfortable.

However, the work of water mills began to disappear with the beginning of industrialization resulting in debt and loss of the mill. Both Francois and Louise then pursued odd jobs. Louise helped support the family doing laundry and other jobs for wealthy families and assisting with harvesting. Bernadette was once seen by one of her relatives bringing an infant to her mother, who was working in the field, to be nursed. When Bernadette was ten, in 1854, a cholera epidemic scourged Lourdes and she almost died. She was left with asthma and palpitations of the heart. That same year, the family of six had to leave the Boly mill. They change homes several times, eventually living free of charge in the single dark and unsanitary room in the city's former prison, the Cachot. In 1856 famine gripped the countryside and many starved.

167

In 1857, when she was thirteen years old, she was again sent to Bartres, 5 km from home where Marie Lagues promised to teach her the catechism so that Bernadette could make her First Holy Communion. There she helped Marie Lagues in the home, in the fields and tended a small flock of sheep. Unfortunately the catechism was in French and Marie could barely read or write and Bernadette spoke only patois, a local dialect. In addition, after all day in the fields tending the sheep Bernadette was too tired to understand a word. Three weeks before her fourteenth birthday she walked back to Lourdes never to go back to Bartres. There, Father Peyramale had promised that he would prepare her for her First Holy Communion.

Back in Lourdes, Bernadette attended school taught by the Sisters of Charity of Nevers, a teaching and nursing order whose mother-house was in Nevers, south of Paris. The sisters operated a hospice, day school and boarding school in Lourdes and were unusually well trained. Under Abbot Peyramale, Bernadette prepared for her First Holy Community. Her family now lived in Le Cachot which had previously been the local jail and was now their home.

Soon after Bernadette had turned 14, the Blessed Virgin Marry appeared to her on February 11, 1858, at the grotto of Massabielle on the Gave River. Our Lady would appear to Bernadette eighteen times in 1858, the last appearance on July 16, 1858. A brief summary of these visits are as follows:

Thursday 11th February 1858: the first meeting. Accompanied by her sister, Toinette, age eleven, and a friend, Jeanne Abadie, Bernadette went to gather firewood for her mother. Her companions crossed the river while she sat down to take off her stockings. Bernadette heard a noise like the sound of a storm. She looked at the trees near the river, but nothing was moving. She was frightened, and stood up straight. Bewildered, she looked across the mill-stream to a niche above a cave in the rock of Massabielle. A rosebush on the edge of the niche was swaying in the wind. It was all that moved. All else was still. In Bernadette's own words:

> *A golden cloud came out of the cave and flooded the niche with radiance. Then a lady, young and beautiful, exceedingly beautiful, the like of whom I had never seen,*

168

stood on the edge of the niche. She smiled and smiled at me, beckoning me to come closer as though she was my mother, and she gave me to understand in my soul that I was not mistaken. The Lady was dressed in white, with a white veil on her head, and a blue sash at her waist. A Rosary of white beads on a golden chain was on her right arm. On that cold winter's day, her feet were bare, but on each foot was a golden rose radiant with the warmth of summer. I went upon my knees and took my Rosary from my pocket. The Lady took the Rosary from her arm and I began to cross myself. My arm could not move until the Lady herself made a beautiful Sign of the Cross. The Lady let me pray the Rosary on my own. She passed the beads through her fingers, she did not say the words. She signed for me to come closer but I did not dare. She smiled at me, she bowed to me. She disappeared into the niche, the golden cloud faded and I was alone.[2]

Sunday 14th February 1858: holy water. Bernadette felt an inner force drawing her to the Grotto in spite of the fact that she was forbidden to go there by her parents. At her insistence, her mother allowed her; after the first decade of the Rosary, she saw the same lady appearing. She sprinkled holy water at her. The lady smiled and bent her head. When the Rosary ended she disappeared.

Thursday 18th February 1858: the Lady speaks. For the first time, the Lady spoke. Bernadette held out a pen and paper asking her to write her name. She replied; "It is not necessary" and she added: "I do not promise to make you happy in this world but in the other. Would you be kind enough to come here for a fortnight?"

Friday 19th February 1858: the first candle. Bernadette came to the Grotto with a lighted blessed candle. This is the origin of carrying candles and lighting them in front of the Grotto.

Saturday 20th February 1858: in silence. The Lady taught her a personal prayer. At the end of the vision Bernadette is overcome with a great sadness.

Sunday 21th February 1858: "Aquero". The Lady appeared to Bernadette very early in the morning. About one hundred people were present. Afterwards Police Commissioner, Jacomet, questioned her. He wanted Bernadette to tell what she saw. Bernadette would only speak of *"AQUÉRO"* ("that thing" in local dialect)

169

Tuesday 23th February 1858: the secret. Surrounded by 150 persons, Bernadette arrived at the Grotto. The Apparition reveals to her a secret "only for her alone".

Wednesday 24th February 1858: «Penance!». The message of the Lady: "Penance! Penance! Penance! Pray to God for sinners. Kiss the ground as an act of penance for sinners!"

Thursday 25th February 1858: the spring. Three hundred people were present. Bernadette relates; *"She told me to go, drink of the spring(....) I only found a little muddy water. At the fourth attempt I was able to drink. She also made me eat the bitter herbs that were found near the spring, and then the vision left and went away."* In front of the crowd that was asking "Do you think that she is mad doing things like that?" she replied; *"It is for sinners."*

Saturday 27th February 1858: silence. Eight hundred people were present. The Apparition was silent. Bernadette drank the water from the spring and carried out her usual acts of penance.

Sunday 28th February 1858: the ecstasy. Over one thousand people were present at the ecstasy. Bernadette prayed, kissed the ground and moved on her knees as a sign of penance. She was then taken to the house of Judge Ribes who threatened to put her in prison.

Monday 1st March 1858: the first miracle. Over one thousand five hundred people assembled and among them, for the first time, a priest. In the night, Catherine Latapie, a woman from Loubajac, 7 kilometer away, went to the Grotto, she plunged her dislocated arm into the water of the spring: her arm and her hand regained their movement.

Tuesday 2nd March 1858: message to the priests. The crowd becomes larger and larger. The Lady asked her: "Go and tell the priests that people are to come here in procession and to build a chapel here." Bernadette spoke of this to Fr. Peyramale, the Parish Priest of Lourdes. He wanted to know only one thing: the Lady's name. He demanded another test; to see the wild rose bush flower at the Grotto in the middle of winter.

Wednesday 3rd March 1858: a smile. From 7 o'clock in the morning, in the presence of three thousand people, Bernadette arrived at the Grotto, but the vision did not appear! After school, she heard the inner invitation of the Lady. She went to the Grotto and asked her again for her name. The response was a smile. The Parish

170

Priest told her again: *"If the Lady really wishes that a chapel be built, then she must tell us her name and make the rose bush bloom at the Grotto."*

Thursday 4th March 1858: the day all were waiting for! The ever-greater crowd (about eight thousand people) waited for a miracle at the end of the fortnight. The vision was silent. Fr. Peyramale stuck to his position. For twenty days Bernadette did not go to the Grotto, she no longer felt the irresistible invitation.

Thursday 25th March 1858: the name they waited for! The vision finally revealed her name, but the wild rose bush, on which she stood during the Apparitions, did not bloom. Bernadette recounted: *"She extended her arms towards the ground, then joined them as though in prayer and said,* 'Que soy era Immaculada Concepciou' (I am the Immaculate Conception)". The young visionary left and, running all the way, repeated continuously the words that she did not understand. These words troubled the brave Parish Priest. Bernadette was ignorant of the fact that this theological expression was assigned to the Blessed Virgin. Four years earlier, in 1854, Pope Pius IX declared this a truth of the Catholic Faith (a dogma).

Wednesday 7th April 1858: the miracle of the candle. During this apparition, Bernadette had to keep her candle alight. The flame licked along her hand without burning it. A medical doctor, Dr. Douzous, immediately witnessed this fact.

On June 3, 1858, Bernadette received her First Holy Communion on the Feast of Corpus Christi (the Feast of the Body and Blood of Christ). When Bernadette was asked,

> "What made you happier, Bernadette, First Holy Communion or the Apparitions?" She answered, *"The two go together. They cannot be compared. I only know I was happy on both occasions. Years later I would write in my prayer book in Nevers, "I was nothing, and of this nothing God made something great. In Holy Communion I am heart to heart with Jesus. How sublime is my destiny."*[2]

Friday 16th July 1858: the final apparition. Bernadette received the mysterious call to the Grotto, but her way was blocked and closed off by a barrier. She thus arrived across from the Grotto to the other side of the Gave. *"I felt that I was in front of the Grotto, at the same distance as before, I saw only the Blessed Virgin, and she was more beautiful than ever!"*

171

For privacy and to protect Bernadette from the town officials, in 1861, Father Peyramale sent her to live with of the Sisters of Charity of Nevers where she was welcomed as an "intern au pair" at the Hospice de Lourdes. There she slowly learned to write and speak French, to sew and embroider. She helped tend to the poor and sick stating in her memoirs, "I love the poor very much. I like caring for the sick, I will stay with the Sisters of Nevers."[2] In April 1862 she collapsed and was anointed. The hospice doctor prescribed medicine but instead, Bernadette requested water from the grotto. She reported that moments after sipping it, she had felt as though a mountain were lifted off her chest.[2]

On July 3, 1866 Bernadette went one last time to the grotto. She said goodbye, turned away and did not look back. Now she would begin her life as a Sister of Charity in Nevers. She crossed the threshold of the Mother House, called Saint-Gillard, in Nevers with two other young girls on July 7, 1866. The day after her arrival at the Mother House, in her Pyrenean costume, Bernadette told the story of the apparitions for the last time in front of the 300 sisters gathered to listen to her. She was told it would be the first and last time she would speak of them. And then she began the period of formation for religious life. Her health remained fragile, and she was given the last sacraments within four months of her arrival. At this time the bishop anointed her and received her Religious Profession. However, when she did not die, the Superior General was angry and stated,

"You are nothing but a little fool. If you are not dead by morning, I will remove your Profession veil and send you back to the Novitiate."[2] Bernadette recovered. Back in the novitiate she was informed that her mother died peacefully on December 8, 1866.

On October 30, 1867, with 43 novices, she professed her vow taking the name of Sister Marie-Bernard. Despite having received the visits from the Blessed Virgin Mary nine years

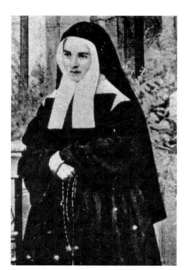

Sister Marie-Bernard
Lourdes-france.org

earlier, Bernadette was not vain or self-important. When treated harshly by the novice-mistress, she responded with perfect humility. The sisters, disappointed by the simplicity of this child of nature made the peasant girl feel bitterly the scant esteem in which they held her; and even her superiors, with the aim of protecting the visionary of Lourdes from the sin of pride, were not sparing in humiliations. With the excuse that she was "stupid, good-for-nothing little thing," her final profession was continually delayed. "God gave to the despised creature, who was punished for 13 years because of her visions, the strength to say: *'You see, my story is quite simple. The Virgin made use of me, then I was put into a corner. That is now my place. There I am happy and there I remain.'"*[3]

Though she would have liked to serve in a community outside of the Mother House taking care of the sick and the poor, her ill health did not allow this. She remained at the Mother House. During her 13 years at Saint-Gildard, Bernadette cared for the sick in the infirmary, was head of the infirmary, sacristan and most often the patient herself. Her life was simple and ordinary. Bernadette had a cheerful character and was available for what was asked of her stating, *"I won't live a moment that I don't spend loving it."*[7] It was noted that her sympathetic manner made her a favorite with sick people. "Her step and touch were light, and her very presence brought comfort."[4] As sacristan she embroidered sacred vestments beautifully which she was able to continue as she became bedridden. Bernadette's father died on March 4, 1871 at the age of 64. Father Peyramale, who had begun the procession at Lourdes and built the chapel, died on September 8, 1877 in Lourdes on the Feast of the Nativity of the Blessed Virgin Mary.

During the last two years of her life (1877-1879), she developed a tumor on one knee which affected the bone causing excruciating pain. She also developed pulmonary tuberculosis which caused much suffering. Sister Marie-Bernard took no part in the consecration of the basilica in Lourdes in 1876. Sister Marie-Bernard made her perpetual and final vows in September 1878, seven months prior to her death.

> On Easter Sunday, Sister Marie-Bernard said, *"This morning after Holy Communion, I asked Our Lord for a respite to talk to Him in comfort. He would not give it. My sufferings will last till death."* On Easter Monday, Bernadette said goodbye to her dear friend Sister Bernard Dalias. "Not that," Sister Bernard had remarked

173

twelve years ago. *"Just that"* said Bernadette as she took her hand. Bernadette took her hand again and said, "Goodbye, Bernard, this time it is the last."

On Easter Tuesday, the chaplain suggested she make the sacrifice of her life. *"What sacrifice?"* Bernadette answered, *"It is no sacrifice to leave this life, where it is so difficult to belong to God."*

On Easter Wednesday, she requested her crucifix to be tied to her, lest her weakening fingers be unable to hold it. She gazed at the statue of Our Blessed Lady and said, *"I have seen her. How beautiful she is, and how I long to go to her."* Sister Nathalie Portat came in about three o'clock, and Bernadette requested, *"Help me to thank to the end."* Taking the crucifix, she prayed, *"My God I love You, with all my heart, with all my soul, with all my strength."* Sister Nathalie began the Hail Mary. Bernadette answered clearly, *"Mother of God, pray for me, poor sinner, poor sinner."* Now was the hour of her death, and like Jesus on the cross, she said, *"I am thirsty."* The Sister brought some water. Bernadette for the last time made the Sign of the Cross as her Lady had taught her in the grotto. Silently she sipped a little water. Peacefully she bowed her head. Gently she surrendered her soul. A sister put the crucifix in her hands and the Rosary through her fingers. Bernadette Soubirous, after thirty-five years on earth, had gone to her God."[5]

Bernadette died on Easter Wednesday, April 16, 1879 at the age of 35 at the Mother House in Nevers, France. In 1909, Mother Josephine Forrestier inaugurated Bernadette's cause of canonization. As part of the formal proceedings, Bernadette's coffin was opened after thirty year in the grave. Her Rosary had rusted, her habit had frayed, but Bernadette was perfectly and beautifully incorrupt. It was as though she had just fallen asleep. Her coffin was opened again in 1919 and 1925 each time the body was discovered incorrupt. In 1925, her body was placed in a reliquary in the Saint Joseph Chapel on 34 rue St. Gildard, in the middle of the garden.

Bernadette

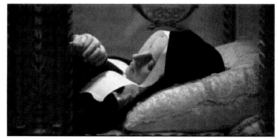

St. Bernadette of Lourdes - Incorrupt
catholicnewsworld.com

was declared venerable with the promulgation of the decree of heroic virtues on November 18, 1923, beatified on June 14, 1925 and canonized on December 8, 1933[6] all by Pope Pius XI. Bernadette was not canonized for her visions but for the humble simplicity and religious trust that characterized her whole life. She is considered the patron saint of shepherds. Website: Some give her two more days: February 18, the day Our Lady promised to make her happy, not in this life, but in the next and February 11th the day the Blessed Virgin Mary first appeared to her which is also the Feast Day of Our Lady of Lourdes).(Memorial per the Vatican Congregation for the Causes of Saints is the day of her death: April 16)

"I love the poor very much.
I like caring for the sick,
I will stay with the Sisters of Nevers"

"Jesus alone for master, Jesus alone for wealth,
Jesus alone for friend"

"God speaks to the heart without any sound of speech"[7]

The Medical Bureau at Lourdes:

In 1883, at the request of Father Remi Sempe, Father of Garaison, the first Rector of the Sanctuary of Lourdes, Dr. Georges-Fernand Dunot de Saint-Maclou established the Bureau des Constations Medicales, so that no one, who thought he had been "cured", would leave Lourdes without having submitted the story of his cure to a rigorous and collegiate medical assessment. And thus formed the Medical Bureau of the Sanctuary. Dr. Auguste Vallet, President of the Bureau from 1927 to 1947, shortly after arrival transformed the bureau into an international multidisciplinary association: Association Medicale Internationale de Lourdes (A.M.I.L.). AMIL includes physicians, pharmacists, dentists, healthcare workers and nurses.[8] Though thousands of miraculous cures have been attributed to the Lourdes water or the Eucharistic procession, as of 11 February 2018, seventy were officially listed.[9] The criteria is stringent and the process arduous to be classified as a miraculous healing. The medical committee must first deem that

175

there is no medical explanation for the cure and this review is conducted over 5 years with annual visits to Lourdes. Subsequently the local bishop of the person cured must approve the report prior to it being submitted to the Vatican.

Our Lady of Lourdes Hospitality, North American Volunteers
The North American Lourdes Volunteers (NALV), staffed with registered nurses, physicians, and lay volunteers, accompanies the sick and suffering, who would otherwise be unable to travel across the Atlantic Ocean on Special Needs pilgrimages to Lourdes.[10]

References:

1) Sanctuaire de Nevers. Sainte Bernadette. Accessed 15 April 2022. https://www.sainte-bernadette-soubirous-nevers.com/fr/pages/bernadette/son -histoire/

2) Catholic Saints. My Name is Bernadette, by Saint Bernadette Soubirous. https://catholicsaints.info/my-name-is-bernadette-by-saint-bernadette-soubir ous/. Accessed 16 April 2022.

3) Katherine I Rabenstein. Saints of the Day, 1998. CatholicSaints.Info. 4 June 2020. Web. 15 April 2022. <https://catholicsaints.info/saints-of-the-day-bernadette-soubirous/>

4) EWTN. St. Bernadette Soubirous. Accessed 15 April 2022. https://www.ewtn.com/catholicism/saints/bernadette-soubirous-494

5) My Name is Bernadette, by Saint Bernadette Soubirous. https://catholicsaints.info/my-name-is-bernadette-by-saint-bernadette-soubir ous/. Accessed 15 April 2022.

6) Hagiography Circle: An Online Resource on Contemporary Hagiography. 1879. Marie-Bernard [Bernadette] Soubirous. Accessed 15 April 2022. http://newsaints.faithweb.com/year/1879.htm

7) Sanctuaire de Nevers. Sainte Bernadette. Accessed 16 May 2022. www.sainte-bernadette-soubirous-nevers.com

8) Lourdes Sanctuaire. Medical Bureau. Accessed 16 April 2022. https://www.lourdes-france.org/en/medical-bureau-sanctuary/

9) Lourdes Sanctuaire. Miraculous healings. Accessed 16 April 2022. https://www.lourdes-france.org/en/miraculous-healings/

10) Our Lady of Lourdes Hospitality, North American Volunteers. Accessed 16 April 2022. https://lourdesvolunteers.org/special-needs-pilgrimage-2022/

St. Giuseppina Vannini, (Italy) (1859-1911)
Foundress of the Congregation of the Daughters of St. Camillus

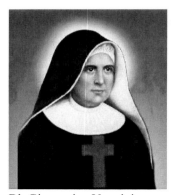

Bl. Giuseppina Vannini
Source: vaticannews.va

Giuditta Adelaide Agata Vannini was born on July 7, 1859 in Rome to Angelo and Annunziata Papi. She was the second of three children. Giuditta was baptized at the Church of Sant' Andrea delle Fratte. Her father died when she was four years old on August 18, 1863. Three years later her mother died on November 6, 1866. At the age of seven she was left orphaned along with her two siblings who were then separated from each other forever.

Giuditta was raised in an orphanage run by the Daughters of Charity of St. Vincent de Paul called the Torlonia Conservatory. At the conservatory she learned domestic skills and receives her education. At the age of 13, on March 19, 1873, she received her First Holy Communion and the Sacrament of Confirmation. Completing her education, Giuditta learned to speak and write in perfect French, and eventually obtained her teacher diploma. She experienced a call to religious life.

Giuditta, at age 21, receives permission to enter the Vincentians. Therefore, the first congregation she entered was the Daughters of Charity beginning the novitiate at the central house in Siena on March 3, 1883 at the age of 23. Usually a 6-12 month trial period precedes the novitiate, called a postulancy, where the religious discerns their call to the specific community occurs. However, within two months of beginning the novitiate, Giuditta was sent to Rome for an additional trial period, to live a year with an acquaintance of the sisters and earn a living with doing embroidery work. She again entered the novitiate on September 20, 1884, having returned to the formation house in Siena 6 months on September 20, 1884 made her first profession receiving and wearing the religious habit of the Daughters of Charity. Over the next four years she worked in Rome, Perugia, Montenero, Siena and Bracciano. Unfortunately she was discharged from the Daughters of Charity on June 26, 1888 for reasons of ill health.

178

Giuditta returned to Rome and there she took the veil of the Sacramentine Sisters. She did not feel that this was the place for her. Leaving this second religious order, she obtained a position teaching kindergarten in Portici, Naples, Italy. Again she is restless, feeling this is not her vocation. She returned to Rome to live with her maternal aunt Anna Maria Papi, who was also her godmother.

Fortuitously, there in Rome, at the age of 32, she met a Camillian priest, Blessed Luigi Tezza, who was then the Procurator General of the Ministers of the Sick (Camillians), while on a retreat sponsored by the religious of Our Lady of the Cenacle for French-speaking ladies. There she discussed with him her challenges with discerning God's will for her life. He suggested to her several other religious orders, each of which she dismisses. Finally he shares with her his desire to re-establish a Camillian Order for women and asks if she would consider being a founder. *[On March 23, 1852, His Holiness Pope Pius IX had granted Oblate Nursing Sisters founded by Blessed Maria Domenica Bruns Barbantini the name of "Ministers of the Sick" and officially decreed the spiritual communion between the Order of Camillian religious and the Congregation of Maria Domenica. However, at the time of their founders death on May 22, 1868, the women's order was small and operated mostly in the city of Lucca. This was also during a time when the secular world opposed the church and religious orders.]* The meeting between Fr. Tezza and Giuditta, was providential because Fr. Tezza was not scheduled to preach at the retreat. He only did so because the priest scheduled had cancelled and he was known to the sisters having spoken at the retreat the year prior. It appears that Divine Providence ordained their meeting.

Giuditta replied, "Father! Let me pray and think and in a few days I will give an answer."At the end of the retreat exercises, Giuditta informs father the following: "I am not capable of anything (...). However, I trust in God who helps those who abandon themselves to Him. Guided by your wisdom and goodness, I do not despair of being able, with holy grace, to accomplish the work to which I feel called by heaven." Thus in collaboration with Fr. Luigi Tezza, Giuditta embarks on a mission for which she does not feel wholly qualified placing, instead, her trust in God and Fr. Tezza.

179

On February 2, 1892, in the room where St. Camillus had died, Giuditta and two other women receive the cape with the red cross of St. Camillus as aspirants from Father Giovanni Mattis, Superior General of the Ministers of the Sick (Camillians). They were housed on Via Merulana, near the hospital. On March 19, 1895, at the age of 35, Giuditta received the religious habit and took the name of Sister Maria Giuseppina. A year later on March 19, 1893, she privately made the vows of poverty, chastity, obedience and the fourth vow of service to the sick even at the risk of her own life. On December 8, 1895, she made her perpetual vows before God and Cardinal Vicar, Lucido Maria Parocchi. Elections were held by a secret ballot and Mother Giuseppina was officially elected Superior General. St. Camillus had invited his religious to serve the sick with the heart of a mother. He had the insight that care of the sick appealed to those qualities and attitudes that are typical of the "female soul": receptivity, readiness to help, tenderness, welcome, a capacity for listening, insight, sensitivity in understanding situations, an aptitude for taking responsibility for other people's problems, an inclination to offer help (Angelo Brusco in Camilliani/s, n. 80 Year VIII - September-October 1994). These gifts along with the philosophy to "always see in the sick the image of the suffering Jesus," Giuditta Vannini and her companions put into practice every day in their care for the sick.

Difficulty arose in 1892 and 1893 when the Holy Father, Pope Leo XIII, refused to sanction the religious order twice because he had decided not to allow the foundation of new religious communities. The local ordinary, through the intercession of Cardinal Vicar, Lucido Maria Parocchi, elevated the religious family to a Conservatory dependent upon the Ordinary on January 24, 1894. Another great difficulty arose when his brother and a friend, P. Ferrini, made false accusations against Father Luigi Tezza. He was forbidden to confess the sisters or enter the sisters' community. He faced the unjust accusations in silence. Fr. Tezza received an assignment to move to France in May 1899. A year later on May 3, 1900, he was instructed to leave for Lima, Peru. There he remained until his death on September 26, 1923. The Congregations of the Daughters of Saint Camillus received official approval in 1909.

As the young Institute was developing rapidly, Mother Giuseppina as they left the mange the new community. Mother Giuseppina was wholly dedicated to teaching the religious to serve Jesus in the person of their neighbor. Her vision of charity was: care for the sick; charity towards the poor; prayer and atonement for the sins of men. She often recommended to the sisters the virtue of humility. She would state that, "the only basis of holiness is humility." The mission of the sisters was the physical and spiritual care of the sick at home, in hospitals, leprosariums and nursing home. In addition to providing nursing care to the sick in Rome, Mother Giuseppina and the Daughters expanded in Italy to Cremona (1893), Mesagne (1894), Brescia, Rieti; Bonsecours, France; in Italy: Monticelli d'Ongina, Capriola and Buenos Aires, Argentina. Many women religious gave their lives in the exercise of this ministry because of he hard work and contagion that occurred when helping the sick.

In 1909, two years prior to her death, Mother Giuseppina Vannini reported to the diocesan ecclesiastical authority in Rome that the Congregation of the Daughters of St. Camillus had 124 religious sisters and 16 houses. That year the "Rules and Constitutions of the Daughters of St. Camillus" were approved by the Cardinal Vicar in Rome on June 21, 1909. This elevated the Pious Conservatory to a Congregation of diocesan right.

Mother Giuseppina led the Institute for eighteen years. She died on February 23, 1911 in Rome at the age of 51 from heart disease. By then, the congregation she founded had 156 professed religious and 16 religious houses between Europe and America. Twenty years after her death on June 17, 1931, the decree of papal approval was conferred. Blessed Giuseppina Vannini is buried in the Generalate of the Daughters of St. Camillus located on via Anagnina in Grottaferrata, Rome, next to that of the co-founder, Father Luigi Tezza.

The decree of heroic virtue was issued by His Holiness Pope St. John Paul II on March 7, 1992. Mother Giuseppina Vannini was beatified by Pope St. John Paul II on October 16, 1994. She was canonized by Pope Francis on Sunday, October 13, 2019 in St. Peter's Square. (Memorial - February 23).

"Always see in the sick the image of the suffering Jesus."

References:

1) Ministers of the Infirm, Camillian Religious. Saints and Blessed. Accessed 17 June 2022. https://www.camilliani.org/en/saint-and-blessed/

2) Dicastero delle Cause dei Santi. Giuseppina Vannini. Accessed 16 June 2022. http://www.causesanti.va/it/santi-e-beati/giuseppina-vannini.html

3) Hagiography Circle. 1911. Accessed 17 June 2022. http://newsaints.faithweb.com/year/1911.htm

St. Maria Domenica Mantovani (Italy) (1862-1934)

As a young girl, visited and assisted the poor and sick
Co-founder, Institute of the Little Sisters of the Holy Family
Served the poor and needy, provided religious instruction,
assist sick and elderly in their homes,
worked with children in nursery schools

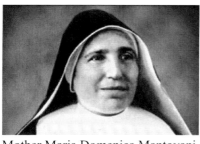

Mother Maria Domenica Mantovani
Source: mantovauno.it

Maria Domenica Mantovani was born on November 12, 1862 in Castelletto di Brenzone (VR), Italy to Giovanni Battista Mantovani and Prudenza Zamperini. She was the eldest of four children. She was confirmed on October 12, 1870 and received her First Holy Communion on November 4, 1874.

She was unable to complete primary school due to the poverty of her family but she had good common sense. She also had an active prayer life.

When Maria Domenica was 15 years old, Blessed Giuseppe Nascimbeni entered Castelletto, first as a teacher and cooperator (1877-1885) and later as the parish priest (1885-1922). He served as her spiritual director and they collaborated in many church activities. She taught catechism to the children and visited and assisted the poor and sick. She enrolled in the Daughters of Mary and served as a roll model for her companions.

On December 8, 1886, at the age of 24, she made a vow of perpetual virginity to her spiritual director and parish priest, Fr. Nascimbeni. She had a great devotion to the Blessed Virgin Mary, Jesus and the Holy Family. She had a great intimacy with Jesus and the contemplation of the Holy Family gave her great strength.

Together with Blessed Fr. Nascimbeni, she collaborated to found the Congregation of the Little Sisters of the Holy Family to serve in humility of life for love of Christ the poor, orphans and the sick. On November 6, 1892, at the age of 30, she became the congregation's first Superior General. The constitution of the order was based upon the rule of the Third Order Regular of St. Francis.

Upon the death of Blessed Father Nascimbeni, on January 21, 1922, Blessed Maria Domenica continued to lead the Institute.

183

At that time, there were approximately 1200 sisters, in 150 branch houses in Italy and abroad.

Mother Maria Domenica Mantovani died on February 2, 1934, after a few days of illness. Mother Maria Domenica was declared venerable with the promulgation of the decree of heroic virtue on April 24, 2001 and beatified on April 27, 2003 both by Pope St. John Paul II. She was canonized on May 15, 2022[2] by Pope Francis. (Memorial - February 2)

Miracle #1 - The first miracle required for her beatification was the miraculous instantaneous cure of an infant who suffered severe brain injury and was in a coma after she fell from a bed the day after her birth. One of the Little Sisters of the Holy Family, a nurse at the hospital touched a medal-relic of Mother Mantovani to the child's head who instantly shook and was healed in a very short time with no sequella. This miracle occurred in the Italian hospital of Bahia Blanca in Argentina.

Miracle #2 - The second miracle required for her canonization occurred in 2011. A twelve year old girl who had been born with a myelomeningocele and paraplegic lower limbs,, was rushed to "Privado del Sur" hospital in Bahia Blanca for severe "Reynaud Syndrome," which affected her lower limbs. During anteriography, she suffered convulsions, cardiac arrest, and respiratory failure. She subsequently developed a lung and urinary tract infection from pseudomonas. The attending physician, who had witness the first miracle, invoked the intercession of Mother Maria Domenica. The mother and relatives joined in prayer. The parents of the sick child were given an image with a relic of Venerable Maria Domenica. The relic was applied to the young girl on June 10, 2011 an she began to improve and was extubated on June 12, 2011. In a short time, with rehabilitation, she returned to a normal life.

References:

1) Congregazione delle Cause dei Santi. Accessed 30 May 2022. http://www.causesanti.va/it/santi-e-beati/maria-domenica-mantovani.html

2) Hagiography Circle: 1934. Domenica Mantovani. Accessed 17 June 2022. http://newsaints.faithweb.com/year/1934.htm

St. Agostina Livia Pietrantoni (Italy) (1864-1894)

Nurse at the Holy Spirit Hospital near the Vatican in Rome.
Joined Sisters of Charity and worked with the critically ill.
Contracted typhus, malaria and tuberculosis.
Stabbed to death during a rape attempt by a patient and
died praying for his forgiveness.[3]

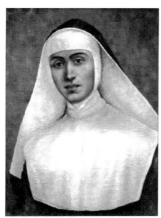

St. Agostina Pietrantoni
reflexionchretienne .e-
monsite.com

Livia Pietrantoni was born on March 27, 1864 in Pozzaglia Sabina, a small town between Rieti, Orvinio, and Tivoli. Known as Livia, she was the second of eleven children born to Francesco Pietrantoni and Caterina Costantini. Her parents were hardworking, religious farmers. She was influenced by the wisdom of her grandfather, Domenico, in a household where everyone took care to do well and prayed often."[1]

She was baptized soon after birth, received the sacrament of confirmation at age 4 and made her First Holy Communion around age 12. Being the second eldest, she helped care for her brothers and sisters. She also worked in the field and care for the animals. She irregularly attended school but managed to learn to such an extent that the other students gave her the title, "professor."

When she was seven she was employed, along with other children, transporting buckets of gravel and sand for the construction of the Orvinio-Poggio Moiano Road. At twelve she traveled to Tivoli to work with other girls in the olive harvest. She took moral and religious responsibility for her younger companions and stood up against some overbearing and unscrupulous persons.

Feeling the call to religious life, Livia traveled to Rome with her uncle but was refused admission. A few months later Mother Giuseppina Bocquin, the Superior General of the Sisters of Charity of St. Jeanne (Giovanna) Antide Thouret and notified her of her acceptance at the Provincial House at Via S. Maria in Cosmedin.

At the age of 22, Livia became a postulant on March 23, 1886. She entered the novitiate and was given the name Sister Agostina after the illustrious St. Augustine.

185

Her first assignment was to work at Holy Spirit Hospital which had served the sick for seven hundred years. Saints who preceded her working there included St. Charles Borromeo, Giuseppe Calasanzio, John Bosco, Camillus de Lellis and others.

Unfortunately at this time, the hospital has been secularized and was even hostile to religion. The Capuchins were forced to leave and crucifixes and other religious articles removed and banned. The sisters would have been expelled also but the Romans feared repercussions. The sisters were forbidden to speak of God. "Sister Agostina, however, did not need a mouth to "cry out to God" and no gag could prevent her life from proclaiming the Gospel!"

Working on the pediatric and later the tuberculosis ward, she showed total dedication to the care of the patient. She contracted tuberculosis and was miraculously cured. During the anti-religion fervor, Sister Agostina found a secret corner in which to place a small statue of the Blessed Virgin Mary, to whom she prayed for graces and for conversions, especially for the obstinate Romanelli.

Romanelli was a difficult, violent and obscene which caused Sister Agostina to multiply her kindness to both him and his blind mother who came to visit. Romanelli annoyed everyone and was subsequently expelled from the hospital by the Director, after he pulled a stunt against the women of the laundry. In his anger, he threatened to kill Sister Agostina. She was killed by Romanelli on November 13, 1894, her lips uttered nothing but invocations to the Virgin Mary and words of forgiveness.

Sister Agostina Pietrantoni was beatified on November 12, 1972 by Pope Paul VI and canonized on April 18, 1999 by Pope St. John Paul II at St. Peter's Basilica.[1] (Memorial - November 13).

References:
1) Congregazione delle Cause dei Santi. Agostina Livia Pietrantoni. http://www.causesanti.va/it/santi-e-beati/agostina-livia-pietrantoni.html. Accessed 16 May 2022.

2) Hagiography Circle: An Online Resource on Contemporary Hagiography. Canonizations after 1558 (4). Accessed 19 April 2022. http://newsaints.faithweb.com/CCS_Saints4.htm

3) "Saint Agostina Petrantoni". CatholicSaints.Info. 11 May 2020. Web. 8 December 2021. <https://catholicsaints.info/saint-agostina-petrantoni/>

4) Vatican News Service. Agostina Livia Pietrantoni (1864-1894), virgin, Congregation of the Sisters of Charity of Saint Jeanne-Antide Thouret. http://www.vatican.va/news_services/liturgy/saints/ns_lit_doc_19990418_pietrantoni_en.html. Accessed 31 May 2022.

St. Maria de Jesus Sacramentado Venegas de la Torre (Mexico) (1868-1959)

*Daughter of the Sacred Heart of Jesus dedicated to
the care of the sick, elderly and abandoned.
For 54 years cared for the poor and sick in the small
Sacred Heart hospital in Guadalajara, Mexico
As the Congregation's leader for 35 years opened hospitals and clinics.
Kept Sacred Heart hospital open during
the repression of Catholicism and persecution
during the Cristero War caring for both soldiers and Cristeros.[1]
1st canonized Mexican saint*

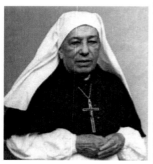

Maria Natividad Venegas de la Torres served as a nurse, Religious Sister and founder of the Daughters of the Sacred Heart of Jesus of Guadalajara, who took the name of *Maria of Jesus in the Blessed Sacrament.*

She was born into a pious Bible-reading, rosary-praying family on September 8, 1868 in La Tapona, Zapotlanejo, Jalisco, Mexico. She was the youngest of 12. Her mother died when she was 16 and her father when she was 19. She was raised by her paternal uncle and aunt. At age 30, on December 8, 1898, she joined the Association of the Daughters of Mary, was active in parish life and taught local children to read. Maria Navidad grew in her interior life, had a great love for Jesus in the Eucharist and attended the Holy Sacrifice of the Mass daily.

She discerned a religious calling at age 37. She was invited by her spiritual director to participate in Spiritual Exercises in the city of Guadalajara. There in 1905 she joined a small community of young ladies dedicated to the care of the sick in the Sacred Heart Hospital.

> She practiced as a nurse with self-denial, was helpful and exquisitely charitable; she distinguished herself for her humility, simplicity for affable ways with her sisters, the sick and people in general. She had a particular way of dealing with bishops and priests in which she saw the continuation of Jesus Christ, the Eternal High Priest.[2]

She worked the next 54 years with the poor and sick in the small Sacred Heart hospital in Guadalajara, Mexico serving as a nurse, pharmacist, housekeeper and the community's accountant and hospital's bookkeeper. On January 25, 1921 she was appointed the Superior General of the Daughters of the Sacred Heart of Jesus. She is considered the founder of the Congregation having written the formal constitution of the Order in 1924 and obtained diocesan approval in 1930. With the diocesan approval of the constitution, she made her Perpetual vows taking the name Mary of Jesus in the Blessed Sacrament. During the 35 years that she served as the leader of the congregation, they increased vocations, opened hospitals and clinics and founded several houses.

In 1926, President Plutarco Elias Calles began enforcing anti-clerical laws, seizing Church property, shutting down Church institutions including schools, hospitals, orphanages and homes for the elderly. The Holy Sacrifice of the Mass was prohibited, religious education outlawed, and all bishops were exiled from Mexico; this persecution started the Cristero War (1926-1928). Mother Natividad managed to keep Sacred Heart hospital open during the repression; when Soldiers arrived to close it down, she overwhelmed them with kindness. She and her sisters treated both Soldiers and Cristeros, so the military held off enforcing the order to shut her down. Mother Natividad insisted that the Eucharist not be removed from the hospital, and to prevent the Soldiers from committing sacrilege, it was often hidden in bee hives on their property.

Mother Nati continued working with the patients until her last days, even when she had to get around in a wheelchair. Her final, bed-ridden days were spent in prayer for them, her hospital and her sisters. She is the first canonized Mexican saint.

Miracle: her canonization miracle involved the healing of Anastasio Ledezma Mora whose heart stopped during surgery, who went into a coma following resuscitation, and was healed following the prayers by the family for the intercession of Mother Nati.[1]

Mother Nati was declared venerable by decree of heroic virtue on May 13, 1989. She was beatified on November 22, 1992 and canonized on May 21, 2000[3] at St Peter's Square in Rome both by Pope St. John Paul II.[4] (Memorial - July 30)

Reference:

1) "Saint María Natividad Venegas de La Torre". CatholicSaints.Info. 4 July 2021. Web. 8 December 2021. <https://catholicsaints.info/saint-maria-natividad-venegas-de-la-torre/>

2) Congregation for the Causes of Saints. Maria de Jesus Sacramentado Venegas de la Torre. Accessed 16 May 2022. http://www.causesanti.va/it/santi-e-beati/maria-de-jesus-sacramentado-venegas-de-la-torre.html

3) Hagiography Circle. Accessed 31 May 2022. http://newsaints.faithweb.com/year/1959.htm

4) "The List of Popes." The Catholic Encyclopedia. Vol. 12. New York: Robert Appleton Company, 1911. 31 May 2022 <http://www.newadvent.org/cathen/12272b.htm>.

St. Mary Elizabeth Hesselblad (Sweden/USA/Italy) (1870-1957)
Studied nursing at Roosevelt Hospital in Manhattan, New York.
Worked as a nurse and provided home care for the sick and aged.
Converted to Catholicism
Joined Carmelites, House of St. Bridget of Sweden.[1]
Re-established the ancient Brigettine Order[3]

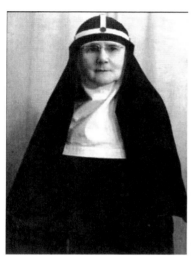

St. Mary Elizabeth Hesselblad
Source: catholic.org

Mary Elizabeth Hesselblad was born on June 4, 1870 at Faglavik, Alvsborg province, Sweden. She was the fifth of fifteen children born to Augusto Roberto Hesselblad and Cajsa Pettesdotter Dag. In July 1870 she was baptized into the Reformed Church of Sweden (Lutheran) in her parish in Hundene. Due to economic hard times, the family moved regularly. She emigrated to New York at the age of 18 to seek work to support her family back in Sweden.

Mary studied nursing at Manhattan's Roosevelt Hospital where she worked as a nurse from 1888 and did home care for the sick and aged. Her work took her into the large Catholic population of New York; her interest in Church grew, and she came to see it as the place closest to Christ. She converted to Catholicism, received conditional baptism on August 15, 1902 by the Jesuit priest Giovani Hagen at the Convent of the Visitation in Washington, District of Columbia (D.C.). In late 1902 she received the Sacrament of Confirmation in Rome while on pilgrimage. There she clearly dedicated herself to the unity of Christians. For the first time, she visited the church and house of Saint Bridget of Sweden. She returned briefly to New York but then sailed back to Rome and settled in the Casa di Santa Brigida on March 25, 1904, the Solemnity of the Annunciation, where she lived with the Carmelite nuns.

In 1906 she received permission from Pope Pius X to take the habit of the Brigittines (Order of the Most Holy Savior of Saint Bridget). In 1911, she was joined by three young English postulants

191

whose particular mission was to pray and work, especially for the unity of the Scandinavian Christians and the Catholic Church. She was ecumenically minded desiring to unite Sweden with the Church, "one fold under one shepherd."

In 1923, St. Maria Elizabeth Hesselblad returned to her homeland, ministered to the poor and tried to revitalize the Brigittine movement there. She established a house in Djursholm, Stockholm, Sweden in 1923. The first monastery and Mother house of the Order that St. Bridget of Sweden founded, in 1369, was situated on Lake Vattern in Vadstena, Sweden. As a results of the Reformation, then the Thirty Year's War and the French Revolution, and general secularism, most of the old institutions in time ceased to exist. The nuns of the Mother house in Vadstena had fled Sweden in 1595 after the Reformation law was passed forbidding Catholicism in all its forms under pain of death. They fled to Gdansk [Danzig].

St. Maria Elisabeth Hesselblad established a foundation in Switzerland in 1924. She received control of the original Rome's Brigittine house and church in 1931 and also established a foundation in England that same year. Finally after 350 years, she established a foundation in Vadstena, Sweden in 1935, the home of the Brigittines (originally founded by St. Bridget of Sweden, Mystic [1303-1373]). Between 1935 and 1963, St. Maria Elizabeth Hesselblad founded a rest home and guest house in Vadstena and in 1968 a convent in Falun, Sweden. In 1963, nuns from the "old order' from Uden, The Netherlands returned to Vadstena and live in an independent Abbey, in a convent opposite the original Abbey Church, which is now Lutheran and still contains the mortal remains of St. Bridget.[4]

In 1937, St. Maria Elizabeth Hesselblad established a Brigittine foundation in India in 1937. During World War II, she saved Jews and others persecuted by the Nazis by giving them refuge in Rome. In 2004, she was recognized by Yad Vashem as one of the *Righteous Among Nations* for this work.

She died on April 24, 1957 in Rome, Italy of natural causes. She was declared venerable by the decree of heroic virtue on March 26, 1999 and beatified on April 9, 2000 both by Pope St. John Paul II. She was canonized by Pope Francis on June 5, 2016.[4] (Memorial - June 4).

We must nourish a great love for God and our neighbors;
a strong love, an ardent love, a love that burns away imperfections,
a love that gently bears an act of impatience, or a bitter word,
a love that lets an inadvertence or act of neglect pass without
comment, a love that lends itself readily to act of charity.[1]

Pray constantly that there be only one flock and one shepherd.
This is the prime goal of our vocation.

Miracle for canonization: The miracle worked by God through the intercession of Blessed Maria Elizabeth Hesselblad was the miraculous healing of a two year old child from a cerebellar desmoplastic (or nodular) medulloblastoma causing extrinsic compression complicating removal by neurosurgery.[2]

References:

1) "Saint Mary Elizabeth Hesselblad". CatholicSaints.Info. 21 September 2021. Web. 8 December 2021. <https://catholicsaints.info/saint-mary-elizabeth-hesselblad/>

2) Congregation for the Causes of Saints. Accessed 31May2022. http://www.causesanti.va/it/santi-e-beati/maria-elisabeth-hesselblad.html

3) Order of the SS Salvatore di Santa Brigida. Santa M. Maria Elisabetta Hesselblad. Accessed 31 May 2022. https://www.brigidine.org/santa_maria_elisabetta.php

4) The Brigettine Order, United Kingdom. St. Bridget of Sweden. Accessed 31 May 2022. https://www.bridgettine.org/st-bridget-of-sweden.html

5) Hagiography Circle. 1957. Maria Elisabeth [Maria Elisabetta] Hesselblad. http://newsaints.faithweb.com/year/1957.htm

6) Marguerite Tjader. (1987). *The Most Extraordinary Woman in Rome.* Vatican Polyglot Press: Rome.

7) Vatican News Service. Maria Elisabetta Hesselblad (1870-1957). https://www.vatican.va/news_services/liturgy/saints/ns_lit_doc_20000409_beat-Hesselblat_en.html. Accessed 31 May 2022.

St. Maria Bertilla Boscardin (Italy) (1888-1922)

*Sister of St. Dorothy, Daughters of the Sacred Heart.
Trained as a nurse in 1907 and
worked on the children's ward in their hospital in Treviso, Italy.
Cared for wounded Italian soldiers during World War I,
noted for staying with patients in 1917 during bombardments.[1]*

Anna Francesca Boscardin was born on October 6, 1888 in Gioia

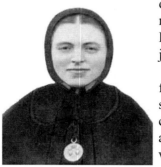

di Brendola, a village near Vicenza in northern Italy to a poor farming family. Her father was an alcoholic, prone to jealousy and violently abusive.

Maria quit school to work in the fields and help at home. With little schooling, she was simple and innocent, considered mentally slow and referred to as "the goose." In her youth, she also worked as a house servant.[1]

In 1904, at age 16, she joined the Sisters of St. Dorothy and worked in the kitchen, bakery and laundry. She received nursing training around 1907 and displayed a special gift for worked with children suffering from diphtheria. She also cared for the very ill and disturbed children.

During World War I, the hospital was taken over by the military. Sister Maria Bertilla cared for the wounded Italian Soldiers, and was noted by local authorities, in 1917, for staying with patients while the area was being bombed. Angry at Sister Bertilla's growing reputation, a supervisor assigned her to the hospital laundry. When her congregation mother-general heard of this vindictive treatment, she transferred Sister Maria Bertilla back to nursing, making her the supervisor of the children's ward in 1919.

St. Maria Bertilla Boscardin died in 1922 at Treviso, Italy after suffering for many years from a painful cancerous tumor.

She was declared venerable with the promulgation of the decree on heroic virtue on July 31, 1949 and beatified on June 8, 1952 both by Venerable Pope Pius XII.[2] She was canonized on May 11, 1961 by Pope St. John XXIII,[3] with some of the patients for whom she had provided nursing care were present. A statue of Santa Bertilla is on the facade of Church of Sts Peter and Paul in Cagnano, Italy.[4] (Feast Day: October 20).

194

"Here I am, Lord, to do you will, whatever comes."[5]

References:

1) "Saint Maria Bertilla Boscardin". CatholicSaints.Info. 31 October 2021. Web. 8 December 2021.
<https://catholicsaints.info/saint-maria-bertilla-boscardin/>

2) Hagiography Circle: An Online Resource on Contemporary Hagiography: 1922.Anna Francesca Boscardin (Maria Bertilla). Accessed 18 April 2022. http://newsaints.faithweb.com/year/1922.htm

3) Matthew & Margaret Bunson (2014). Encyclopedia of Saints (2nd ed). Huntington, Indiana: Our Sunday Visitor, Inc., 169.

4) Franciscan Media. (26 February 2021). St. Maria Bertilla Boscardin https://www.franciscanmedia.org/saint-of-the-day/saint-maria-bertilla-boscardin (accessed 17Oct2021).

5) A.J. Valentino (20Oct2020). Oct. 20: St. Maria Bertilla Boscardin. Accessed 19 April 2022.
https://www.mountcarmelblessedsacrament.com/oct-20-st-maria-bertilla-boscardin/l 2020.

St. Nazaria Ignacia March y Mesa
(Spain/Mexico/Argentina/Bolivia) (1889-1943)

Religious Sister, Institute of Sisters of the Abandoned Elders. Served as a nurse, cook, housekeeper and occasional beggar to support the poor and neglected for twelve years in the Institute's hospice in Oruro, Bolivia. Founded the Congregation of the Sisters of the Pontifical Crusade. Mother Nazaria and sisters cared for and brought sacraments to soldiers on both sides during the war btw. Bolivia and Paraguay

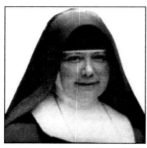

St. Nazaria Ignacia March y Mesa

Source: www.es.catholic.net/

Nazaria March y Mesa was born on January 10, 1889 in Madrid, Spain, to Jose Alejandro March y Reus and Nazaria Mesa Ramos in Arcos de Santa Maria. She was the fourth of eighteen children and had a twin sister Ignacia and ten brothers who survived infancy. She was baptized on April 11, 1889 in the Parish Church of San Giuseppe. Nazaria made her First Holy Communion at the age of nine, on 21 November 1898 and made a personal vow of consecration to God. She actually heard our Lord call, ***"You, Nazaria, follow me."*** To which she responded, *"I will follow you Lord, as closely as possible to a human creature."*[2]

Unlike many children who are drawn to religious life at an early age, her family was indifferent to the faith, and grew so tired of her of her devotions that they once "grounded" her from going to the Holy Sacrifice of the Mass. On August 15, 1890, at the age of 11, she consecrated her virginity to the Lord. She was confirmed at the age of 13, on March 15, 1902, the feast of Blessed Marcelo Spínola y Maestre. By that time, her family had grown used to her piety, and allowed her to join the Franciscan Third Order and more actively practice her faith. She succeeded in getting several of them to return to the Church.

Nazaria tried to enter the Institute of the Sisters of the Cross in Seville, Spain. However, Mother Angelita and Father Tarin had a premonition that she would go to America and return from there with her companions.[2]

In late 1904, business failures led the family to move to Mexico. On the trip, Nazaria met sisters in the Instituto de

196

Hermanitas de los Ancianos Desamparados (Institute of Sisters of the Abandoned Elders), and was so inspired by their charism that on 7 December 1908, at age 19, she followed a calling to religious life, and entered the Institute in Mexico City, Mexico. After her postulancy, she was sent to Palencia, Spain to complete the novitiate. There she made her first profession on October 15, 1911, taking the name Sister Nazaria de Sainte-Thérèse (Sister Nazaria Ignacia of St. Theresa of Jesus).

A year later she was sent to Bolivia with nine sisters, to the Oruro Foundation. She made her perpetual vows on 1 January 1915. Her diaries of the time show a deep devotion to her calling, but struggles with her vows of obedience to her superiors. She was assigned to the Institute hospice in Oruro, Bolivia where she worked as a nurse, cook, housekeeper, and occasional beggar to support the poor and neglected for twelve years.

The region around Oruro was not entirely Christian, many Protestant groups were establishing missions, and the few priests in the area were often lax or lived scandalous lives. Beginning in 1920 Sister Nazaira began to feel a call to found a new congregation devoted to missionary work, evangelization and religious education. On 18 January 1925, the feast of the Chair of Saint Peter, Sister Nazaria made a special vow of obedience to the Pope, and on Pentecost that year she made a vow to work for the union and extension of the Holy Catholic Church. On 16 June 1925, with six other sisters, she founded the Pontifical Crusade, later renamed the Congregation of the Missionary Crusaders of the Church, and began service as their superior. The mission of the Congregation was to catechize children and adults, support the work of priests, conduct missions, and to print and distribute short religious tracts. In addition to the three vows of poverty, chastity and obedience, the sisters took two others: the first of love and obedience to the Pope, and the second of working with all their strength for the union and extension of the Kingdom of Christ.[4]

With the blessing of the Nuncio and the Bolivian hierarchy, Sister Nazaria began the foundation of a missionary institute with only 40 cents in her pocket. Monsignor Felipe Cortesi, while in Bolivia, worked to help Mother Nazaira to found the Congregation. On February 12, 1927, the diocesan religious congregation of the Sisters of the Pontifical Crusade was canonically erected. This was the first legitimate congregation formed in the Bolivian Church according to the Bishop of Oruro. It was to serve all men but especially the poorest and most needy.

When Monsignor Felipe Cortesi was assigned to be the apostolic nuncio of Argentina in 1930, he asked Mother Nazaria to open a Missionary Crusader house in Buenos Aires. She established "social canteens, and worked tirelessly for the promotion of women and for the education of children.

The Congregation received an early test under fire during the war between Bolivia and Paraguay (1932-1935). Mother Nazaira and the sisters cared for and brought the sacraments to soldiers on both sides, and helped establish homes for war orphans. In 1934 she founded the first magazine in Bolivia for women in religious life, *Al Adalid de Cristo Rey*, and the first female trade union, Sociedad de Obrera Católicas

In early 1934, Monsignor Cortesi asked the Vatican Congregation of Religious to approve the rules for the Crusaders that Nazaira had written, based on Ignatian spirituality. Later that year, Mother Nazaria traveled to Rome with an Argentinian pilgrimage group to work for the approval of her Rule. She made pilgrimages to several sites, and had a private audience with Pope Pius XI during which Nazaria said that she was willing to die for the Church; the Pope told her that she must, instead, live and work for the Church.

Leaving Italy for her native Spain, Mother Nazaira founded a retreat center for spiritual exercises in Madrid under the flag of Uruguay; the sisters there survived the Spanish Civil War (1936-1939) as Franco did not wish to risk the international incident killing them would cause. With the help of the Bolivian government, Mother Nazaria was able to leave the persecutions in Spain and return to the Americas. She summoned a general chapter of the Congregation in 1937 to strengthen the unity and zeal of her sisters. She labored for the spiritual formation of new sisters, and set an example by her pious, simple life. To the superiors of the Congregation houses she always recommended a maternal approach to the sisters in their care, to remember their role as Mother of the house.

When the Spanish Civil War ended, Nazaira returned to Spain to check on the sisters she had left behind, then returned to the Americas for the final time. The Congregation spread throughout

South America and began to work in Portugal, Spain, France, Italy and Cameroon. Though Nazaira did not live to see it, the Congregation received Vatican recognition on June 9, 1947 by Pope Pius XII.

Mother Nazaira died on July 6, 1943 in the Rivadavia Hospital in Buenos Aires, Argentina from complications from pneumonia and tuberculosis. She is buried in Chacorita cemetery in Buenos Aires on July 8, 1943. Her relics were moved to the Congregation house at Buenos Aires on June 14, 1957. Relics were enshrined in the crypt of the mother house of the Congregation in Oruro, Bolivia in 1972.

She was declared venerable (decree of heroic virtues) on September 1, 1988, beatified on September 27, 1992 and canonized on October 14, 2018[3] by Pope St. John Paul II at St. Peter's Basilica in Rome, Italy. She is considered the patron of Missionary Crusaders of the Church. (Memorial - July 6).[1]

References:

1) "Saint Nazaria Ignacia March y Mesa". Accessed 21 January 2022. CatholicSaints.Info.<https://catholicsaints.info/saint-nazaria-ignacia-march-y-mesa/>

2) Congregation for the Causes of Saints. Nazaria Ignazia di Santa Teresa di Gesu (1889-1943). Accessed 31 May 2022. http://www.causesanti.va/it/santi-e-beati/nazaria-ignazia-di-santa-teresa-di-gesu.html

3) Hagiography Circle. Nazaria Ignacia March Mesa. Accessed 31 May 2022. http://newsaints.faithweb.com/year/1943.htm

4) Misioneras Cruzadas de la Iglesia. Saint Nazaria Ignacia. Accessed 31 May 2022. https://misionerascruzadasdelaiglesia.net/en/identity/

BLESSED

Beatification

Bl. Teuzzo of Razzuolo (Italy) (early 11th c -1095)

Benedictine Monk
Assigned to the office of nurse
As abbot, built a hospital and hospice staffed by the monks

Teuzzo was born in the early part of the 11th century. He was one of the first students of St. Giovanni Gualberto who broke away from Saint Miniato to start a monastic life more adherent to the Benedictine rule and spirit.

Teuzzo entered the Benedictine Monastery in Vallombrosa, Italy founded by St. Giovanni Gualberto. There the monks strictly adhered to the Benedictine Rule. He served as a nurse for the monastery.

Shortly after 1047, San Giovanni Gualberto had the third Vallombrosan Abbey built in Razzuolo, between Tuscany and Romagna and dedicated it to San Paolo. With eight brother monks, Teuzzo was entrusted with the governance of the Abbey as its first abbot.

He promptly built a hospital and hospice which was staffed by the monks. He wrote about the life and work of Saint Giovanni who had been his spiritual advisor and mentor. Teuzzo also wrote about the meaning and application of the Benedictine Rule. He died in 1095. (Memorial - August 7)

References:

1) "Blessed Teuzzo of Razzuolo". CatholicSaints.Info. 18 April 2022. Web. 6 June 2022. <https://catholicsaints.info/blessed-teuzzo-of-razzuolo/>

2) Mauro Bonato. Blessed Teuzzo of Razzuolo, Abbot. Santi e Beati. Accessed 6 June 2022. http://www.santiebeati.it/dettaglio/99469

201

Bl. Benvenute of Gubbio (Italy) (d. 1232)

First Order, Confessor, Franciscan Brother
Beloved nurse assigned to care for lepers at his own request.[1]
Mystic, Jesus descended into his arms in the form of a child[2]

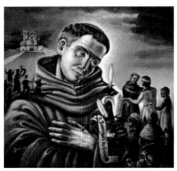

Blessed Benvenute of Gubbio
Source:anspiascolisatriano.it

Benvenute was born in the 12th century in Gubbio, Italy, a town north of Assisi. He served as a knight and was known for his valor. Benvenute heard St. Francis speak in Gubbio in 1222 and was so inspired that two days later, he presented himself to St. Francis in full military attire and asked for admittance as a Franciscan lay brother. Recognizing him as a true soldier of Christ St. Francis received Benvenute into the order.

Benvenute showed himself a worthy Franciscan choosing the poorest clothing, food and dwelling. He was perfect in obedience showing almost no will of his own.

Benvenute was assigned to care for the sick at the leper hospital which he did with great compassion. The Franciscan Book of Saints describes his care for the patients

> There he had, in truth, daily and hourly opportunities to practice heroic charity and self-denial. But Benvenute was always seen to wait upon the patients, even the most repulsive among them, with such cheerful devotion and care as if he were serving his Divine Lord. Otherwise very serious and reserved, he was very sociable when he spoke to the sick and the depressed in order to cheer them up.[2]

He was contemplative and would spend many hours in prayer. Sometimes he spent whole nights pleading for the conversion of sinners. He had a great devotion to the Eucharist and to the Blessed Virgin Mary. So ardent was his devotion to the Eucharist that Jesus would descent into his arms in the form of a charming child.

"The more complete to purify his soul and increase his merit, God allowed him to be seized with a severe illness..."[2] With perfect charity, he submitted himself to God's holy will. Benvenute died ten years after entering the Franciscan Order on June 27, 1232 in Corneto, Italy. He was buried at the parish church in Corneto.

Many miracles occurred at his grave providing evidence of his holiness and attracting pilgrims. This led His Holiness Pope Gregory IX (1227-1241) to give permission for public veneration of Benvenute in Corneto and the surrounding country. This devotion was extended to the whole Franciscan Order in 1697 by His Holiness Pope Innocent XII (1691-1700)[3] at which time the concession of mass and office (C.M.O.) was held conferring on Benvenuto the title of Blessed.[4]

His relics were translated to Deliceto, in the Diocese of Bovino, Italy in 1243. (Memorial - June 29).

"St. Francis considered soldier training
(obedience, self-denial, fearless courage)
good preparation for religious life."[2]

References:

1) "Blessed Benvenutus of Gubbio". CatholicSaints.Info. 22 June 2017. Web. 8 December 2021.
<https://catholicsaints.info/blessed-benvenutus-of-gubbio/>

2) Marion A. Habig, O.F.M. (1979). The Franciscan Book of Saints. Franciscan Herald Press: Chicago, 473-475. Also:
https://www.roman-catholic-saints.com/blessed-benvenute-of-gubbio.html

3) The List of Popes. (1911). In The Catholic Encyclopedia. New York: Robert Appleton Company. Retrieved June 2, 2022 from New Advent:
http://www.newadvent.org/cathen/12272b.htm

4) Hagiography Circle. Accessed 2 June 2022. Concession of Mass and Office. Bd. Benvenuto from Gubbio (? - 1232) c.m.o. 1697.
http://newsaints.faithweb.com/concession_mass.htm

Bl. Jutta of Thuringia (modern Germany) (1220-1260)
Noble woman, widow, hermit, cared for sick, particularly lepers
Prayed for the conversion of Prussia

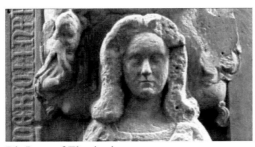

Bl. Jutta of Thuringia
Source: franciscanmedia.org

Jutta von Sangerhausen (Judith) was born around 1220 in Sangerhausen in Saxony-Anhalt (now Sachsen-Anhalt).
She was married at fifteen to Baron Johannes Konopacki von Bielczna and had several children with him.

She lived amidst luxury and power, both being of noble rank, though virtue and piety, were always of prime importance to both Jutta and her husband. When they were making their way on a pilgrimage together to the holy sites in Jerusalem, Jutta's husband died. Jutta was now a widow and single mother. Each of her children entered a monastery upon reaching a suitable age which left Jutta to pursue a more austere religious way of life.

Jutta wanted to lead a life following Christ in evangelical poverty but without entering an order. After providing for her children, she disposed of her costly clothes, jewels, and furniture and became a Secular Franciscan. Jutta wore a simple garment of a religious. She lived in the vicinity of the Ulrichkirche in Sangerhausen and devoted herself to nursing according to the model of Elisabeth of Thuringia. She was also in contact with Mechthild of Magdeburg. She devoted her life to contemplation and caring for the sick, particularly lepers and tending to the poor whom she visited in their hovels. She helped the crippled and blind with whom she would share her home.

She was mocked by the towns people who laughed at how this once distinguished woman now spent her time. However, Jutta saw the face of God in the poor and felt honored to render whatever services she could.

In 1256, Jutta moved to the frontier of Christian Europe with her relative Anno von Sangerhausen, Grand Master of the Teutonic Knights Order. She chose as her base a derelict building in

Bildschon (now Bielczyny), near Kulmsee (today's Chelmza) in Prussia, part of the Monastic State of the Teutonic Order, the area governed by the Teutonic Knight. There she lived as a hermit.

At the cathedral church of Kulmsee she met her patron and confessor Johannes Lobedau. He was succeeded by the Dominican Provincial Heidenreich of Kulm, who had previously been the Archbishop of Armagh in Ireland. There people approached her for counsel and prayers and she earned the reputation of holiness. She said that there were three things that can bring one near God: painful sickness, exile from home and poverty voluntarily accepted for God. She prayed unceasingly for the conversion of the non-Christian population of the region.

Jutta died around 1260 at Kulmsee in the Monastic State of the Teutonic Order (now Chelmza, Kuyavian-Pomeranian Voivodeship, Poland). She was buried according to her wishes in Kulmsee (Chelmza). When her bones were to be raised in 1637, they were lost. However, Jutta Chapel has been preserved at the cathedral in Kulm. A cultus developed around her immediately and the Kulmsee cathedral and Bielczyny became a destination for pilgrims. In Sangerhausen the Jutta von Sangerhausen-Platz commemorates her today. She has been venerated for centuries as the special patron of Prussia.

Canonization: The procedure of the canonization of Jutta by the local bishop was carried out already 15 years after her death, the canonization in Rome did not take place, so she is considered blessed. Patroness of Prussia. (Memorial: May 5).

> *There were three things that can bring one near God:*
> *painful sickness, exile from home and*
> *poverty voluntarily accepted for God.*

References:
1) Franciscan Media. Blessed Jutta of Thuringia. Accessed 2 May 2022.
https://www.franciscanmedia.org/saint-of-the-day/blessed-jutta-of-thuringia

2) Catholic Online. St. Jutta. Accessed 2May2022.
https://www.catholic.org/saints/saint.php?saint_id=4154

Bl. Lukarda of Oberweimar (Germany) (1275-1309), Stigmatic
Infirmarian / Nurse
Miraculous healer. Deep Mystical Prayer Life
Stigmatic[1]

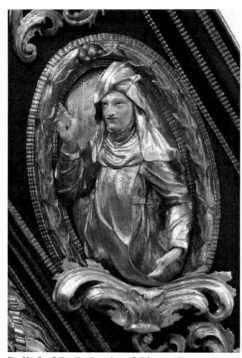

Relief of St. Lukarda of Oberweimar on pulpit at Parish Church of the Assumption of the Virgin Mary, former Cistercian Collegiate Church, Baumgartenberg Abbey, Upper Austria
Public Domain

Lukarda was born in 1276 in Thuringia (modern Germany). When she was twelve, she entered the Cistercians of the Abbey at Oberweimar, near Weimar. She was assigned as the infirmarian of the monastery where she devoted herself with great diligence and compassion to the nursing care of the sick.

She endured many sufferings with patience and perseverance. She was comforted by the Blessed Virgin Mary and Saint John the Baptist. She was devoted to the Passion of Jesus Christ. She received the stigmata during a vision of Jesus. She informed the nuns that she would only live to the age of 33.

She had the gift of healing and many miracles were attributed to her during her lifetime. These included two blind men regaining their sight after cloths stained with the blood of St. Lukarda's wounds were placed on their eyes.[2] A biography on the monastery website which is now a Lutheran Church reports, "She experienced the death of her mother in spirit, had conversations with the deceased and foresaw two fires in the monastery. Christ often appeared to her, comforting and encouraging."[3]

Sister Lukarda of Oberweimar died on Palm Sunday, March

22, 1309 at the Oberweimar Abbey in Weimar, Thuringia (modern Germany) from natural causes. She was buried in the side chapel of the monastery. Many people immediately honored her and through her intercession many obtained extraordinary healings. The veneration of Blessed Lukarda was suppressed in the area by Protestant officials during the Reformation. The cult of Saint Lukarda disappeared and was never resumed.
(Memorial - March 22)

References:

1) "Blessed Lukarda of Oberweimar". CatholicSaints.Info. 13 April 2022. Web. 6 June 2022.
<https://catholicsaints.info/blessed-lukarda-of-oberweimar/>

2) Santi Beati. Blessed Lukarda of Oberweimar, Cistercian nun. Accessed 6 June 2022. http://www.santibeati.it/dettaglio/99560

3) Evangelisch-Lutherische Kirchengemeinde. Oberweimar-Ehringsdorf. Blessed Lukardis of Oberweimar (1276-1309). Accessed 6 June 2022. http://www.kirche-oberweimar.de/83_lukardis.html

Bl. Bonaventure of Barcelona (Spain) (1620-1684)
Infirmarian[1]

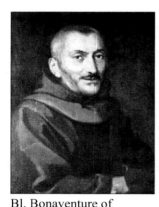

Bl. Bonaventure of Barcelona.
Source: catholicsaints.info

Miguel Baptista Gran Peris (widower, lay Franciscan brother) was an only child in a farm family, born on November 24, 1620 in Riudoms, Tarragona, Catalonia (modern day Spain). He worked as a shepherd and married at age 18 in accordance with his father's wishes. He lived with his wife in perfect chastity both remaining a virgin. Upon her early death, 16 months following their marriage, Miguel followed his calling and joined the Franciscans as a lay brother entering the convent of San Miquel d'Escornalbou taking the name of Bonaventure. He made his religious profession on July 14, 1641 at age 20 and was assigned to the convents in Mora d'Ebre, Figueres, la Bisbal d'Emporda and Terrassa where he worked as a infirmarian, cook, beggar, and porter for 17 years. Blessed Bonaventure of Barcelona received his name for his extensive work in the Diocese of Barcelona.

Brother Bonaventure was sent to Italy in 1658 at age 38, where at San Damiano at Assisi he heard a voice saying to him, *"Go to Rome, and there fill my house with joy!"* In Rome he founded the convent of St. Bonaventure on the Palatine where the rule of St. Francis was strictly observed. Reportedly it was Our Lord Himself who said, *"This rule which Francis adopted was not dictated and composed by his human intellect and prudence, but by Me, according to My will. Every word written in it was inspired by My Spirit."* He founded four monasteries and was commissioned to write the constitutions. Upon the Pope's command, he assumed the office of superior.

He was assigned to houses in Aracaeli and Capranica in Sutri and served as porter at Saint Isidore's College. In 1662 at age 42, he founded the *Riformella*, a reform movement of retreats and spiritual meditation for his brother friars to bring them back to the original Franciscan spirituality. The Pope gave pontifical approval to his writings about "Retreats." He was known for his supernatural

208

wisdom and served as advisor to many pope including Pope Alexander VII, Pope Clement IX, Pope Clement X and Pope Innocent XI.

When he was sixty-four years old, Bonaventure was attacked by a fever. Blessed Bonaventure died on September 11, 1684 at the age of 64 at the friary of St. Bonaventure on the Palantine Hill in Rome, Italy. He was buried on the Gospel side of the little church of St. Bonaventure in Rome. In 1972 his relics were transferred to Riudoms, Spain and enshrined in the tabernacle chapel in the church of Saint James the Apostle in Riudoms.

Bonaventure was declared a venerable Servant of God by Pope Pius VI in 1775. Pope Pius X officiated his beatification ceremony on June 10, 1906. His beatification miracles included the healing of a woman in 1790 from injuries sustained in a fall from a horse. (Memorial - September 11).[2][3]

References:

1) "Blessed Bonaventure of Barcelona". CatholicSaints.Info. 13 September 2021. Web. 8 December 2021.
<https://catholicsaints.info/blessed-bonaventure-of-barcelona/>

2) Marion A. Habig, OFM. Roman Catholic Saints: Blessed Bonaventure of Barcelona. Accessed 13Mar2022:
https://www.roman-catholic-saints.com/blessed-bonaventure-of-barcelona.html. From The Franciscan Book of Saints.

3) Blessed Bonaventure of Barcelona. Accessed 13Mar2022
http://www.2hearts1love.org/bonaventure_b.htm

Bl. Marie-Catherine de Saint-Augustine (France) (1632-1668)
*Served in the Hotel-Dieu (hospital) in Bayeux, France and
in 1648 helped establish the Hotel-Dieu de Quebec in New France.
Honored as one of the six founders of the Catholic Church in Canada.[1]*

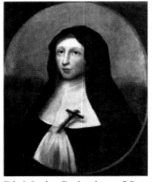

Bl. Marie-Catherine of St.
Augustin Source: cccb.ca

Catherine de Longpre was born on May 3, 1632 in Saint Saveur le Vicomte near Cherbourg, Normandy, France to Jacques Simon de Longre and Francoise Jourdan. She was raised primarily by her grandparents. Her maternal grandfather, M. De Laune-Jourdan was known as "a man of prayer and a grand almoner, whose virtue was appreciated by everyone."[2] "As early as three years of age, Catherine de Longre showed a precocious inclination to follow the will of God absolutely... At age five, she had strong mystical prayer experiences where she felt direct contact with God. When she was only eight, she understood that the Holy Spirit was calling her to be a saint, and at age 10 she wrote a note to "Lady Mary."[3] Catherine was well educated by her relatives, had an affectionate disposition and was very ardent. Advised by St. John Eudes, she became a postulant in the Hospital of Hotel-Dieux, the hospital that the Hospitaler Sisters of Saint Augustine operated in Bayeux, France.

On October 24, 1644, at the age of 12, she received the habit of the Augustinian Hospitaller Sisters of the Mercy of Jesus and took the name Marie Catherine de Saint Augustine. She made her solemn profession at age 16, on May 4, 1648, in Nantes.[4] and set sail for New France on May 27 of that same year.

Though opposed by her family, she volunteered for the mission of her community in Quebec. Her father went so far as to petition the courts to stop her but later accepted her mission there. She set sail for New France (Canada) on May 27 and on the voyage, contracted the plague.[5] She attributed her cure to the intercession of the Blessed Virgin Mary. Blessed Marie-Catherine arrived in Quebec on August 19, 1648 at age 16. At the new hospital she served as treasurer and nurse and oversaw one of the expansions of the Hotel-Dieu de Quebec which provided health care to the region around Quebec in New France (Canada). She devoted her life to

210

serving the sick and the poor in her adopted country. She learned the language of the people in order to better care for them.

Catherine offered herself as a victim for sinners, hiding from everyone a debilitating illness which she bore patiently. In addition, "for sixteen years she also suffered period of spiritual dryness and abandonment, temptation and extreme destitution. It was only after her death that the extent of her suffering and the depth of the holiness became known, even to the sisters of her community." She also served as Novice mistress and was known to spend her spare time in prayer and penance in support of the hospital mission.

In the circular letter notifying the sisters in France of Catherine's death, the superior of the Quebec mission stated, *"Her outward bearing had a charm that was the most attractive and winning in the world: it was impossible to see her and not love her. Her nature was one of the most perfect that could have been desired; prudent, with simplicity, keen of perception, without curiosity, sweet and gracious, without flattery, invincible in her patience, tireless in her charity, amiable to all, without undue attachment to any, humble without being mean-spirited, courageous, without any haughtiness."*[6]

Blessed Marie-Catherine de Saint Augustine died on May 8, 1668 in the Hotel-Dieu de Quebec, Quebec City, New France. She was 36 years old. Her relics are enshrined at the Centre Catherine de Saint Augustine next to the Hotel-Dieu de Quebec. She is considered one of the founders of the Catholic Church in Canada.

Her cause for canonization was introduced on September 11, 1980. Due to her heroic virtues, Sister Marie Catherine de Saint Augustine was declared a venerable Servant on God on June 9, 1984 and five years later beatified on April 23, 1989[7] by Pope St. John Paul II. (Memorial May 8).

"I offered myself to the Divine Majesty to serve Him as a victim whenever it pleased Him; I took no care for my life or my possessions. I only wanted God to dispose of them according to His holy will."[3]

211

References:

1) "Blessed Marie-Catherine de Saint-Augustin". CatholicSaints.Info. 12 November 2021. Web. 8 December 2021. <https://catholicsaints.info/blessed-marie-catherine-de-saint-augustin/>

2) University of Toronto (2015). Simon de Longpre, Marie-Catherine de Saint Augustin. Accessed 13 March 2022 http://www.biographi.ca/en/bio/simon_de_longpre_marie_catherine_de_1F.html

3) Canadian Conference of Catholic Bishops. Blessed Catherine of Saint Augustine (Catherine de Longpre, 1632-1668). Accessed 13 March 2022 at https://web.archive.org/web/20151218194047/http://www.cccb.ca/site/images/Blessed_Catherine_of_St_Augustine-EN.pdf

4) Canadian Conference of Catholic Bishops (2015). The Life and Spirituality of Blessed Catherine of Saint Augustine. Accessed 13 March 2022. https://web.archive.org/web/20151218230901/http://www.cccb.ca/site/eng/media-room/announcements/4189-the-life-and-spirituality-of-blessed-catherine-of-saint-augustine

5) Midwest Augustinians. Blessed Catherine of Saint Augustine. Accessed 13Mar2022 https://www.midwestaugustinians.org/bl-catherine-of-st-augustine from John Rotelle, Book of Augustinian Saints, Augustinian Press, 2000.

6) Province of St. Augustine-Augustinians of the Western United States. Accessed 13Mar2022 https://web.archive.org/web/20160807060505/http://osa-west.org/blessed-marie-catherine-of-saint-augustine.html

7) Hagiography Circle. 1668. Marie-Catherine Simon de Longpre [Symon de Longprey] [Marie-Catherine of Saint Augustine]. Accessed 2 June 2022. http://newsaints.faithweb.com/year/1668.htm

Bl. Maria Rafols Bruna (Spain) (1781-1853)

Dedicated to serving the most helpless: the sick, the mentally ill,
abandoned children and the disabled.
During Napoleonic wars she worked in bombed ruins
to save the sick and children.
Begged enemy camp French generals,
for help with the sick and wounded.[1]
Imprisoned and exiled during the Carlist Wars.[2]

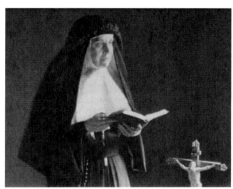

Bl. Maria Rafols-Bruna
Source: chcsa.org

Maria Rafols-Bruna was born November 5, 1781 in the Molino d'en Rovira, 1 km from Vilafranca del Penedes and 64 km from Barcelona, Spain to Cristobal Rafols and Margarita Bruna. Maria was the 6th of ten children. Her parents were poor and simple peasants. On November 7, 1781 she was baptized with the names of Maria Josefa Rosa. She received the Sacrament of Confirmation at the age of four (along with her sisters Margarita and Josefa, the latter two months old) from the Bishop of Barcelona, Don Gabino Valladares, in the convent of the Carmelitas Calzadas de Vilafranca. The family was constantly changing residences due to financial difficulties. Five of her little brothers died. Her father died of exhaustion at the age of fifty leaving her mother to raise five children. These early childhood difficulties enabled Maria to understand the difficulties of the poor, the sick and the dying.

Accompanied by Venerable Father Juan Bonal, twelve religious sisters and twelve Brothers of Charity travel to Zaragoza, Spain on December 28, 1804 to care for patients at the Royal and General Hospital of Our Lady of Grace. There they cared for the sick, insane, abandoned children who availed themselves of the charity hospital. The motto of the hospital was *Domus Infirmorum Urbis et Orbis,* House for the sick of the city and the world.

At sunset upon their arrival, they make their first visit to *Pilar,* to put that new risky mission in the hands of the Lady. And

213

from there they went to the Hospital of Our Lady of Grace founded in 1425 by Alfonso V. *(Pilar refers to the Church of Our Lady of the Pilar in Zaragoza, Spain which houses the infamous pillar on which the Blessed Virgin Mary stood as she encouraged the Apostle St. James the Great in his preaching to convert the people of what is now modern day Spain in 40AD. "Becoming the apostle of what today is Spain, St. James was having a hard time evangelizing the northern region of Zaragoza. One night, as he prayed asking help for his plight, he suddenly beheld a great light in the midst of which he saw Our Lady surrounded by a multitude of angels. The interesting thing is that Mary was still living in Jerusalem at the time.").*[3]

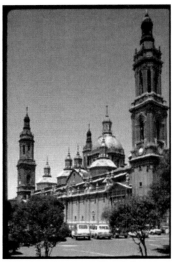

Church of Our Lady of the Pilar, Zaragoza, Spain. Source: americaneedsfatima.org

From there they went to the Hospital of Our Lady of Grace founded in 1425 by Alfonso V. Maria Rafols was made superior of the religious sisters at the age of 23. She had to face the challenge of bringing order, cleanliness and respect to the group and above all, a spirit of dedication compassion to the poor in their care. The women became known as the Sisters of Charity of St. Anne. After three years, the brothers had disappeared but the sisters stayed and increased in number. Maria Rafols knew how to circumvent the pitfalls with prudence, tireless charity and a heroic temperament. She was a determined and brave woman willing to take risks. She demonstrated her and her sisters ability to perform the bloodletting operation, frequently used in medicine at the time, before the entire Hospital board. At this time, and by a woman, this ability was inconceivable.

Soon after arriving, the first sisters endured the bombs of the War of Independence, in the Sieges of Zaragoza. The hospital was bombed and burned by the French. Between the bullets and ruins, she exposed her life to save the sick, begs for them and deprives herself of her own food. When the city lacked food, medicine and

214

water, she went to the French camp and petitions Marshal Lannes and receives from him care for the sick and wounded. She attended the prisoners and interceded for them and in some cases achieved their freedom.

In 1813 Mother Maria Rafols cared for the orphaned or homeless children, the poorest of the poor. Her presence kept order and peace in this department, one of the most difficult in the Hospital. She followed the children in their adoptive homes and removed them if they were not cared for and treated well by the families.

During the First Carlist War (1833-1840), despite the fact that she was declared innocent at her trial, Sister Maria Rafols was imprisoned for two months and spent six years of exile at the Hospital of Huesca with an order founded in 1807, similar to the one in Zaragoza. At the slightest suspicion or slanderous denunciation, she like so many others suffered the same fate. Throughout her prison term and in exile, through humiliation and slander, she suffered with peace and without a complaint. Upon her return, she simply resumed her work with the children. [The Carlist Wars were Spanish civil wars fought by contenders to claim the throne following the death of King Ferdinand VII - Queen Maria Crista became regent on behalf of their infant daughter Queen Isabella II (Christinos). His brother Infante Carlos of Spain, Count of Molina also claimed the throne (Carlists).][4]

Sister Maria Rafols died on August 30, 1853, about to turn seventy two in Zaragoza, Spain of natural causes. She had been a Sister of Charity for forty-nine years. Her death was a reflection of her life: serene, peaceful showing affection and gratitude to the Sisters.[2]

Blessed Maria Rafols-Bruna was recognized for her heroic virtue on July 6, 1991 and declared venerable. She was beatified on October 16, 1994 both by Pope St. John Paul II.[5] (Memorial - August 30)

References:

1) "Blessed María Rafols-Bruna". CatholicSaints.Info. 12 November 2021. Web. 8 December 2021.
<https://catholicsaints.info/blessed-maria-rafols-bruna/>

2) Hermanas de la Caridad de Santa Ana. Fundadores - Maria Rafols. Accessed 13 March 2022 https://www.chcsa.org/identidad/4/fundadores

3) Andrea F. Phillips (1998). Our Lady of the Pillar. America Needs Fatima. Accessed 13 March 2022
https://www.americaneedsfatima.org/stories/our-lady-of-the-pillar

4) Wikipedia: The Free Encyclopedia. Carlist Wars. Accessed 13 March 2022. https://en.wikipedia.org/wiki/Carlist_Wars.

5) Hagiography Circle: An Online Resource on Contemporary Hagiography. 1953 - Maria Rafols Bruna. Accessed 13 March 2022.
http://newsaints.faithweb.com/year/1853.htm#Rafols

6) Carmelites Philippines. Memorial of Blessed Maria Rafols. Accessed 16 June 2022. https://carmelitesph.org/memorial-of-blessed-maria-rafols.

216

Bl. Maria Domenica Brun Barbantini (Italy), (1789-1868)[1]

Foundress, Sister Ministers of the Infirm of St. Camillian (Camillian Sisters)

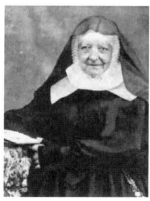

Mother Maria Domenica
Source: camillians.org

Maria Domenica Brun was born on January 17, 1789 in Lucca, Italy to Pietro Brun and Joan Granucci. Her father was a native of Lucerne, Switzerland and served in the Swiss Guards stationed in Lucca. Her mother was from the small town of Pariana in the province of Lucca. Though they were not rich, since the salaries of the Swiss Guard were not high, they were privileged to live in a quarter in the Ducal Palace.

Maria Domenica had a great love for the Blessed Virgin Mary. It is also reported that during the consecration at the Holy Sacrifice of the Mass at Chiesa di Miracoli, Maria saw the Precious Blood overflowing from the chalice elevated by the priest. This incident she only revealed to her confessor. Other than that, she had an ordinary childhood. Unfortunately, her teen years were marked by tragedy. She lost her father and three siblings in a short time period.

Maria Domenica's mother was now left care for the family. Three years after her father's death Maria Domenica suffered a psychological crisis. She recovered presumably due to the firm education she received during her childhood and with the help of her mother's patience and guidance. At the age of fifteen she adopted an austere lifestyle, devoted to study and forgoing the pleasures of youth. As she grew into an attractive woman, she had plenty of suitors and admirers. At the age of eighteen, Salvatore Barbantini, a young man, of Lucca, who had inherited a fabric store from his father, proposed to Maria Domenica. He was not rich but they could live comfortably. Her mother was not happy about his prospects desiring for her daughter a more secure position. For four years, mother and daughter disagreed until eventually her mother capitulated. Domenica and Salvatore were married on April 22, 1811, in the cathedral of St. Martin in Lucca.

Tragedy soon struck when suddenly, five months after their wedding, Salvatore died leaving Domenica alone and with child. As

217

a 22-year-old widow, she faced the raising of her child without his father. On February 14, 1812, Lorenzo Pietro Barbantini was born. Though still grieving the loss of her husband and now perpetually wearing a simple black dress, Maria Domenica lived to provide for her son. She provided him an exceptional religious and secular education such that at age four he was able to answer questions about the Holy Scriptures and at age seven he wrote correctly in Latin and knew some French. During this time, she also devoted her time to the care of poor and sick women. She assisted them at night in their homes. Tragedy again struck the life of Maria Domenica when Lorenzo Pietro died at the age of eight from a sudden serious illness. She was yet again grief stricken.

Instead of closing upon herself in grief, Maria Domenica dedicated her time to the care of the poor and lonely sick, the abandoned and the dying. Now, in both the day and night, she walked the narrow and dark streets of Lucca, sometimes with her lantern-lit to go to the bedsides of the most serious and lonely infirmed. She was not stopped by a hurricane, arriving at a home with her clothes soaked. Disregarding her needs, she provided assistance caring about "Jesus, present in the sick body of that sick person."[2] Some people were cruel and attempted to thwart her efforts such as the time a person put soap on the steps that Maria Domenica had to climb to arrive at a sick person's home. This caused her to slip and fall. She was not intimidated by unknown ill-intentioned people who would at times pursue her at night. Some nights she worked through the night caring for others to the point of exhaustion. She used the little money she had to care for the sick, to help alleviate some of their misery.

Some miraculous event occurred through her intercession.

"One day she put on the body of a poor pregnant woman, who seemed about to die, a flower taken from the altar on which the Blessed Sacrament was exposed. The woman gave birth to twins and recovered her health.

Another sick woman could not feed her newborn. Maria Domenica prayed to the Blessed Virgin venerated at the altar of a church familiar to her. At the end of the prayer, Brun Barbantini ran to the woman, told her to pray to Our Lady and to take the baby to her breast. The woman obeyed and, to her surprise, could feed her baby."[2]

218

Realizing that she could not deal on her own with all the sick in Lucca, Maria Domenica formed a group of women who committed themselves to care for the sick poor. In 1819, they were called the "Pious Union of the Sisters of Charity" and were placed under the patronage of Our Lady of Sorrows. Archbishop Sardi officially approved the Pious Union and Monsignor Del Prete became their confessor and spiritual father, helping them write basic rules. Monsignor Del Prete also directed to Maria Domenica two women who wanted to "leave the world," live together in community and devote themselves to prayer and the apostolate. He encouraged Maria Domenica to purchase a home where the two postulants could live. This she did and it became the foundation of the Oblates of St. Francis de Sales.

After establishing these first two foundations, the clergy of Lucca entrust Maria Domenica with the establishment of a "Monastery of the Visitation" for the education of youth. She was docile to the requests of the clergy and sensitive to the needs of the Church. However, this third endeavor took six years to accomplish and still exists today in Lucca.

Maria Domenica then returned to her original vocation and established a religious Congregation of Oblate Nursing Sisters to serve Christ in the sick and suffering. On January 23, 1829, the first community of Oblate Nursing Sisters was established to perform authentic charity "at the bedside of the sick and dying, in poor dwellings, where even the dying lay alone and abandoned."[2] She taught the sisters to serve the sick, even at the risk of one's own life. In the rule she wrote, "They will serve Our Lord Jesus Christ in the persons of the sick with generosity and purity of intention, always ready to lay down their lives for love of Christ who died on a cross for us."[2]

The Rules and the Institute were approved by Monsignor Domenico Stefanelli, Archbishop of Lucca on August 5, 1841. Eleven years later, the Holy Father conferred upon them the name: "Congregation of the Ministers of the Infirmed." Maria Domenica entrusted the institute to the protection and guidance of Our Lady of Sorrows whom she referred to as "Our Superior." "Just as the Mother of Jesus assisted her crucified Son and shared His pain, torment and abandonment, so Maria Domenica invited her daughters to live "compassion" alongside the sick and suffering of every age.[2]

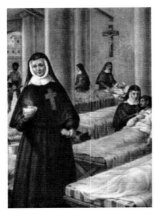

Fortuitously, Maria Domenica met members of the Camillians founded by St. Camillus de Lellis. Fr. Antonio Scalabrini saw the similarity in charisms of both founders. On March 23, 1852, His Holiness Pope Pius IX conferred on the institute the *Decretum Laudis*, the pontifical document through which he granted the daughters of Maria Domenica the name of "Ministers of the Sick" and officially decreed the spiritual communion between the Order of Camillian religious and the Congregation of Maria Domenica. Three years later, in August 1855, the daughters wore the red cross on St. Camillus when they responded to the cholera epidemic claiming victims throughout Tuscany.

As seems to occur with many founders, Maria Domenica experienced accusations, backbiting and perhaps envy. There was a misunderstanding between her and Archbishop Giulio Arrigoni, who was an intelligent and open person. She approached these trials with the armor of HUMILITY, by praying for, forgiving and loving her persecutors.

Maria Domenica fell seriously ill in 1866 but was cured through the intercession of St. Camillus de Lellis. Realizing her strength was diminishing, she made efforts to leave everything in order. Her prayer life intensified. This was a time in which a united Italy was taking shape and in which an anti-clerical and hostile wave to religious congregations was rising. Afflicted by an undiagnosed illness, her face swelled and she was weakened by illness. Mother Maria Domenica Brun Barbantini died on May 22, 1868 leaving the Institute with a small number of sisters, strong in spirit and generous in the service to the sick.

Maria Domenica Brun Barbantini was declared venerable by the promulgation of the decree of heroic virtue on March 26, 1994. She was beatified by His Holiness Pope St. John Paul II on May 17, 1995[4] in Rome, Italy. (Memorial - May 22).

Just as the Mother of Jesus assisted her crucified Son
and shared His pain, torment and abandonment,
so Maria Domenica invited her daughters to live "compassion"
alongside the sick and suffering of every age.

References:

1) Ministers of the Infirm, Camillian Religious. Saints and Blessed. Accessed 17 June 2022. https://www.camilliani.org/en/saint-and-blessed/

2) Camillian Sisters, Philippine Mission. Biography of Maria Domenica Brun Barbantini. Accessed 16 June 2022. https://camilliansisters.org/our-foundress/biography/

3) Dicastero delle Cause dei Santi. Maria Domenica Brun Barbantini. Accessed 17 June 2022. http://www.causesanti.va/it/santi-e-beati/maria-domenica-brun-barbantini.html

4) Hagiography Circle: 1868. Accessed 17 June 2022. http://newsaints.faithweb.com/year/1868.htm

Bl. Gertrude Prosperi (Italy) (1799-1847)
Served as a nurse, sacristan, camerlenga, novice mistress and abbess.[1]

Gertrude Prosperi was born August 19, 1799 in Fogliano di Cascia, Perugia, Italy and was baptized on the same day at the parish church of San Hippolytus in Fogliano di Cascia. Her parents were the wealthy and pious Dominic and Maria Diomedi. When she was 20 years old, Gertrude joined the Benedictines at the Monastery of Sante Lucia di Trevi on May 4, 1820 and took the name Sister Maria Luisa Angelica. There she served as a nurse, sacristan, camerlenga (four times) and novice mistress. She meticulously carried out her duties in order to be able to devote herself intensely to prayer, often inviting sisters

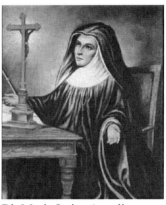

Bl. Maria Luisa Angelica (Gertrude) Prosperi Source: ilpopolotortona.it

to join her. Testimonies are unanimous in describing her as lovable, well-liked by the pupils and nuns.

This was not always considered the case as she experienced considerable suffering. After the arrival of the first spiritual director, Sister Maria Luisa was forced to come out of silence and tell what happens to her in prayer. She saw *"Jesus carrying the cross on His shoulder... He told her, 'this is how I want you, you will be the opprobrium of all. You will see yourself oppressed and you will also suffer from demons, you will suffer because of the Confessors. They will want to help you, but they will not be able to. Oh God, what pain!'"*[2] and He informed her that she would also have to carry hers." She was, therefore, made the object of monastic sanction and misunderstood by the sisters.

However, 17 years into religious life, at the age of 38, she was elected abbess on October 1, 1837. Sister Maria Luisa served as abbess for the last 10 years of her life. She revived full observance to the Benedictine Rule and served as an example in action. She overcame residual mistrust through a personal practice of total humility, so much so as to surprise the nuns on many occasions. She had an attractive way of governing, not authoritarian, but with a strong personal charisma. Sister Maria Luisa was devoted to

Eucharistic adoration. She infused the monastery with a new spirit, in which the sisters saw her as a nun who loved interiority and recollection and who did not tolerate sloppiness or little attention in prayer. Her capacity for introspection was often decisive, especially in her ability to inspire new vocations to the monastic life. Under the management of Sister Maria Luisa, the monastery passed from narrowness to abundance. It became a source of alms for many and the abbess gave to the poor who knocked on the door of the monastery in Trevi where life for many was very hard. In order not to leave someone empty-handed, she even took food from the warehouse without warning the camerlenga.

Though desiring to keep her mystical experiences secret, her new spiritual director, the Archbishop of Spoleto Monsignor Ignazio Giovanni Cadolini, obliges her to write periodic reports. They are overwhelming experiences of encounters with the beloved, the Christ. Beginning in 1838, Sister Maria Luisa begins to sign "Maria Luisa of God's will." It is suffering for her to write about these things but Mons. Cadolini obliges her to do so on a regular basis. In all, she will send the Bishop over three hundred pages. In the visions she sees the Sacred Heart of Jesus which was a popular piety in the 19th century. Often they happen to her close to the moment when she is about to receive the Eucharist and become a unitive moment with Christ. She reports dialogues between her and Christ as loving dialogues similar to the Song of Songs. The union of the hearts necessarily means participation in the pains contained in the heart of Christ who in one visions tells her, *"behold daughter your dwelling, here you will rest, ask for what you want, put here your hearts that I have accepted them, just to love me more, sinners to convert, the infidels to return to My Church."* The vision of a suffering cardinal in Purgatory serves to introduce a discourse of unexpected criticism of the internal situation of the Church.

In the last four years of her life she experienced great personal suffering. The Holy Week of 1847 on Palm Sunday she falls ill seeming to suffocate. On Holy Thursday she lies as if paralyzed in bed, she does not move and has very strong pains. She lives the Passion of Christ in all its moments. She recorded for the bishop, "Around the head He has like signs in the form of a thorn crown, near the heart He has an open wound full of living blood, in His hands appeared a paonazzo sign in the middle." After Easter

Sister Maria Lusia's condition improved. Unfortunately an infection returned with a violent fever and headache. From August 1847 she remained ill in bed getting up very little.

A few weeks before her death she was described as continuing to oversee the monastery, until the last --- sick in bed, dying — but always abbess. The last moments of her life were a sign of serenity. She prepared to die by lying in the position of the Crucified One. Sister Maria Luisa Angelica died September 13, 1847 in Trevi, Perugia, Italy of natural causes and is buried in the church of Santa Lucia in Trevi.[1]

The diocesan process for the recognition of the heroic virtues of Sister Maria Lucia was started in 1914 by the Bishop of Spoleto Pietro Pacifici. They were suspended for the war events of the 1900's. It was officially reopened by Archbishop Ottorino Pietro Alberti on December 13, 1987 and closed on December 13 by Archbishop Antonio Ambrosanio. Pope Benedict XVI issued the decree of heroic virtue declaring her venerated on July 1, 2010. Pope Benedict XVI signed the decree recognizing her miracle: the healing of an Umbrian woman seriously ill in the brain. She was beatified on November 10, 2012 by Pope Benedict XVI at the cathedral of Spoleto. (Memorial - September 12).[1]

References:

1) "Blessed Gertrude Prosperi". CatholicSaints.Info. 28 July 2020. Web. 8 December 2021. <https://catholicsaints.info/blessed-gertrude-prosperi/>

2) Santi Beati. Beata Maria Luisa Angelica (Gertrude) Prosperi, Benedettina. http://www.santiebeati.it/dettaglio/95646. Accessed 16 June 2022.

Bl. Giovannina Franchi (Italy) (1807-1872)

*Laywoman, established Pious Union of nurses to care for sick, poor and
dying in their homes. Utilized inheritance to establish initial home
After her death, this became: Suore Infermiere dell' Addolorata
Founder, Congregation of Nursing Sisters of Our Lady of Sorrow*

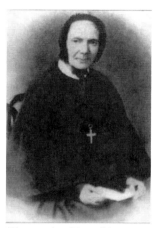

Giovannina Franchi
Source: santodelgiorno.it

Giovannina Franchi was born on June 24, 1807 in Como, Italy to a wealthy family. She was the second of seven children having 4 sisters and two brothers. She was educated for 10 years at a boarding school run by the nuns of the Monastery of the Visitation from 1814-1824. With the other girls, she shared the cloister with the nuns and was almost completely separated from her family from ages 7 to 17. During this time at age 11, she received her First Holy Communion on November 5, 1818. When she departed the monastery in 1824, she was given regulations for piety, a spiritual and behavioral manual to guide her.

Her parents was not much involved in politics and led a somewhat secluded life. They did not attend theaters or other worldly events. Instead they participated in parish life and functions held in the sanctuary of the Crucifix of Como. From 1836-1843, Giovannina, her mother and sister, Carolina, were enrolled as Daughters of Mary in the central oratory of St Dorothy and St. Provino. They were registered as leaders of a small group in this association of ladies dedicated to teaching catechism to girls.

Giovannina was engaged to be married and greatly in love. Unfortunately, in 1840, her fiancee died of an incurable illness, causing her much suffering and making plans of marriage vanish. After his death it was a time of introspection. She did not much think about marriage nor did she discuss religious life, though she continued to keep alive her relationship with the Monastery of the Visitation. She did reflect upon the material misery and moral degradation in the Cortesella district, located close to the Duomo and the palaces of noble and wealthy families. In 1842 she was willed 3000 lire from her Uncle Carlo Andrea Franchi's estate who died having no children.

When she was 42, her mother died. He father followed in death 3 years later. She inherited from his estate the furniture existing in the room in which she lived and 32,000 lire. She was entrusted to the custody of her brothers Andrea and Pietro, as long as she lived in the family.

The next year at age 46, on March 24, 1853, Giovannina Franchi purchased a building located on via Vitani in the center of the Cortesella district. With three other women, she established a pious house for their sanctification and the bodily and spiritual assistance of the sick under the direction of Don Giovanni Abbondio Crotti, canon of the Cathedral. From 1853 to 1856 the women follow a simple rule of life. They lived in community but did not wear a religious habit nor did they make vows. Each was free to dispose of their own assets and to continue to be associated with groups to which they belonged prior to entering the Pious Union.

They cared for people with a variety of needs in the Pia Casa. These include a person who was mentally ill, another affected by paralysis, women who needed safe asylum. Two catechumens came to be educated in the Catholic religion. At this time, they were called the Sisters of S. Nazaro because they were close to a church by the same name. They were known in the community for their charitable activity for the spiritual and temporal relief of the poor and the sick. Still, for the first three years (1853-1856), the Sister Nurses were known as a group of women, not yet a religious order.

During this time, in March 1854, Giovannina was granted the permission of the Congregation of Rites to open a private oratory in the house on via Vitani. The Holy See granted permission for the Holy Sacrifice of the Mass to be celebrated there twice daily where the women and their guests could receive Holy Communion and the Sacrament of Reconciliation. In the oratory was a statue of Our Lady of Sorrows, a gift from the Mother Superior of the Visitation nuns.

On July 27, 1954, Giovannina deeded the building in the name of the Archpriesthood of the Cathedral for the women at the service of the poor and the sick. The building was to continue to be used for the relief of the poor should she die. From 1855 to 1857 Giovannina had the house enlarged to house additional sisters and accommodate the poor and sick in considerable numbers. During this time on October 7, 1856, Dom Giovanni Abbondio Crotti died.

On November 11, 1856, Don Giovanni Bernasconi became

226

their director. Giovannina Franchi and Dom Giovanni Bernasconi screened new aspirants. Between 1857-1872 they defined the basic charism and spirituality of the Pious Union. Since 1859, the Pius Union, conducted dedicated spiritual exercises. With Dom Bernasconi the religious habit, Method of Life, presence of the Eucharist in the oratory of the house, first community chapter and the beginning of a trial period for aspirants were established.

Giovannina Franchi was strongly influenced by Salesian spirituality. In addition she promoted in the women: devotion to the Blessed Sacrament, a great love for the Crucifix and Our Lady of Sorrows, of which the sick were the living image. The patron saints of the community included: the Guardian Angel, St. Camillus de Lellis, the founders of the order of the Visitation: St. Francis de Sales and St. Jane Frances di Chantal and the patron saint of the diocese: St. Abbondio. They were strongly influenced by the Ignatian Spirituality enabling them to unite a profound spiritual life with an active apostolate caring for the sick, poor and dying.

On April 4, 1858, at age 51, after 5 years in the Pious Association, Mother Franchi began wearing a religious habit with a silver crucifix identical to the one worn by the Visitation nuns. The community wears the distinctive habit beginning in November 21, 1858. Earlier that year Bianchi Giuseppa Curiori left her house on Croce di Quadra 15 to "the establishment of Ms. Franchi Giovannina" which has some changes made to it to fit the purpose of the Pious Union.

In February of 1862, Giovannina obtained the permission of the Holy See, now, to keep the Blessed Sacrament in the oratory of the house. The oratory was enlarge and decorated in preparation to receive Jesus in the Blessed Sacrament into their house. It was a joyous occasion. On July 8, 1862, the Method of Life described the rule which was simple and similar to that of St. Frances de Sales and the Visitations. It included home visit to poor sick people and a sober and familiar internal structure: a right balance between work, rest and prayer. Women of all age were accepted, even some with delicate health and some widows. All had to be willing to dedicate themselves to the physical and spiritual assistance of the poor and of the sick, especially the dying.

This same year, in 1862, the Sisters celebrate the feast of Our Lady of Sorrows for the first time. And happily, on January 8,

227

1863, the Vicar General and the Archpriest of the Cathedral, Mons Carlo Zafferani approved the Method of Life. Two years later in 1865 the women solemnize the month of May dedicated to the Blessed Virgin Mary and that of June dedicated to the Sacred Heart of Jesus.

In 1866 as Mother Giovannina's health began declining, she drew up a will appointing canon Giovanni Bernasconi as universal heir. In her writings on January 23, 1869, Mother Giovannina Franchi wrote to the Provincial Prefecture of Como regarding the Pious Union defining it as follows:

> The Pious Union is an Establishment, nothing more than a small union of women, who wish to take care of the poor sick at home, linked between of them only by the bond of charity, and possessing in their own right what little substance they have.

She does not believe by action to ask for the erection of a moral body of said Establishment. This will however, occurred after her death. In January 1870, Mother Giovannina purchase the building next to the house of the Pious Union and transferred the boarders and the long-term patients to it.

In 1871 a smallpox epidemic affected the walled city of Como. The nurses, including Giovannina provided heroic assistance to the sick. On February 23, 1872 Mother Giovannina Franchi was struck by smallpox. At 5:30 a.m. she died at age 65, after serving the sick, poor and dying in Como, Italy for 19 years. The house doctor wrote on her death certificate, "ruin," a generic term alluding to the terrible state of the diseased, rather that publically acknowledging that she had smallpox. A smallpox diagnosis would have required that the Pia Casa be placed in quarantine. Giuseppina Pozzi communicated Mother Giovannina's death to her sister writing:

> ...today, February 23, a seed fell that was the support of all of us and of all the poor of the city. Yes, a precious seed that fell to the ground, a seed that made the whole earth sprout with its good works, today it fell extinct never to sprout again in this mortal life. Yes, our respectable and Reverend Mother disappeared like this seed, charged with virtue and good works, from this earth to the glory of Heaven.
>
> After a serious and burdensome illness that she endured with great patience combined with resignation to the will of God,

228

however, we have the beautiful consolation that she received all the Sacraments with full feelings; which was dear, how sorry her death is...

Mother Giovannina Franchi was buried in a tomb of the Pious Union, one she had purchased 17 years earlier, in 1855, where five sisters had already been placed along with a Sister of Charity of Maria Child who died in 1866 in via Vitani.

After her death Giuseppina Pozzi was elected the new superior on July 8, 1872. The community had built a modern and efficient "Health House" into which the whole community moved in 1879. The Rules of the Institute were approved on January 8, 1928 and "The Pious Union" became a religious congregation taking the name Congregation of the Nursing Sisters of Our Lady of Sorrows in 1935 and His Holiness Pope Pius XII definitively approved the Congregation and the Constitutions of the Nursing Sisters on June 8, 1942.

When Mother Giovannina Franchi's body was exhumed in 1935, they found the remains of the first ten sisters arranged in two chests without any distinction. Thus it was impossible to identify the remains of Giovannina.[1]

Mother Giovannina Franchi was declared venerable with the promulgation of the decree of heroic virtue on 20 December 2012 and the miracle for beatification approved on 9 December 2013. She was beatified on 20 September 2014 by His Holiness Pope Francis. (Memorial: February 23).

The postulator for the cause of her canonization is Fra Giovangiuseppe Califano, OFM, Suore Infermiere dell-Addolorata, Via Dante Alighieri, 11, 22100 Como, Italy.[2]
Website: www.suoreinfermieredelladdolorata.org

Serve the sick with respect for their person, perform all activities with delicacy and attention full of love for others, dedicating our whole life to them selflessly Serve the sick but with care, with a big heart.

229

References:

1) Suore Infermiere dell' Addolorata. Biography of Mother Giovannina Franchi. Accessed 2 May 2022.
http://www.suoreinfermieredelladdolorata.org/note_biografiche.html

2) Hagiography Circle: 1872. 1) Giovannina Franchi. Accessed 1 May 2022. http://newsaints.faithweb.com/year/1872.htm

Bl. Maria Luisa Merkert (Silesia / Poland) (1817-1872)

*Dedicated herself to assisting the sick and poor and
collected alms for their needs.*
*Co-Foundress and first Superior General of
the Congregation of the Gray Sisters of St Elizabeth*

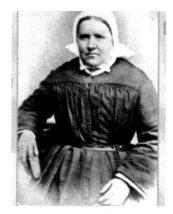

Bl. Maria Merkert
Source: https://www.
zwiastowaniepanskie.com.pl/

Maria Luisa Merkert , religious sister of St. Elizabeth, "was born on 21 September 1817 at Nysa in Silesia, Poland, then part of the Breslau Diocese and in German territory. Maria was the second daughter born to Karol Antoni Merkert and Maria Barbara Pfitzner, from a strongly Catholic and German middle-class family. She was baptized the next day in the church of St. James and St. Agnieszka (Agnes).

Maria's father died when she was just nine months old which resulted in the family being impoverished. Maria and her older sister Matilde graduated from the Catholic school for girls in Nysa. Their mother educated both girls in a spirit of faith and love and in the practice of authentic Christian values. The religious atmosphere at home influenced the girls' formation and sowed the desire to serve the Lord in religious life and their neighbour through charitable works.

Maria assisted her mother during the illness prior to her death on 11 July 1842. After their mother's death, they both sold their modest fortune and, together with Franciska Werner and Klara Wolff (a Third Order Franciscan), devoted themselves to helping the abandoned sick and homeless in Nysa.

After the Holy Sacrifice of the Mass on September 27, 1842 (this day was a memorial of Saints Cosmas and Damian, doctors-martyrs from the 3rd century), they laid down in front of the painting of the Sacred Heart of Jesus in the church of St. James and St. Agnieszka, making an act of devotion to help those in need, regardless of religion, nationality and gender. Thus began the "Association of Sisters for the Assistance of Abandoned Sick, under the Protection of the Most Sacred Heart of Jesus." The parish priest,

231

Fr Francis Xavier Fischer, gave them his blessing.

Maria dedicated herself to assisting the sick and poor and collected alms for their needs. On 31 July 1844 the first five Sisters signed the Statutes of the young Association. By 8 May 1846 their number dropped to four with the death of Matilde Merkert, who had contracted typhus while caring for the sick.

Discerning the young Sisters' need for religious formation, Fr Fischer encouraged them to enter the novitiate of the Sisters of Mercy of St Charles Borromeo in Prague, and on Christmas Day 1846 they began this period of religious formation.

On 30 June 1850, grateful for the formation they had received, Maria and Frances left the Sisters of Mercy to dedicate themselves to their original project of serving the homebound sick and needy. On 19 November 1850, Feast of St Elizabeth of Hungary, with full trust in God, the Sisters again took up their works of mercy at Nysa. They were known as the Grey Sisters of St Elizabeth. They focused their concern on people who had no one to care for tem with a desire to keep them in their own environment. It was typical of the first Elizabethan women to keep people in their homes.

In December 1850, Maria submitted the names of her companions as well as the Association's Statutes to the local magistrate. On an ecclesiastic level the Institute was approved by Bishop Henry Förster of Breslau on 4 September 1859. The first General Chapter was held on 15 December 1859 and Maria Merkert was elected Superior General, a position she held for 13 years until her death.

On 5 May 1860 Mother Maria and 25 Sisters professed the religious vows of poverty, chastity and obedience, along with a fourth vow to assist the sick and most needy. The Motherhouse was built in Nysa during the years 1863 to 1865. Under her leadership 90 religious houses, 12 hospitals, and many nursing homes were established in 9 diocese (Chelmno, Gniezno-Poznan, Warmia, Wroclaw, Fulda, Olomouc, Osnabruck, Prague, Paderborn) and 2 apostolic vicariates (Saxony and Sweden). On June 7, 1871, Pope Pius IX approved the congregation she founded. In 1887 the definitive approval as a Congregation of Pontifical Right was granted by Pope Leo XIII.

The life and work of Mother Maria Merkert was animated by a spirit of ardent charity for the suffering members of the

Mystical Body of Christ. Her sequella Christi was marked by a radical and creative dedication to the sick and the most needy by putting into practice Jesus' words, "As you did it to one of the least of my brethren, you did it to me" (Mt 25: 40).

Mother Maria's maternal solicitude was also directed toward her Sisters, to whom she gave a lofty spiritual and moral formation characterized by a profound spirit of humility.

Mother Maria died in the odor of sanctity on 14 November 1872 in Nysa at the age of 55. At the time of her death, the congregation had 465 sisters in 87 houses. She was buried at the local Jerusalem Cemetery.

On 16 July 1964 her mortal remains were placed in the crypt in the Church of St James and St. Agnieszka in Nysa, and on 19 September 1998 they were translated to a marble sarcophagus in a side chapel of the same Church.

Mother Maria Merkert was declared venerable with the promulgation of the decree of heroic virtue on 20 December 2004 by Pope St. John Paul II.[1] Pope Benedict XVI in June 2007 approved the decree on the miracle through the intercession of Maria Merkert which was the healing of tuberculosis of one of the Elizabethan women, Mira's sister.[2] She was beatified on 30 September 2007 in the Cathedral of Saints James the Apostle and Agnes, Nysa (Poland), presided by Cardinal José Saraiva Martins,[3] prefect of the Congregation for the Causes of Saints. (Memorial November 14).

As you did it to one of the least of my brethren, you did it to me.

References:

1) Vatican News Service. Blessed Maria Luisa Merkert (1817-1872). https://www.vatican.va/news_services/liturgy/saints/ns_lit_doc_20070930_merkert_en.html. Accessed 6 April 2022.

2) Parafia Rzymskokatolicka pw. Zwiastowania Panskiego. Parish Announcement - Memorial of Bl. Maria Luisa Merkert. https://www.zwiastowaniepanskie.com.pl/2017/11/12/14-listopada-wspomnienie-bl-marii-luizy-merkert/. Accessed 6 April 2022.

3) Hagiography Circle: An Online Resource on Contemporary Hagiography Saints of 2007. Accessed 6 April 2022. http://newsaints.faithweb.com/2007.htm

Bl. Jose Olallo Valdes (Havana, Cuba) (1820-1889)

Nurse at Brothers Hospitallers of Saint John of God
hospital in Puerto Principe in April 1835.
Appointed head nurse of the hospitals in 1845.
Cared for people during cholera epidemic.
Treated wounded on both sides in the
Ten Years War in Cuba from 1868-1878.[1]

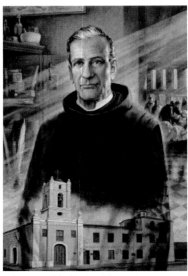

Bl. Jose Olallo Valdes
catholicsaints.info

Jose Olallo Valdes was born on February 12, 1820 in Havana Cuba. He was abandoned as an infant at the age of one month at the St. Joseph orphanage in Havana, Cuba.

A Cuban site relates:
His origin is a compelling argument for LIFE. A young woman, probably seduced and deceived, heartbroken with pain, is forced to part with her son from her womb. She does not want to abandon him, she leaves him in the arms of God, trusting that He will take care of him. This is how Father Tato Karel tells it: On March 15, 1820, while a persistent fog barely allowed people to be distinguished, a woman, wrapped in her shawl, as if she wanted to hide her face and a bundle, which she carried in her arms, headed towards Calle de Los Oficios. She stopped before a large wooden gate, at number 59. She raised her eyes clouded with tears and could read on the pediment: Real Casa Cuna. She signed deeply and pulled from under her cloak her bulk wrapped in a woolen scarf. She looked around and deposited the package on the turnstile by the door, placing a sealed envelope on top of it. With trembling hands, she picked up the bundle again. She clasped him in her arms, parted the scarf and placed a long kiss on him and then left him on the lathe again while she murmured: 'My God, I don't know what I'm going to do, but you know, Lord, that I can't do anything else. His father didn't even want to see him; if they find out in my house, they are capable of killing me. I can't raise him by myself. I put him in Your

234

hands. You take care of him and help him to be good." She tugged on the call cord. In the distance two timid chimes sounded. The woman let go of the cord as if it burned her hand. She took one last look around her. She crossed herself. She covered her face with her cloak and left quickly, getting lost in the narrow streets of the city. An hour later, Father Antonio Eusebio Ramos contemplated before him an almost newborn baby, with a white face and well dressed. Inside the envelop was a piece of paper written with a women's trembling hand, which said: *"The child was born on February 12. He is unbaptized"* With the name of Jose Olallo Valdes, he was baptized on March 15, 1820 by the priest Antonio Eusebio Ramos in the chapel of the Casa Cuna del Patriarca San Jose, which was run by the Daughters of Charity of Saint Vincent de Paul in Havana.[2]

Jose lived at Casa Cuna de San Jose in Havana until age seven when he moved to the Benefencia orphanage which was also located in Havana. Seeing the frequent death of children in the almshouses, almost a daily occurrence Olallo decided to consecrate his life to remedy human pain. At age 13-14 he was admitted to the Hospitaller Order of San Juan de Dios, in the community of the hospital of Saints Felipe and Santiago in Havana.[3]

That year he was assigned to work in the hospital in Puerto Principe (today Camaguey) where he completed his nursing training. He served as an assistant nurse, then at age 25 became a "Senior Nurse" at the San Juan de Dios Hospital. A cholera epidemic decimated the population soon after he had completed training during which Brother Olallo was observed to be an efficient, humble, accommodating, and self sacrificing nurse. He would take on the most difficult tasks served the sick in an efficient, humble manner. He took on the most unpleasant tasks such as cleaning dirty chamber pots (bedpans), washing bloody cloths and carrying corpses. Despite his youth people testified that he was the heart of the hospital.

He was chosen Prior of the Brother in Camaguey in 1856. The Archbishop of Santiago de Cuba recommended that he become a priest, which he declined, desiring, instead, to continue his work in the hospital. He treated war wounded (1868-1878) during the Ten Years War in Cuba. He prevented the massacre of civilians ordered by Spanish forces. From 1876 upon the death of his last brother in the community and due to the suppression of religious orders by the

235

Spanish government, he was the only surviving member of the Hospitallers in Cuba for the last 13 years of his life.

For 54 year, from 1835-1889, Brother Olallo worked in a hospital for poor and elderly, in the midst of lack of means, hunger, war, epidemics, slavery, political and social rivalries..." In those 54 years he was absent from the hospital for one night only, and this was through no fault of his own. Upon the beatification of Blessed Jose Olallo-Valdes on November 29, 2008, in his homily, Cardinal Jose Saraiva Martins stated,

> I would also like to mention his fearless intervention before the military authorities, defending the care of the weakest in the hospital and preventing at any given moment that the bells gave the signal of attack, as was decided, thus saving the population from a real and proper carnage. His charity to care for the sick in prison before, during and after the war was also impressive. Father Olallo is also distinguished by his enthusiastic fidelity to the hospitable vocation as a diligent and careful nurse, caring and close to all, dedicated in particular to the marginalized and the sickest, for their physical and social, psychological and spiritual healing, at a historical moment in which Camaguey society suffered great poverty and misery. He was, therefore, as has rightly been defined, "*a champion of Christian charity*", in solidarity with those whom he called "*his favorite brothers*", with all kinds of help...In his funeral monument there is a phrase that says: "Father Olallo, the poor who have died comforted by you await you, those you left without consolation prays for you... Father Olallo is a person who *trusted God completely*, aware that the presence of the Lord in history wants the good of all people.[4]

Blessed Jose Olallo-Valdes died on March 7, 1889 in Camaguey, Cuba from natural causes. He is buried at the chapel of the Brothers Hospitallers of Saint John of God hospital in Camaguey. He was declared venerable on December 16, 2006 and beatified on November 29, 2008[5][6] both by Pope Benedict XVI. His beatification miracle involved the healing of three-year-old Daniela Cabrera Ramos. His beatification was celebrated at the Plaza de La Caridad, Camaguey in Cuba presided over by Cardinal Jose Saraiva Martins.[7][8] (Memorial - March 7)

References:

1) "Blessed José Olallo Valdés". CatholicSaints.Info. 22 May 2020. Web. 8 December 2021. <https://catholicsaints.info/blessed-jose-Olallo-valdes/>

2) Javier's Catholic Web. Accessed 15 March 2022. http://webcatolicodejavier.org/JoseOlallo.html

3) Vatican News Service. Jose Olallo Valdes (1820-1889). www.vatican.va/news_services/liturgy/saints/2008/ns_lit_doc_20081129_olallo_sp.html. Accessed 4 April 2022.

4) Congregazione delle Cause dei Santi. (29Nov2008). Homily by Cardinal Jose Saraiva Martins. http://www.causesanti.va/it/archivio-della-congregazione-cause-santi/interventi-del-card-jose-saraiva-martins/beatificacion-jose-olallo-valdes-29-novembre-2008-camagueey.html

5) Hagiography Circle. Jose Olallo Valdes. Accessed 3 June 2022. http://newsaints.faithweb.com/year/1889.htm

6) Congregazione delle Cause dei Santi. Jose Olallo Valdes (1820-1889) http://www.causesanti.va/it/santi-e-beati/jose-olallo-valdes.html

Bl. Luigi Maria Monti (Italy) (1825-1900)

Layman, Studied nursing. Worked with the sick in the cholera epidemic in Brescia, Italy in 1855. Founded The Congregation of the Sons of the Immaculate Conception, men who served in hospitals and as travelling nurses to the scattered, impoverished farmers.[1]

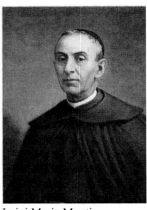

Luigi Maria Monti
(1825-1900) Source:
vatican.va/news_services

Luigi Maria Monti, layman, founded The Congregation of the Sons of the Immaculate Conception with Father Luigi Dossi.

Luigi was born on July 24 1825 at Bovisio, Masciago, Diocese of Milan, Italy, the eighth of eleven children. When he was 12 years old his father died. He helped to support the family by making wood craft items. He formed a prayer group with other devout craftsmen and farmers calling themselves The Company of the Sacred Heart of Jesus. The people of Bovisio referred to them as "The Company of Friars." In addition to praying together, this group cared for the poor and sick. In 1846, at the age of 21, Luigi took private vows of chastity and obedience, dedicating his life to God.

Not everyone in the town was able to grasp the spirituality of Luigi. Some people in the small town, together with the parish priest, mounted a campaign of opposition which led to slanderous charges of political conspiracy against the Austrian occupation authorities. In 1851 the men were arrested for conspiracy and imprisoned in Milan. They were released 72 days later at the end of the formal investigation, the authorities realizing they were a religious, not a political group.

Docile to his spiritual director, Fr. Luigi Dossi, Luigi Monti joined the Sons of Mary Immaculate, the congregation founded by Blessed Ludovico Pavoni only five years earlier. He spent six years in this congregation as a novice. He studied and loved the constitution written by Blessed Pavoni. Here he gained experience as an educator and learned both the theory and practice of nursing care, which he placed at the service of the community and those stricken by cholera during the epidemic of 1855 in Brescia. At this time he

238

willingly accepted to be isolated in the local asylum with the sick.

At age 32, a miraculous event occurred as he continued to search for the concrete realization of his own consecration as related in Vatican documents:

> In a letter dated 1896, four year prior to his death, he evoked the nighttime of the spirit which he had lived at that time: "I would spend hours before Jesus in the Blessed Sacrament, but they were all hours without a drop of heavenly dew; my heart remained arid, cold, and unmoved. I was on the verge of abandoning everything, when, alone in my room, I heard a clear and distinct inner voice saying to me: 'Luigi, go to the choir in church and present your tribulations once again to the Blessed Sacrament.' I heeded this inspiration and hastened to follow it. I knelt down and after a short time—what wonder!—I saw two personages in human form. I recognized them. It was Jesus with His Most Holy Mother, who approached me and in a loud voice said to me: 'Luigi, much indeed will you still have to suffer; other varied and greater battles will you face. Be strong; you will emerge victorious from everything; never lacking to you will be our powerful help. Continue the way you began.' Thus did they speak and then disappear."[2]

Inspired to start a congregation for the care for the sick, Luigi Maria Monti traveled to Rome with the idea of establishing a congregation to care for the sick in Rome called the Congregation of the Sons of the Immaculate Conception. His colleague Pezzini, met with the Commendatore, the highest ranking authority at Santo Spirito Hospital where the Capuchin chaplains were also in the process of creating a sort of Third Order of St. Francis for the bodily assistance to patients. When Luigi arrived, he was humbly admitted to this group and was initially assigned tasks reserved today to practical nurse assistants. He also worked as a phlebotomist and was certified, receiving a diploma from La Sapienza University in Rome.

In 1877, at the age of 52, following the unanimous wish of his confreres, His Holiness Pope Pius IX placed him at the head of his own Congregation, where he remained until his death in 1900. As Superior General, Luigi Monti prepared for the Congregation a rule of life. The community of Santo Spirito Hospital lived this rule, "Nourished by the Eucharist and meditation upon the privilege of the "Lady all Pure," the Brothers dedicated themselves with heroism to the care of the sick. They served at times of mass admissions due to epidemics of malaria and typhoid and also in the aftermath of armed conflict. The Brothers did not hesitate to surrender their own beds for the comfort of the sick and infirmed.

Luigi founded small communities throughout the region where men served in hospitals and as traveling nurses to the scattered, impoverished farmers. In 1882, a Carthusian monk came to see him at the Santo Spirito Hospital and said he had been inspired by Mary Immaculate to do so. The monk came from Desio and presented Monti with the pitiful case of his four nephews who had lost both their parents. This was a sign from the Spirit of God, and Luigi Monti expanded their mission and founded orphanages with attached schools.

Luigi Monti died prior to receiving ecclesial approbation for the congregation he founded. Thus, though he was known as "Father" by members of the Congregation and those whom he helped, Luigi Maria Monti remained a layman all his life. He died at the age of 75, on October 1, 1900 in Saronno, Varese, Italy of natural causes and is buried there. In 1904, Pope St. Pius X approved the new model of community foreseen by the Founder, granting the ministerial priesthood as an essential complement for carrying out an apostolic mission addressed to the whole man in both assistance to the sick and safe haven for youth in need. In this community served both ordained and lay 'Brothers' in equality of rights and responsibilities, where elected as superior of the community was to be the Brother deemed best suited.[2]

His beatification miracle involved the rapid, instantaneous, and permanent healing of Giovanni Luigi Iecle, a farmer from Bosa, Sardegna who had three operations including a subtotal gastrectomy, multiple fistulas and an intestinal occlusion and was in a septic state. This miraculous cure occurred on December 26, 1961 in Bosa, Nuoro, Italy. Luigi Maria Monti was declared venerable with the promulgation of the decree on heroic virtues on April 24, 2001 and beatified on November 9, 2003 both by Pope St. John Paul II.

In his homily for the beatification, Pope St. John Paul II stated, "Blessed Luigi Maria Monti was entirely dedicated to healing the physical and spiritual wounds of the sick and the orphaned. He loved to call them "Christ's poor ones," and he served them, enlivened by a living faith and sustained by intense and continual prayer. In his evangelical commitment, he was constantly inspired by

240

the example of the Holy Virgin and placed the Congregation he founded under the sign of Mary Immaculate..."[4]
 (Memorial - October 1)

References:

1) "Blessed Luigi Maria Monti". CatholicSaints.Info. 11 January 2020. Web. 8 December 2021.
<https://catholicsaints.info/blessed-luigi-maria-monti/>

2) Vatican News Service. Luigi Maria Monti (1825-1900). www.vatican.va/news_services/liturgy/saints/ns_lit_doc_20031109_monti_en.html. Accessed 4 April 2022.

3) Hagiography Circle: An Online Resource on Contemporary Hagiography. 1900. Luigi Maria Monti. Accessed 4 April 2022. www.Newsaints.faithweb.com/year/1900.htm#Monti.

4) Homily of John Paul II at the Beatification of Five Servants of God, Feast of the Dedication of the Lateran Basilica, Sunday, 9 November 2003. Accessed 4 April 2022.
www.vatican.va/content/john-paul-ii/en/homilies/2003/documents/hf_jp-ii_hom_20031109_beatifications.html.

241

Bl. Francisco Garate Aranguren (Spain) (1857-1929)

*Infirmarian at La Guardia college in 1877 and
subsequently at Jesuit Duesto college in 1888.[1]*

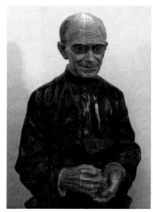

Francisco Garate
Aranguren
Source: jesuits.global

Francisco Garate Arauguren, Jesuit, was born on February 3, 1857 in Azpeitia, Guipuzcoa, Kingdom of Spain to Francisco and Maria Aranguren. He was the second of seven brothers. At the age of 14, he left home to work as a domestic servant at the newly opened Jesuit College of Nuestra Senora de la Antigua in Orduna, Spain. At the age of 17 in 1874, he felt the calling to enter the Jesuit order. He traveled with two companions on foot to Poyanne, France to begin the novitiate. The Spanish Jesuit had been expelled from Spain following the revolution of 1868 and had opened their novitiate in France.

His initial vows as a Jesuit brother were made on February 2, 1876. He then left the town on October 29, 1877 to be a sacristan and a nurse in the La Guardia college near the Atlantic where he was in charge of the care of 200 young men. He was noted for his encouragement and tender care to the needs of students in his care. He made his final vows on August 15, 1887 (Feast of the Assumption). In late March, he was assigned to the Jesuit Duesto college as doorkeeper, sacristan and infirmarian, where he served for the next 40 years. He was known for his prayer life and simple living, his kind care and charity for the students, and as a source of wisdom and advice. He prayed constantly, carried a rosary everywhere and was a beloved example of living an ordinary life of piety. He lived a simple life in terms of his room, clothes and even the foods that he ate. Following his example, two of his brothers also became professed Jesuit brothers.

He experienced sharp abdominal pains following the Holy Sacrifice of the Mass on September 8, 1929. After finishing his chores, he agreed to remain in bed where he asked for Viaticum. His discomfort was so bad that a nurse alerted the doctor who operated on his blocked urethra after which he continued to decline. Francisco Garate Aranguren died on September 9, 1929 (the Feast of Jesuit

242

Saint Peter Claver) in Deusto, Bilbao, Vizcaya, Spain. Students processed by his coffin touching their rosaries and crucifixes thereupon for his posthumous blessing.[1][2]

Francisco Garate Aranguren was declared venerable with the promulgation of the decree on heroic virtues on February 11, 1982 and beatified on October 6, 1985 both by Pope St. John Paul II.[3] In his homily for the beatification, Pope St. John Paul II stated,

Brother Garate lived his religious consecration as a radical openness to God, to whose service and glory he gave himself (cf. Lumen Gentium, 44), and from where he received inspiration and strength to bear witness to a great goodness towards all. This could be confirmed by so many people who passed through the gate of the affectionately called "Brother Kindness," at the University of Deusto: students, teachers, employees, parents of the young residents, people in the end of all kinds and conditions, who saw in Brother Garate the welcoming and smiling attitude of those who have their hearts anchored in God. He gives us a concrete and current witness to the value of the *interior life as the soul of every apostolate* and also of religious consecration. In fact, when one is devoted to God and one focuses one's life on Him, the apostolic fruits are not long in coming. From the door of a house of studies, this Jesuit Brother coadjutor made present the goodness of God through the *evangelizing power of his quiet and humble service*.[4]

Francisco Garate was beatified on October 6, 1985 by Pope St. John Paul II. (Memorial - September 9).

*To the extent that it is possible for me to do everything well,
I do it. Our Lord does the rest.
With His help, everything becomes easy and beautiful
because we have a Good Lord.*

References:

1) "Blessed Francisco Gárate Aranguren". CatholicSaints.Info. 18 November 2021. Web. 8 December 2021.
<https://catholicsaints.info/blessed-francisco-garate-aranguren/>

2) Francisco Garate Aranguren. Accessed 4 April 2022.
https://en.wikipedia.org/wiki/Francisco_Garate_Aranguren#Life.

243

3) Hagiography Circle: An Online Resource on Contemporary Hagiography. 1929. Francisco Garate Aranguren. Accessed 4 April 2022. www.newsaints.faithweb.com/year/1929.htm#Garate.

4) Homily of the Holy Father John Paul II, Mass of Beatification of Three Servants of God: Diego Luis de San Vitores-Alsonso, Jose Maria Rubio Peralta and Francisco Garate Aranguren, Sunday, October 6, 1985. https://www.vatican.va/content/john-paul-ii/es/homilies/1985/documents/hf_jp-ii_hom_19851006_beatificazione-tre-gesuiti.html. Accessed 4 April 2022.

Bl. Enrico Rebuschini (Italy) (1860-1938)
Dedicated to the care of the sick.
Ministered to the sick in Verona, Italy 1889-1899,
then served at the San Camillo di Cremona nursing home
until his death in 1938.[1]

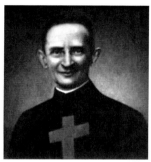

Bl. Enrico Rebuschini
Source: pgvcamillianiroma.it

Enrico Rebuschini, professed priest, Camillian, was born on April 28, 1860 at Gravedona, Como, Italy to Domenico and Sophia Rebuschini. He was second of five children. His father was an administrative clerk and then became the head tax official for Como province. Though his father accompanied his mother to the church door, he was not in favor of religion, therefore, he remained outside.

Enrico graduated from Como High School. His father opposed his entering the priesthood so he studied mathematics at the University of Padua. He studied there only one year because the anti-clericalism aroused in him bitterness and disgust. As part of compulsory military service, he graduated from the non-commissioned officer's school in Milan as a Reserve Second Lieutenant. His superiors encouraged him to make the Army a career. Enrico opted, instead, to study accounting. In 1882 he received an accounting diploma and started working in the administration of a silk business located 45 km north of Como that was managed by his sister Dorina's husband. After three years, it was clear he was depressed and troubled. He confided to his father that this work in industry and commerce didn't suit him. He wrote his brother-in-law, *"The thought of forever remaining a burden rather than being a good assistant,... the fact of knowing at the same time, that my parents will never be at peace, as long as I remain in a path that doesn't suit my nature (and which makes me unhappy), has finally persuaded me that I have to give it up, for my Mom and Dad's good, for your good and for mine. I am telling you this with a painfully heavy heart."* (9 August 1884).[2]

Three months later Enrico enrolled in the Gregorian University in Rome to pursue ecclesiastical studies. His professors noted, "Edifying conduct, with a very good spirit of the Church." A visit from his parents and Aunt Magdalena found content and at

245

peace. Unfortunately from March 1886 to May 1887 he was overcome by a profound nervous depression. This may have been caused not only by his temperament but also by excessive mortifications. Enrico returned to his family and spent some time at a clinic. Eight years later when recalling this episode, Enrico wrote, *"I was sent to a spa. There God restored my health by giving me total confidence in His infinite goodness and mercy."* In May 1887 Enrico fully recovered his health though he did experience relapses which were less prolonged and less serious. The trial was overcome by a progressively more correct understanding of God, which brought about a filial relationship based on trust. The best feature of Blessed Enrico's spirituality would, from then on, be the consideration of the infinite ocean of mercy found in the Heart of Jesus, of the maternal tenderness of our Mother, the Most Blessed Virgin Mary, whom the Church invokes by the consoling title of Health of the Sick.

During the summer of 1887, Enrico worked as an accountant at the civil hospital in Como but was dismissed after a few weeks because he was rarely in his office. Instead he went to the wards to visit the sick. He assessed their needs, helped solve their problems and supported them both morally and materially sacrificing his last dime and even his own clothes. His aunt Lena, who was president of the St. Vincent de Paul Society, recommended that he visit the sick and poor at home which he found very rewarding. During this time he wrote in his notebook as he practiced the spiritual exercises of St. Ignatius of Loyola, *"The Most Blessed Virgin, to whom I have abandoned myself in order that she might find me a task suited to my weakness, obtained a position for me in the administrative department of the civil hospital, where I was working several hours a day. I spend the rest of the time alone, in pious exercises... Seeing as how I could not continue in this way and feeling called to embrace religious life, my spiritual father (when I revealed to him my attraction to the religious family of Saint Francis) suggested to me that of Saint Camillus, which seemed to him more suited to my circumstances and also because he feared for my health. I did it without discussion — I embraced it immediately."*

Enrico entered the Camillian religious order in Verona at the age of 27 on September 27, 1887. Taking into consideration the studies he had already undertaken in Rome, he was ordained to the priesthood during his novitiate on April 14, 1889 by Bishop Sarto of Mantua, the future Pope St. Pius X. In 1890 Father Enrico was named Chaplain for the military and civil hospitals in Verona. The clerics, religious and soldiers considered him a saint.

He made his perpetual profession on December 8, 1891. He again suffered depression and spiritual trial in the years 1890-1891 — a perfectionist nature, he took on spiritual exercises that did not take into account his nervous frailty. He was too concerned about thought of eternity. As Chaplain of the hospital, however, he was able to recover his balance and calmness by attending to the afflictions of his neighbors. In 1895 he was named Vice-Novice master and Professor of Theology resulting in a state of constant tension. When relieved of these responsibilities his depression abated. One last bout of depression occurred in 1922 when he was again overloaded with work. This he overcame in a few month.

Though plagued with bouts of depression, Father Enrico admirably took upon himself heavy responsibilities with great generosity for over 25 years between the attacked of 1895 and 1922. And then from 1922 to his death in 1938, for over 16 years, he more than ever showed a stable equilibrium and complete serenity. A colleague, Fr. Joseph Moar, who worked alongside him during the last seven years only learned of the depressions Father Rebuschini had experienced during the beatification process of collecting and reviewing documents. He wrote, "When I knew him, he was utterly balanced and always his same old self. It had never occurred to me that he might have been able to suffer from depression."

In summary, Blessed Enrico Rebuschini ministered to the sick in Verona for 10 years from 1889 to 1899. He then served at the San Camillo di Cremona nursing home the rest of his life - almost 40 years. He served as treasurer for the community for 34 years and superior for eleven. He carried out these offices honestly, integrity and accuracy. Every day he carved out time for a daily visit to the sick guests and for frequent visits to the sick in the city. The Decree from the Congregation of Saints states, "as an extension of the inexhaustible mercy and patience and goodness of Jesus, who bent over all the miseries of humanity wounded by sin through the care of painful bodies and gave peace and salvation to souls."

Father Enrico Rebuschini died on May 10, 1938 in Cremona, Italy from pneumonia. He was declared venerable with the promulgation of the decree on heroic virtues on July 11, 1995 and beatified on May 4, 1997 both by Pope St. John Paul II.[3] (Memorial - May 10)

In his homily for the beatification, Pope St. John Paul II stated:

> Throughout his life, Bl. Enrico Rebuschini walked resolutely towards that "perfection of charity" which is the dominant theme of this Sunday's Liturgy of the Word. In the footsteps of the founder, St Camillus de Lellis, he witnessed to merciful love, practising it wherever he worked. His firm resolution "to commit his own life to giving God to his neighbour, seeing in him the Lord's own face", involved him in a demanding ascetic and mystical journey, marked by an intense life of prayer, extraordinary love for the Eucharist and constant dedication to the sick and the suffering. He became a sure reference point both for the Clerics Regular, Servants of the Sick, as well as for the Christian community of Cremona. His example is a pressing invitation to all believers to be attentive to the suffering and the sick in body and in spirit.[4]

> *" 'To love him with the same love that God loves him.'*
> *'To love him as a creature of God;' to be in his spirit*
> *'His lowest servant;' to love his neighbour 'before God so that my*
> *only thought about them is to pray for their needs*
> *and to do the little that I can in the spirit of a lowest servant,*
> *because this is my duty. '"*[5]

References:

1) "Blessed Enrico Rebuschini". CatholicSaints.Info. 10 May 2021. Web. 8 December 2021. <https://catholicsaints.info/blessed-enrico-rebuschini/>

2) Saint of the Day - 10 May - Blessed Enrico Rebuschini MI (1860-1938) posted May 10, 2020. Accessed 4 April 2022. https://anastpaul.com/2020/05/10/saint-of-the-day-10-may-blessed-enrico-rebuschini-mi-1860-1938/

3) Hagiography Circle: An Online Resource on Contemporary Hagiography. 1938. Enrico Rebuschini. Accessed 4 April 2022. www.newsaints.faithweb.com/year/1938.htm#Rebuschini.

4) Pope St. John Paul II, Sunday, 4 May 1997. Homily for the Eucharistic Celebration for the Beatification of Five New Blesseds:...Enrico Rubuschino https://www.vatican.va/content/john-paul-ii/en/homilies/1997/documents/hf _jp-ii_hom_19970504.html. Accessed 5 April 2022.

5) Ministers of the Infirm, Camilian Religious. Enrico Rebuschini: a Gift and a Model (10/05/2017). Accessed 4 April 2022. www.camillianiorg/en/enrico-rebuschini-a-gift-and-a-model/

Bl. Marta Wiecka (Poland/Ukraine) (1874-1904)
Daughter of Charity
Nurse, worked in present day Ukraine
Served the sick and suffering in the
Vincentian spirit of humility, simplicity and love

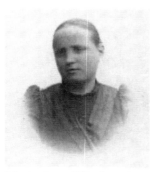

Marta Anna Wiecka prior to entering religious life
martawiecka.pl

Marta Anna Wiecka was born on January 12, 1874 in Nowy Wiec, Koscierzyna district in Pomerania (Poland) to Marceli Wiecki and Paulina nee Kamrowska. She was the third of thirteen children. Marta was baptized on January 18, 1874 in the parish church in Szczodrow.

The region of Poland in which she lived was governed by Prussia. During a program called the Kulturkampf, Prussia's leadership attempted to destroy the national and Catholic identity of Poland. In spite of these efforts by the Germans, the Wiecka household remained deeply religious and patriotic. In the home the family prayed together, read pious books and shared the content of Sunday sermons in common.

When she was two years old, Marta was miraculously healed through the intervention of the Blessed Virgin Mary, Our Lady of Piaseczno. (In the 14th century a "Beautiful Lady" appeared to the paralysed son of a tar producer, healing him. Piaseczno is a traditional place for pilgrimage of the Pomerania.[1]) Thereafter, Marta had a great devotion to Mary and turned to her often for help.

Marta also admired St. John Nepomucen (1345-1393), the patron saint of Czechoslovakia and the "martyr of the confessional" because he was killed by the King Wenceslaus IV because he would not divulge the Queen's sins from confession. As a young girl, Marta was often observed standing in prayer by his wayside shrine which was erected at her request.

After receiving her First Holy Communion on October 3, 1866, Marta attended the Holy Sacrifice of the Mass at every opportunity. This required that she walk to the parish church in Skarszewy, 12 kilometers away. She looked after her siblings due to her mother's frequent illnesses earning her the name "second mother."

250

She attempted to enter the local Daughter of Charity in Chelmno at age 16. She was instructed to wait two more years. At the age of 18 Marta entered the Daughters of Charity at the Provincial House at 8 Warszawska Street in Krakow on April 26, 1892. She entered in Krakow because her friend, Monika Gdaniec, had been denied entry at Chelmno and they both accepted in Krakow. It was not the sisters who denied her entrance but the "invaders," the Prussian government who imposed restrictions on the religious order. After a four month postulancy, Marta began the novitiate on August 12, 1892.

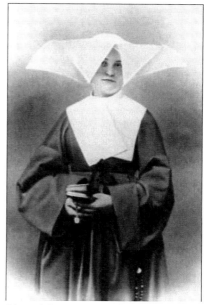

Sister Marta Anna Wiecka
Source. Vatican.va

After eight months, on April 21, 1893, Marta received the habit of the Daughters of Charity of Krakow and was sent to her first assignment to the General Hospital in Lviv, Ukraine. She had a reputation for serving the patients with great love and devotion. On November 15, 1894, she was transferred to the hospital in Podhajce (Pidhaitsi). Here she served for five years and made her first profession on August 15, 1897, committing to serve God in the person of the poorest of the poor.

In 1899 Sister Marta was assigned to the Daughter of Charity house in Bochnia. Here she had a vision of Jesus on the cross in which He urged her to "patiently endure adversity and promised that she would be with Him soon."[2]

The adversity soon began. A demoralized man began spreading rumors that she was pregnant. He was a student and relative of the parish priest. Her superior, Sister Maria Chablo kept her in Bochnia so that her innocence would become apparent. Sister Marta endured these insults with serene patience relying solely upon God. After this situation calmed, she was assigned to the hospital in

251

Sniatyn, Ivano-Frankivs'k (then in Poland; now in Ukraine).

There she ensured that no one in her department died without first receiving the sacrament of reconciliation. She took equal care of her patients regardless of their ethnicity or religion. "She had a unique gift of helping people be reconciled with God."[3] "The local parish priest sent parishioners to her with various problems and spiritual matters that she successfully solved for the good of their souls."[2] She helped where ever she was needed. She loved caring for her patients and did so with extraordinary kindness bringing healing to both the body and soul. Her whole life was an act of love.

During a typhoid epidemic, she volunteered to disinfect a room of a person who had been ill with typhoid in place of a fellow nurse, a man who was a father whose assignment this was. She contracted typhoid. Crowds of people prayed for her healing, including Jewish people who prayed for her in their synagogue. After receiving Viaticum (the Holy Eucharist given to the dying, "food for the journey") she was observed to be deep in prayer. Sister Marta died peacefully on May 30, 1904 in Sniatyn, Poland (now Ukraine). Many people flock to her grave convinced that "Matuszka" will answer their requests.

Sister Marta Anna Wiecka was declared venerable with the promulgation of the decree on heroic virtues on December 20, 2004 by Pope St. John Paul II. She was beatified was approved for May 24, 2008 by Pope Benedict XVI.[1] The beatification ceremony was held at the Bogdan Chmielnecki Park in Lviv, Ukraine and presided by Tarcisio Cardinal Bertone.[4] (Memorial May 30)

Prayer to obtain favors through the intercession of Blessed Sister Marta Wiecka:[2]
Lord God, You called Sister Marta Wiecka
to the Congregation of the Sisters of Mercy,
so that, following Your Son, she would serve the poor and the sick.
Obedient to your call,
she followed the path of a Vincentian vocation,
devoting herself entirely to service,
to the point of giving her life for a human being.
Lord, my God, I adore you for all the favors
you deigned to grant Blessed Sister Marta Wiecka.

I am begging you, please show through her intercession
the power of your love and grant me the grace ……… ..
for which I am asking you with humility and trust,
if it agrees with Your will.
Through Christ our Lord. Amen.

Our Father, Hail Mary, Glory be to the Father,
O Mary conceived without sin,
pray for us who have recourse to You.

Reference:

1) Opanuj Gniew. Piaseczno. Accessed 15 Mary 2022.
https://www.gniew.pl/919,piaseczno

2) Biography Blessed Sister Marta Wiecka (1874-1904). Accessed 15 May
2022. https://martawiecka.pl/

3) Hagiography. 1904-Marta Anna Wiecka. Accessed 15May2022.
http://newsaints.faithweb.com/year/1904.htm

4) Hagiography. Saints of 2008. Accessed 15 May 2022.
http://newsaints.faithweb.com/2008.htm

5) Congregation of the Mission. Marta Wiecka. Accessed 15 May 2022.
https://cmglobal.org/en/2020/10/02/marta-wiecka/

Bl. Maria Troncatti (Italy/Ecuador) (1883-1969)

Red Cross nurse in an Italian military hospital during World War I.[1]
From a simple and poor clinic, she managed to establish a hospital and
prepared the nurses herself.[2]

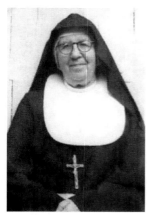

Bl. Maria Troncatti
sbnews.blogspot.com

Blessed Maria Troncatti, religious sister of the Daughters of Mary Help of Christians (Society of Salesian Sisters), was born on February 16, 1883 in Corteno Golgi, Brescia, Italy to a large farm family. She cared for her younger brothers and sisters and regularly attended catechism in her parish, developing a deep Christian spirit. She delayed her entry into religious life in obedience to her parish priest. When she was twenty-five, in 1908, Maria made her first profession with the Institute of the Salesian Sisters at Niza Monferrato.

The FMA was a woman's Salesian order founded collaboratively by St. Mary Mazzarello and St. John Bosco in 1872 in Mornese, Italy. Their aim and program was the same as the Salesian male order: the religious perfection of each member by means of observance of the vows, and by an apostolate among the young, especially the more needy. The three guiding lights of their sanctity: the Holy Eucharist, Our Lady, Help of Christians and the Pope. The order received temporary approval in 1911 and definitive approval in 1921.[3]

During the 1st World War (1914-1919), the FMA assisted the military at the front and sisters worked as nurses in military hospitals, where the Salesian style was comforting.[4] Maria took a course in health care in Varazze and worked as a Red Cross nurse in the military hospital. This expertise proved valuable in her future work in the Amazon forest in Ecuador. Following a violent flood, Maria promised the Madonna that if she saved her life she would leave for the missions. Grace obtained, Sister Mary asked the Mother General to go among the lepers.

At the age of 39, in 1922, Mother Caterina Daghero assigned her to the missions of Ecuador where she will work with the Shuar tribe in the Amazon forest. Together with two other Sisters, she began the difficult work of evangelizing, while providing

254

health care. There were many real dangers they faced: beasts of the forest, fast flowing rivers that had to be crossed on fragile bridges made from vines or on the shoulders of the Indians. She earned the esteem of the Shuar when she operated on the chief's daughter wounded by a bullet with a penknife. The sisters lived in Macas, a village of settlers surrounded by the collective housing of the Shuar.

Blessed Maria Troncatti was called Madrecita. Very successful as a catechist and evangelizer, her faith patience and fraternal love results in hundreds of new Christian families, formed

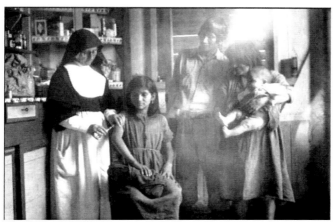

Sister Maria at work in her clinic.
Source: sdnews.blogspot.com

for the first time by free personal choice of young spouses. Initially establishing a simple and poor clinic, she managed to establish a hospital and there prepared nurses.[2] She continued this work in Ecuador for 47 years until her death at age 86 in 1969. Blessed Maria Troncatti died on August 25, 1969 in a tragic airplane crash in Sucua, Morona-Santiago, Ecuador. She was buried at Macas, in the Province of Morona, Ecuador.[5]

Blessed Maria Troncatti was declared venerable with the promulgation of the decree on heroic virtues on November 12, 2008 and beatified on November 24, 2012 both by Pope Benedict XVI.[6] The Holy Sacrifice of the Mass for her beatification was celebrated at Macas, Morona Santiago, Ecuador presided by Cardinal Angelo Amato, prefect of the Congregation for Causes of the Saints.[7] (Memorial - August 25)

255

"A glance at the Crucifix gives me life and courage to work."

References:

1) "Blessed Maria Troncatti". CatholicSaints.Info. 3 February 2019. Web. 8 December 2021. <https://catholicsaints.info/blessed-maria-troncatti/>

2) Agenzia Info Salesiana (ANS).. (23Aug2019). Accessed 5 April 2022. https://www.infoans.org/en/sections/special-reports/item/8646-rmg-25-august-50th-anniversary-of-blessed-maria-troncatti-s-death

3) The Daughters of Mary Help of Christians (FMA). https://salesianmissions.org/about-us/who-we-are/about-st-john-bosco/our-history/the-salesian-family/the-daughters-of-mary-help-of-christians-fma/ Accessed 5 April 2022.

4) IFMA. Daughters of Mary Help of Christians and times of Crisis. (11April2021). Accessed 5 April 2022. https://www.cgfmanet.org/en/ifma-en/daughters-of-mary-help-of-christians-and-times-of-crisis/

5) Salesians of Don Bosco. Blessed Maria Troncatti (1883-1969). (25Aug2015). Accessed 5 April 2022. https://www.salesians.org.uk/news/2015/08/blessed-maria-troncatti-1883-1969.

6) Hagiography Circle. Maria Troncatti. Accessed 5April2022. http://newsaints.faithweb.com/year/1969.htm#Troncatti

7) Catholic New Agency. Ecuador to celebrate beatification of religious missionary. Accessed 5 April 2022. https://www.catholicnewsagency.com/news/25997/ecuador-to-celebrate-beatification-of-religious-missionary

Bl. Maria (Corsini) Beltrame Quattrocchi (Italy) (1884-1965)
Volunteer Red Cross nurse, World War I.[1]
First married couple to be beatified

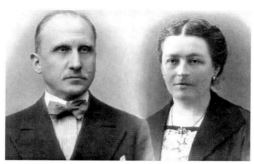

Blesseds Luigi and Maria Beltrame-Quattrocchi.
Source: testimoniospersonales.blogspot.com

Maria Luisa Corsini, laywoman, was born on June 24, 1884 in Florence Italy, the only daughter of Army Captain Angiolo Corsini and Giulia Salvi. Her father was an officer of the Sardinian grenadiers. His career caused the family to move frequently. By the time she was nine, Maria had lived in Pistioa, Florence, Arrezo and Rome, Italy. Maria was intelligent, enthusiastic and she studied languages. She also became a prolific writer.

In Rome, Maria met Luigi Beltrame Quattrocchi, a young lawyer who had graduated in July 1902. Maria and Luigi were married on November 25, 1905 in the Basilica of St. Mary Major in Rome. They had four children. Filippo (in 1906), Stefania (1908), Cesare (1909) and Enrichetta (1914). All their children would later enter religious life. Enrichette was declared "Venerable" by Pope Francis, on August 30, 2021. Luigi and Maria provided a pious example regularly receiving the Sacrament of Reconciliation and daily Communion and praying the Holy rosary every evening.

Maria served as a volunteer Red Cross nurse during World War I (1914-1918). Together Luigi and Maria assisted soldiers, the wounded and families in need. In 1919 when it was thought she might die, Maria wrote *Voce di Madre*, about the riches of her faith and her mother's heart. Maria recovered and lived into her 80's. During this time, Father Matthew Crawley, the great apostle of the Sacred Heart of Jesus and reparation for sins of the world, enthroned the picture of the Sacred Heart of Jesus in their home and left them a command: "Be apostles!"

On November 5, 1924, the family went to an audience with Pope Pius XI and then accompanied Filippo to the Capranica Seminary and Cesare to the Benedictine Monastery of San Paolo. In

257

October 1927 Stefania entered a convent in Milan, becoming Sister Cecilia. Enrichetta later consecrated herself to God in a secular Institute.

Maria served as a catechist and taught women in the parish. Luigi and Maria were involved in the lay apostolate, Catholic Action, supporting the Catholic University, various initiatives at the service of young people, workers and the poor. During World War II Luigi and Maria sheltered refugees in their home.

Maria (Corsini) Beltrame Quattrocchi died on August 26, 1965 at the age of 81 in the arms of her daughter Enrichetta as soon as the Angelus was recited at noon.

Blessed Maria Corsini Beltrame Quattrocchi and her husband Luigi were declared venerable with the promulgation of the decree on heroic virtues on July 7, 2001 and beatified on October 21, 2001 both by Pope St. John Paul II. Blessed Maria's beatification miracle involved the healing of a young man with a severe circulatory disorder. He subsequently became a neuro-surgeon in Milan, Italy.[2]

The Quattrocchis are the first married couple to be beatified together. Their daughter Enrica received the title Venerable Servant of God in 2021. They were beatified upon the occasion of the celebration of the 20th anniversary of the promulgation of the Apostolic Exhortation "Familaris consortio" (On the Role of the Christian Family in the Modern World). Pope St. John Paul II held them up as a couple who lived an ordinary life in an extraordinary way stating:[3]

> This couple lived married love and service to life in the light of the Gospel and with great human intensity. With full responsibility they assumed the task of collaborating with God in procreation, dedicating themselves generously to their children, to teach them, guide them and direct them to discovering his plan of love. From this fertile spiritual terrain sprang vocations to the priesthood and the consecrated life, which shows how, with their common roots in the spousal love of the Lord, marriage and virginity may be closely connected and reciprocally enlightening.
>
> Drawing on the word of God and the witness of the saints, the blessed couple lived an ordinary life in an extraordinary way. Among the joys and anxieties of a normal family, they knew how to live an extraordinarily rich spiritual life. At the centre of their life was the daily Eucharist as well as devotion to the Virgin Mary, to whom they prayed every evening with the Rosary, and consultation

with wise spiritual directors. In this way they could accompany their children in vocational discernment, training them to appreciate everything "from the roof up", as they often, charmingly, liked to say.

The riches of faith and love of the husband and wife Luigi and Maria Beltrame Quattrocchi, are a living proof of what the Second Vatican Council said about the call of all the faithful to holiness, indicating that spouses should pursue this goal, *"propriam viam sequentes"*, "following their own way" (Lumen gentium, n. 41). Today the aspiration of the Council is fulfilled with the first beatification of a married couple: their fidelity to the Gospel and their heroic virtues were verified in their life as spouses and parents.[4]

The relics of Luigi and Maria are in a crypt in the Shrine in Divino Amore (Divine Love) in Rome, Italy.

Maria condensed her whole life with Louis and their children in only three word drawn from the deepest roots of the Heart of Jesus and the Immaculate Heart of Mary Most Holy: (Memorial - 26 August)

> *"Thy Will be done." "Thy kingdom come."* and
> *"My soul magnifies the Lord."*
> (Fiat, Adveniat and Magnificat)[5]

References:

1) "Blessed Maria Corsini Beltrame Quattrocchi". CatholicSaints.Info. 14 January 2018. Web. 8 December 2021. <https://catholicsaints.info/blessed-maria-corsini-beltrame-quattrocchi/>

2) Hagiography Circle: An Online Resource on Contemporary Hagiography. 1965. 14) 26 August in Serravalle, Bibbiena, Arezzo (Italy). Accessed 8 April 2022. http://newsaints.faithweb.com/year/1965.htm

3) Paul Zalonski (25Nov2016). Blesseds Luigi and Maria (Corsini) Beltrame Quattrocchi. Communio. Accessed 8 April 2022. https://communio.stblogs.org/index.php/2016/11/blesseds-luigi-and-maria-corsini-beltrame-quattrocchi/

4) Pope St. John Paul II. (21 October 2001). Homily upon the Beatification of the Servants of God Luigi Beltrame Quattrocchi and Maria Corsini, Married Couple. Accessed 8 April 2022. https://www.vatican.va/content/john-paul-ii/en/homilies/2001/documents/hf_jp-ii_hom_20011021_beltrame-quattrocchi.html

5) Maria Di Lorenzo (3Dec2016). Santi Beati. Blessed Luigi Beltrame Quattrocchi and Maria Corsini Sposi. Accessed 8 April 2022. http://www.santiebeati.it/dettaglio/90324

Bl. Edward Joannes Maria Poppe (Belgium) (1890-1924)
Served as a battlefield nurse during World War I.[1]

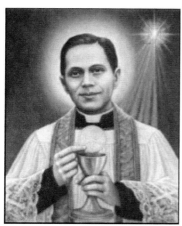

Bl Edward Poppe
Source: vangelodelgiorno.org

Blessed Edward Joannes Maria Poppe, priest of the Diocese of Gent, was born on December 18, 1890 in Temse, Namur, Belgium to Desire and Josefa Poppe. His father was a baker. Edward was one of eleven children, five of whom became nuns and a brother also became a priest.. In 1902, at age 12, he received his First Holy Communion and the Sacrament of Confirmation.

At age 14, his father introduced him to the family bakery business. However, Edward expressed a vocation to the priesthood. Edward's father died in January 1907, when he was 16 years old and Edward thought he should take over the family business. He entered the seminary at his mother's insistence. A few months prior to his twentieth birthday, in September 1910, Edward was drafted into military service. On March 13, 1912, he entered the seminary in Leuven, Belgium and studied in Ghent, Belgium in September 1913. During World War I (1914-1918) he served as a battlefield nurse. His prayers to St. Joseph during that time led to the miraculous freeing of several prisoners of war.

He was finally ordained to the priesthood on May 1, 1916 and assigned as Associate pastor focusing his ministry on the poor, children and the dying. He taught catechism and founded Eucharistic associations. He worked against the secularization of life in the city. When his health suffered, he was transferred to rural Moerzeke, Belgium where he served from 1918 to 1922 as rector of a religious community.

He was transferred to rural Belgium for recuperation after suffering a heart attack on May 11, 1919. This time he spent studying, praying and writing hundreds of articles and thousands of letter against Marxism, secularism and materialism. He developed a devotion of Saint Therese of Lisieux (1873-1897) who had died when he was seven and was declared venerable three years prior to

261

his death on August 14, 1921 and beatified the year prior to his death. He adopted her spirituality: the "little way;" to do all things with love.

Edward organized teachers in an evangelization camp and his home became the center of organization, prayer and spiritual rebirth. He served as the spiritual director for seminarians in military service in October 1922. After suffering another hearth attack on January 1, 1924, his health deteriorated rapidly. He worked tirelessly until his death, a the young age of 33, encouraging both the laity and seminarians.[2]

Blessed Edward Joannes Maria Poppe died on June 10, 1924 at Moerzeke, Hamme, Belgium suffering a stroke only six months after his second heart attack. He was declared venerable with the promulgation of the decree on heroic virtues on June 30, 1986 and beatified on October 3, 1999[3] both by Pope St. John Paul II. (Memorial - June 10).

References:

1) "Blessed Edward Joannes Maria Poppe". CatholicSaints.Info. 10 November 2019. Web. 8 December 2021. <https://catholicsaints.info/blessed-edward-joannes-maria-poppe/>

2) Catholic News Agency (10April2022). Blessed EdwardPoppe. Accessed 10 April 2022. https://www.catholicnewsagency.com/saint/blessed-edward-poppe-503

3) Hagiography Circle: An Online Resource on Contemporary Hagiography. 1924. 11) 10 June in Moerzeke, Hamme (Belgium). 1924. Edward Poppe. Accessed 8April2022. http://newsaints.faithweb.com/year/1924.htm

262

Bl. Aurelia Mercede Stefani (Italy/Kenya) (1891-1930)

Served as a nurse in Kenya treating injured and sick during World War I.
Nicknamed Nyaatha (Merciful Mother)

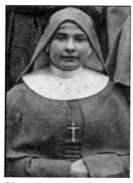

Sister Irene Stefani
Public Domain

Aurelia Jacoba Mercede Stefani was born on August 22, 1891 in Anfo, Brescia, Italy to Giovanni Stefani and Annunziata Massari. At her baptism she was called Aurelia Giacomina Mercede. Aurelia was the fifth of twelve children. She grew up in a pious family and was known for charity at an early age helping the sick, elderly, poor and taking on the hardest jobs. When her mother died at an early age she became the educator and catechist for her brothers and sisters. And although she had expressed, to her parents, a desire to serve as a missionary when she was thirteen, this wish would not be fulfilled until she was twenty.

In 1910, Blessed Giuseppe Allamano founded a religious institute for women missionaries in Turin, Italy, the Consolata Missionary Sisters. Prior to this the Consolata Institute for Foreign Missions only included priests and coadjutor brothers. Aurelia joined the Consolata Missionary Sisters in 1911. After a year postulancy, on January 28, 1912 she took on the religious habit taking the religious name Sister Irene. Completing the Novitiate, she made her religious profession on January 29, 1914 and at the end of that year left for Kenya.

During the First World War (1914-1918), Sister Irene served as a nurse in British military hospitals tending both wounded soldiers and civilians. In 1916 she was appointed to assist the Red Cross and served in a variety of settings including hospitals in Lindi and Dar es Salaam in Tanzania. She washed, medicated and bandaged sores and wounds. She handed out medicine and food, feeding the most serious and the weak with a disconcerting delicacy. Her personal charity was able to sweeten the hearts of unscrupulous doctors, cruel overseers and incredulous Muslims. She learned various languages and was able to speak to the Africans about Jesus, to encourage and console them. She prepared many for Baptism, over three thousand baptisms were administered to those in danger of death. She was called "a nun's angel."[1]

263

After the war, Sister Irene returned to Nyeri, Kenya helping to promote native vocations. Later in Gikondi(1920-1930) at Our Lady of Divine Providence Mission she taught in local schools and taught catechism to parishioners. She invited anyone she met to school and catechism. She took care of the sick, assisted women in labor, and saved abandoned children. She also served as the local superior of her community for eight years.[2] She instructed the young sisters teaching them missionary work. She also took the time to correspond with African "children" who had moved away to cities of Kenya such as Mombasa and Nairobi.

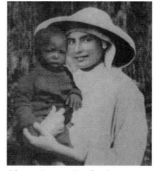

Sister Irene Stefani
Source: angelusnews.com

Sister Irene was fondly called "Nyaatha" which, in the Kikuyu language means, "a woman of compassion, mercy, goodness: or "Merciful Mother." She burned with a desire to make Jesus and the Gospels known. When a fellow teacher, Julius Ngare, incited some students to challenge her work as a teacher, she still cared for him when he was sick. In fact, he died in her arm and that is how she contracted the bubonic plague which would subsequently took her life.

During a course on spiritual exercises on September 14, 1930, with the consent of her superior, she received permission to offered her life for the local bishop and for the missions. She made this offering of her life on October 17, 1930. Nine days later, on Sunday October 26, she was seized by shivers. She died On October 31, 1930 at Gikondi, Mukurweini, Nyeri, at the age of 39.

She was declared venerable with the promulgation of the decree on heroic virtues on April 2, 2011[3] by Pope Benedict XVI. The beatification miracle[4][5] is described as follows:

> The event that took place, on January 10, 1989 in the village of Nipepe, in Mozambique, was examined as a possible miracle to obtain her beatification. Around 6 in the morning, during the celebration of Mass, shots were heard, a sign of the armed struggle between the two contending factions during the civil war; the church was then besieged.

In the church there were the people who took part in the Mass, but also the catechists and the animators of the parish with their families. They were joined by other people, who hoped to take refuge in the building so as not to be killed. For three and a half days, under threat of death, about two hundred and seventy people were barricaded, including many children.

As the hours went by, thirst arose; moreover, in Mozambique, winter is the warm season. At that point, the head of the catechists, Bernard Bwanaissa, granted permission to drink from the baptismal font, given the emergency. The source was actually a basin, the capacity of which could reach a maximum of 12 liters, but there were certainly less, since baptisms had been administered two days earlier. Plus the bowl was full of cracks.

One of the missionaries then invited us to pray asking for the intercession of Sister Irene: in those days, in fact, he was reading her biography. The water was not only sufficient to quench everyone's thirst, but it continued to flow for several days, until, between the afternoon of January 12 and the following morning, the besieged were able to return to their homes.[1]

Servant of God Irene Stefani was declared venerable with the promulgation of the decree of heroic virtue on April 2, 2011 by His Holiness Pope Benedict XVI. She was then beatified on May 23, 2015[6] by Pope Francis.

A 3-day beatification ceremony as held on the grounds of Dedan Kimathi University in Nyeri, Kenya an presided over by Tanzanian Polycarp Cardinal Pengo[7] and John Cardinal Njue. Website: https://missionariedellaconsolata.org/i-nostri-santi-2/ (Memorial - October 31).

References:

1) Gianpiero Pettiti. (13May2018). Santi Beati E Testimono. Blessed Irene (Aurelia Jacoba Mercede) Stefani. Accessed 16 April 2022. http://santiebeati.it/dettaglio/92401

2) Brother Silas Henderson, SDS. Aleteia. Accessed 16 April 2022. https://aleteia.org/daily-prayer/tuesday-october-31/

3) Charles G. Braganza. Hagiography Circle: An Online Resource on Contemporary Hagiography. News 2014. Accessed 16 April 2022. http://newsaints.faithweb.com/news_archives_2014.htm

4) "Blessed Irene Stefani". CatholicSaints.Info. 1 July 2016. Web. 16 April 2022. <https://catholicsaints.info/blessed-irene-stefani/>

5) Elvis Nyakangi (15Oct2022). Miracles performed by Sister Irene Stefani: Aurelia Mercede Stefani beatification in Nyeri, Kenya. Accessed 16 April 2022.
https://kenyayote.com/miracles-performed-by-sister-irene-stefani-aurelia-me rcede-stefani-beatification-in-nyeri-kenya/

6) Consolata Missionary Sisters (23May2015). Beatification of Sr. Irene Stefani. Accessed 16 April 2022.
http://consolatasisters.org/beatification-of-sr-irene-stefani/

7) Hagiography Circle: An Online Resource on Contemporary Hagiography. Saints of 2015. Accessed 16 April 2022.
http://newsaints.faithweb.com/2015.htm

Bl. Maria Restituta Helena Kafka (Czechoslovakia/Austria) (1894-1943), Martyr

Surgical Nurse. Imprisoned during World War II. Cared for prisoners. Beheaded by the Nazis.[1]

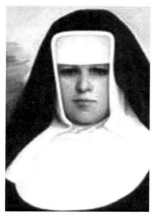

Helena Kafka was from a Czech family and grew up in Vienna, Austria. She was born on May 10, 1894 to Anton and Marie Kafka in Brno-Husovice (aka Brunn-Hussowitz), Brnensky, Czechslovakia (now the Czech Republic), the sixth daughter of a shoemaker. She was baptized 13 days after her birth at the Church of the Assumption in the town of Husovice, located in Austria. The family moved to Vienna where Helena grew up. She received her First Holy Communion in May of 1905 at St. Brigitta Catholic Church and was confirmed there in 1906.

She attended school for 8 years. In 1909, at the age of 15, she left school and worked as a servant and a cook while being trained in nursing. At the age of 19 she became an assistant nurse at the Lainz City Hospital where she met he Franciscan Sisters of Charity. She felt called to religious life with these sisters which her parents initially opposed. Eventually they relented, she entered the Franciscan Sisters in 1914. On October 23, 1915 she made her first vows taking the name of Sister Maria Restituta, after a martyr who had been beheaded. She made her final vows a year later.

By the end of World War I, Sister Restituta was the lead surgical nurse in the Modling Hospital in Vienna. She worked with her hospital's best surgeon who was described as "difficult." She ran his operating room and became a world-class surgical nurse. She worked as a surgical nurse for twenty years during which she gained a particular reputation for her devotion to the materially and socially poor.

On March 12, 1938, the Austrian Nazi Party pulled off a successful coup d'etat taking control of the government. Nazi Germany then annexed Austria which was known as the Anschluss (joining). Sister Restituta voiced her opposition to the Nazi regime occupying Austria. She called Hitler a "madman." She was tough and people called her "Sr. Resolute" because of her stubbornness. She could also be easy-going and funny. After work, she'd visit the local pub and order goulash and "a pint of the usual."

Her first personal encounter with the Nazi regime occurred when Sister Restituta hung crucifixes in every room of her hospital's new wing. The Nazis demanded she remove them or she would be dismissed. She refused. One of the doctors on staff, a fanatical Nazi, denounced her to the Nazi Party and on Ash Wednesday, 1942, she was arrested by the Gestapo as she came out of the operating room. The charge was, *"hanging crucifixes and writing a poem that mocked Hitler."* The Nazis promptly sentenced her to death for *"aiding and abetting the enemy in the betrayal of the fatherland and for plotting high treason."*

Although many nuns and religious sisters lost their lives in the extermination camps, Sister Restituta would be the only Catholic religious sister ever charged, tried and sentenced to death by a Nazi court.[2] The Nazis offered her freedom if she would abandon the Franciscan sisters and she refused. Martin Bormann expressly rejected the requested commutation of her sentence with the words: "I think execution of the death penalty is necessary for effective intimidation." She spent five months in prison caring for other prisoners.[3]

Sister Restituta was beheaded on March 30, 1943, Tuesday of Holy week, in Vienna.[4] She was 48 year old. As she approached the guillotine wearing a paper shirt and weighing just half her previous weight, her last words were, *"I have lived for Christ; I want to die for Christ."* The Nazis buried her in a mass grave fearing the Catholic Christians would promote her as a martyr. The crucifix that hung from Bl. Restituta's belt is preserved in the Basilica of St. Bartholomew on the Tiber River in Rome in a chapel dedicated to the 20th century martyrs.[5]

Blessed Maria Restituta was declared venerable with the promulgation of the decree of martyrdom on April 6, 1998 and beatified on June 21, 1998[6] both by Pope St. John Paul II. Website: www.restituta.at. (Memorial - October 30)

"I have lived for Christ; I want to die for Christ."

References:

1) "Blessed Mary Restituta Kafka". CatholicSaints.Info. 28 May 2020. Web. 8 December 2021.
<https://catholicsaints.info/blessed-mary-restituta-kafka/>

2) Larry Peterson (12April2016). Meet the Only Nun Sentenced to Death by a Nazi Court. Accessed 10 April 2022.
https://aleteia.org/2016/04/12/meet-the-only-nun-sentenced-to-death-by-a-nazi-court/

3) Katherine I Rabenstein. Saints of the Day, 1998. CatholicSaints.Info. 28 May 2020. Web. 10 April 2022.
<https://catholicsaints.info/saints-of-the-day-blessed-maria-restituta-kafka/>

4) Catholic New Agency.
https://www.catholicnewsagency.com/news/17468/martyr-who-refused-to-remove-crucifixes-from-hospital-to-be-honored-oct-29, (accessed 16Oct2021).

5) CatholicSaintsGuy. The Tough Nun Nurse who Stood Up to the Nazis. (30Mar2016). Accessed 3 June 2022.
https://catholicsaintsguy.wordpress.com/2016/03/30/the-tough-nun-nurse-who-stood-up-to-the-nazis/

6) Hagiography Circle: An Online Resource on Contemporary Hagiography. 1943. 10) Helene Kafka (Maria Restituta). Accessed 10 April 2022.
http://newsaints.faithweb.com/year/1943.htm#Kafka

269

Bl. Maria Crescencia Perez (Argentina/Chile) (1897-1932), Incorrupt

Worked with sick children in tuberculosis hospital in Argentina. Also served in a hospital in Chile.[1]

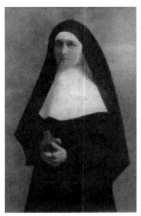

Maria Angelica Perez
(Sister M. Crescencia)
Source: oocities.org/

Maria Angelica Perez was born on August 17, 1897 in San Martin, Buenos Aires, Argentina to Augustin Perez and Ema Rodriguez, immigrants from Spanish Galicia. She was the fifth of their eleven children. She was raised on a farm and helped her parents with the farm work. Her family was a religious one and had the custom of praying the rosary together each day. Maria Angelica was know to be pious. Maria Angelica studied at "Hogar de Jesus", "House of Jesus" in Pergamino and earned a degree as a craft teacher from this school.

Maria entered the novitiate of the Daughters of Our Lady of the Garden on December 31, 1915 in Buenos Aires. She receives the holy habit and her religious name, Sister Maria Crescencia when she professes her vows on September 2, 1918. Soon after, her father died.

Sister M. Crescencia initially taught crafts and was a catechist in various schools, including at Colegio del Huerto in Buenos Aires. From 1924-1928 she worked in a tuberculosis hospital in Mar del Plata (Maritime Sanatorium), with children suffering from tuberculosis of the bone. When her own health began to suffer her superiors moved her to a place where the weather would help her recover. She was moved to their religious house in Vallenar, Republic of Chile. There she assisted at a local hospital. She was loved by her patients because of her joyful spirit and the comfort she gave.[2] She was known as "Sister Sweetness."[3] Blessed Maria Angelica Perez had a great devotion to the Sacred Heart of Jesus and experienced visions and mystical union with Jesus.[4]

In 1928, Sister Maria Crescencia visited Pergamino for the last time to say goodby to her family forever. Returning to Chile with the Provencial Superior, before long, she herself began to need medical attention. She spent 3 months in the hospital in isolation to

270

protect her from potential infection.[5] She then spent the last weeks of her life in her community with the Sisters assisting her and she them, with her serenity and deep inner peace. The Daughters of Our Lady of the Garden chronicles the events surrounding Sister M. Crescencia's death:

God had reserved a very special grace for this moment. According to the chronicles, she received, in a vision, the visit of the Founder, San Antonio Gianelli [1789-1846]. From the image of the painting of Our Lady of the Garden that was next to her bed, the Blessed Virgin Mary blessed her and the Sisters. Baby Jesus made a move to leave the arms of His Mother and Maria Crescencia extended hers to receive Him.

With true piety she received the Holy Viaticum, surrounded by her Superiors and Sisters. While she prayed the prayers of the dying with those present, she sits up and bowing deeply before the picture of the Sacred Heart of Jesus, repeated the words that Jesus Himself taught her: **"Heart of Jesus, for the sufferings of Your divine heart, have mercy on us."**

Then she breaks into a fervent prayer: *"Heart of Jesus bless me and bless my Sisters, give them strength to fight with courage and seek the salvation of souls in these difficult times. Bless our Institute, from which I received so much good and in which, in these moments, I consider myself the happiest creature in the world. I ask You Most Holy Heart of Jesus that You send many and good vocation to our Institute, Oh Heart of Jesus, I ask You a special blessing for Chile and since it is Your will that I die here happy, I offer You this sacrifice for the peace and tranquillity of this nation."*

It seems that the Heart of Jesus made her see the prize that He had prepared for her, because she continues, *"When, Lord, have I deserved that? What are the sufferings of this world compared to the happiness of heaven? I am more than a miserable creature, the smallest of all, I am less than a worm of the earth, where did I come from so much happiness? Heart of Jesus I do not deserve all that. Everything is the work of Your Heart, Jesus. I would like to love you as much as you love Yourself."*

Her desire to join Jesus was vehement, so she exclaims *"Do not stop me anymore...Do not stop me anymore... Yes, let all go to the Most Holy Heart of Jesus, there you will find the salvation of your soul".* Finally she says smiling, *"Father...into your hands I entrust my spirit."* Thus she dies saintly, on May 20, 1932.

271

Shortly after her death, at "Colegio del Huerto" in Quillota, 600 km distant from Vallenar, the Sisters together perceive a fragrance similar to the perfume of violets, which remains several days within the walls of the school. Because of this inexplicable fact, the Superior says, "Sister Crescencia has died." Immediately a telegram arrived announcing her death."[6]

Blessed Maria Angelica Perez (Sister Crescencia) died on May 20, 1932, at age 34 in Vallenar, Atacama, Chile from lung disease. The local community was already so attached to their "little saint" as they called her that even when the congregation left Vallenar, the community would not allow her body to be taken away. It remained in Vallenar, Chile for 35 years. On November 8, 1966, it was decided to transfer her body to Quillota. When the coffin was open her body and habit were perfectly preserved and almost intact. She then rested in the convent crypt in Quillota for 17 years. In 1983 her remained were reinterred in the College Chapel, the Church of the Sisters, in Juerto de Pergamino, Argentina. In 1986 she was transferred again, this time to the Chapel of Our Lady of the Garden school.

She was declared venerable with the promulgation of the decree on heroic virtues on June 22, 2004 by Pope St. John Paul II and beatified on November 17, 2012[7] by Pope Benedict XVI. Her beatification miracle involved the cure of a person from type A hepatitis. The beatification ceremony was officiated by Angelo Cardinal Amato, Prefect of the Congregation for the Causes of Saints, at Pergamino, Argentina. Patron of Nurses. Website: https://sistersfmh.org/history/sr-maria-crescencia/ (Memorial: May 20).

Prayer for the canonization of Blessed Maria Angelica Perez :
Father of Jesus and our Father, through Your Divine Spirit
You make holiness flourish in Your Church.
We give You thanks for Blessed María Crescencia Pérez
who loved You with simplicity. Her example and intercession,
may serve to extend Your Kingdom and to increase vocations to the
religious life. We humbly implore You, that through her intercession
we might be granted the grace for which we ask
(Express your petition) *Through Christ our Lord. Amen.*
Our Father, Hail Mary, Glory Be

Please communicate any favors received to: Sister Josefina, Av. Independencia 2140, zip code 1225 - Buenos Aires - Argentina - or to any House of the Sisters of the Garden.[9] vocationfmh@gmail.com.

Heart of Jesus, by the suffering of Your Sacred Heart, have mercy on us![8]

References:

1) "Blessed María Angélica Pérez". CatholicSaints.Info. 10 November 2019. Web. 8 December 2021. <https://catholicsaints.info/blessed-maria-angelica-perez/>

2) Brother Silas Henderson, SDS. (10April). Blessed Maria Angelica Perez. Aleteia. https://aleteia.org/daily-prayer/monday-may-20/. Accessed 10 April 2022.

3) Born Glorious. Maria Angelica Perez. Accessed 10 April 2022. https://www.bornglorious.com/person/?pi=5790827

4) Ana St. Paul (20May2020). Saint of the Day-20May-Blessed Maria Crescencia Perez FMH (1897-1932 "Sister Sweetness." Accessed 11 April 2022. https://anastpaul.com/?s=Blessed+Maria+Crescencia

5) Zyciorysy.info. Blessed Maria Angelika Perez. Accessed 11 April 2022. https://zyciorysy.info/bl-angelika/

6) Sisters FMH. Bl. Maria Crescencia Perez. Accessed 11 April 2022. https://sistersfmh.org/history/sr-maria-crescencia/

7) Hagiography Circle: An Online Resource on Contemporary Hagiography. 1932. 7) Maria Angelica Perez. Accessed 10 April 2022. http://newsaints.faithweb.com/year/1932.htm#Perez

8) Daughters of Our Lady of the Garden. Bl. Maria Crescencia Perez. Accessed 11 April 2022. https://sistersfmh.org/history/sr-maria-crescencia/

9) Sister Maria Crescencia Perez. Accessed 10 April 2022. http://www.oocities.org/sorcrescencia/oracion.htm

Bl. Liduina Meneguzzi (Italy/Ethiopia) (1901-1941)
Housekeeper, sacristan, nurse and big sister to the girls
at Santa Croce boarding school.
Nurse in the Parini Civil Hospital in Ethiopia, caring for civilians
and then injured soldiers in World War II.[1]

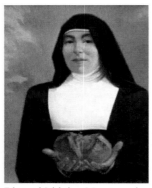

Blessed Liduina Meneguzzi
Source:
vatican.va/news_services

Elisa Angela Meneguzzi (Sister Liduina) was born on September 12, 1901 in Giarre, near Abano Terme, Padua, Italy to a poor farm family who was rich in faith. She was the second of eight children. She began each day with the Holy Sacrifice of the Mass and praying the Rosary, even though she had to walk two kilometers to attend the Holy Sacrifice of the Mass. She frequented and later taught catechism. She shared the faith with her brothers and sisters and, in the evening, prayed with her family.

At age 14, she assisted in supporting her family by working for some well-off families and in some hotels in Abano which had a well-known thermal resort. She was loved by many who appreciated her mild and willing personality. Her father died in 1923, when she was 22 years old, at which time she increased the hours she worked at the Hotel "Due Torri in Abano to help support the family.

In 1917 she had met the Sisters of St. Francis de Sales who began teaching in the local kindergarten and elementary school in Abano. Called to religious life, she joined the Sisters of the Congregation of Saint Francis de Sales on March 5, 1926 taking the name Sister Liduina. She professed her final vows on September 8, 1929.

Sister Liduina worked for 11 years at Santa Croce boarding school in charge of linen, as a sacristan, nurse and among the girls who consider her as a good friend. She was an exceptional listener and she assisted them resolve their concerns imparting wise advice.

On July 16, 1937 her dream to work in the missions was realized when she was assigned to the public hospital "Giacinto Parini" in Dire-Dawa, Ethiopia Fifteen (15) sisters accompanied her from Italy.[2] Here she remained for the last four years of her life. She

274

worked as a nurse in the Parini Civil Hospital which, after the outbreak of World War II, became a military hospital. Thus she cared for both civilian patients and injured soldiers. When the city was bombed, she worked in the streets, carrying the wounded to shelter, baptizing the dying children and leading dying Christians through acts of contrition. Shouts rang out on the street and in the hospital, "Help, Sister Liduina!" She rushed to help, seeing the image of Christ in her suffering brother.[3] The natives call here "Sister Gudda" (Great).

She worked caring for people of many backgrounds, races and religions including Catholic, Copts, Muslims and native pagans. Her work gave her a chance to speak to them about the faith and she would tell any who would listen about the goodness of God the Father. She led many to convert and she became known as the "ecumenical flame."[4]

Sister Liduina died at age 40 on December 2, 1941 in Dire-Dawa, Ethiopia from an abdominal tumor. She underwent a delicate surgical operation which initially seemed to go well but left her intestines paralyzed. She accepted her illness patiently. Upon her death, she abandoned herself to God's will, offering her life for peace in the world. One doctor commented, "I've never seen someone dying with such joy and bliss."

She was initially buried in the military cemetery at the insistence of an injured soldier. Twenty years later, in July 1961, her remains were reinterred at the motherhouse of the Sisters of the Congregation of St. Francis de Sales in Padua, Italy.

Blessed Liduina Meneguzzi was declared venerable with the promulgation of the decree of heroic virtue on June 25, 1996 and beatified on October 20, 2002[5] both by Pope St. John Paul II. (Memorial - December 1).

References:
1) "Blessed Liduina Meneguzzi". CatholicSaints.Info. 12 November 2021. Web. 8 December 2021.
<https://catholicsaints.info/blessed-liduina-meneguzzi/>

2) EWTN. (20Oct2002). Biographies of New Blesseds - 2002. Bl. Liduina Meneguzzi (1901-1941). Accessed 13 April 2022.
https://www.ewtn.com/catholicism/library/biographies-of-new-saints-5251

3) Sr. Liduina Meneguzzi (1901-1941). Accessed 12 April 2022. https://www.vatican.va/news_services/liturgy/saints/ns_lit_doc_20021020_meneguzzi_en.html

4) Angelus (2Dec2021). Saint of the day: Blessed Liduina Meneguzzi. Accessed April 13, 2022. https://angelusnews.com/faith/saint-of-the-day/blessed-liduina-meneguzzi/

5) Hagiography Circle: An Online Resource on Contemporary Hagiography. 1941. 24) Elisa Angela Meneguzzi (Liduina). Accessed 12 April 2022. http://newsaints.faithweb.com/year/1941.htm

Bl. Hanna Chrzanowska (Poland) (1902-1973)

First lay Catholic registered nurse to be beatified
Helped nurse victims of the Polish-Bolshevik war-1917
Graduated in 2nd class from Warsaw School of Nursing-1924
Studied community health nursing in France, Belgium & USA
Liaison officer, Krakow Branch, Polish Welfare Committee &
German authorities. Coordinated social and nursing help for
the poor, displaced and homeless in the Krakow region (WWII).
Head, Department of Community Nursing, Krakow School of Nursing.
During Soviet Occupation - fired from her post as Assistant Director of the
School of Nursing because of her strong Christian values and appointed
Director of the School of Psychiatric Nursing in Kobierzyn-1957
Authorities closed down the Psychiatric School of Nursing
Started Parish Nursing in Krakow Diocese with support of Fr. Machay
Lent 1960, invited Bishop Karol Wojtyla (Pope St. John Paul II) to
accompanied her to visits 35 chronically ill patients in their homes.[6]

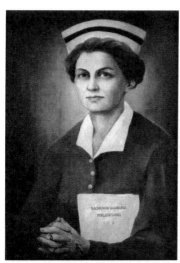

BŁOGOSŁAWIONA HANNA CHRZANOWSKA
(1902–1973)
PIELĘGNIARKA

Hanna Chrzanowska was born on October 7, 1902 in Warsaw, Poland to Ignacy Chrzanowski and Wanda Szlenkier. She was baptized on July 23, 1903 at the Church of St. Adalbert in Wiązowna. She had one brother, Bogdan. Her father was a renowned professor of Polish literature who came from a family of landowners. Her mother was from a wealthy Lutheran family of Warsaw Industrialists. They along with her aunt were known for their extensive charity and philanthropic work.[1] Her maternal Aunt Zofia Szlenkier founded and endowed a pediatric hospital in Warsaw. In 1910 the family moved to Krakow and Hanna attended high school in a school run by the Ursuline sisters graduating with distinction. Having left school she enrolled in a Red Cross course in order to help nurse victims of the Polish-Bolshevik war (1917).

In 1920 she enrolled at the Jagiellonia University studying Humanities in the Department of Philosophy and Philology because

277

as yet, a school of nursing did not exist in Poland. In 1922 her Aunt Zofia was instrumental in establishing of the first professional school of nursing in Poland (Warsaw) after she returned from nursing training in London at St. Thomas School of Nursing where she may have met the aged Florence Nightingale.

Hanna entered the second nursing class at the Warsaw School of Nursing in 1922 and graduated in 1924. In 1925 and 1926 she studied community health nursing in France and Belgium. She taught community health and nursing care of the newborn from 1926-1929. In May 1929 she resigned due to ill health and was treated in Zakopane, Poland and Davos, Switzerland. At this time she wrote the novel "The Key to Heaven," which was published in 1934. From 1929-1939 she was the Editor of "Polish Nurse," the first professional nursing journal. She served as Vice-chair of the Polish Association of Professional Nurses (PNA) and in 1935 actively participated in preparing the 1st Nurse Practice Act. She assisted in the formation of the Catholic Union of Polish Nurses in 1937. She published her second novel, "A Cross in the Sands," in 1938, at which time World War II had begun.

During World War II, in 1939, she single-handedly rescued a friend from advancing German soldiers by transporting her over 50 km on a horse-drawn cart to relatives. Tragedy struck the family in 1939, when her cousin Andrew Chrzanowski died, Aunt Zofia Szlenkier died and her dear schoolmate Zofia Wajda died, all during military attacks in the first days of the war. In addition, in 1939, her father, a retired professor from Jagiellonia University was deported, with his colleagues, to the Sachsenhausen concentration camp by the Nazis where he died in January of 1940. That year, in 1940, her brother was murdered in the Katyn woods by Soviet Troops and buried in a mass grave. Throughout the war she wondered as to his whereabouts and only discovered the horrible truth at the close of the war. Needing the Soviets as allies, a fabrication blamed the Nazis for this mass slaughter, however, a monument in the town square in Krakow testifies to the true brutality of the Soviet communists which would become even more apparent to religious orders and citizens of occupied East Block countries after the war (See "Martyrs from the Congregation of Saint Elizabeth - Soviet Occupation-1945" on future pages).

During the war Hanna worked as a liaison officer between the Krakow Branch of the Polish Welfare Committee and the German authorities. She coordinated social and nursing help for the poor, displaced and homeless in the Krakow region and visited prisoners. In 1942 she worked extra shifts in a neonatal unit to ensure safe care and delivery of Polish infants so that they were not euthanized.

After World War II, in 1945, during the Soviet Occupation, she worked with the United Nations Relief and Rehabilitation Administration (UNRRA) in Krakow organizing help for refugees and distributing aid. At this time she also became the Head of the Department of Community Nursing at the Krakow School of Nursing. She was sent on an UNRRA scholarship to study public and community health nursing at a large Public Health Service on Staten Island, New York. She was later housed at a School of Nursing attached to Columbia Presbyterian Hospital where she visited the poor and indigent in Harlem. She was very impressed by the professionalism and excellent care given by a dark skinned nurse whom she accompanied on visits. Upon her return to the Krakow School of Nursing, she discovered that militia secret police interrogated, threatened and imprisoned, albeit briefly, nursing students. Nursing lecturers were required to attend socialist indoctrination sessions delivered by special education officers of the Communist Party. Hanna emphasized educating young nurses in a spirit of authentic service to the sick, treating patients with dignity and paying attention to physical and spiritual needs.

In 1956 as her faith deepened, she became a Benedictine Oblate of Tyniec Abbey at Benedyktynska 37, 30-398 Krakow, Poland, located on the outskirts of Krakow, Poland. In 1957, while Poland was still under Soviet, communist occupation, she was fired from her post as Assistant Director of the School of Nursing because of her strong Christian values. She was appointed Director of the School of Psychiatric Nursing in Kobierzyn, 10 km outside Krakow. After Hanna allowed students to participate in the 1st annual pilgrimage to Jasna Gora (Czestochowa) to pay homage to the Black Madonna (a picture of the Blessed Virgin Mary and infant Jesus, originally painted by St. Luke the Evangelist), the authorities closed down the Psychiatric School of Nursing. Strangely, in 1957, although they had fired her, the Polish socialist government also

279

awarded her a medal for exemplary activity in promoting Public Health Nursing.

Now in retirement she was even more prolific. She started Parish Nursing in Krakow which subsequently expanded to the whole diocese. She especially focused on the lonely, abandoned, elderly, disabled and chronically sick who were deprived of any kind of nursing and spiritual care. She coordinated Catholic nurses who were employed by the church/diocese, and volunteer religious sisters (Sisters of St. Joseph, Franciscan Sisters from the Congregation of St. Felix of Calisante [Felician Sisters], Sisters of the Sacred Heart and Daughters of Charity of St. Vincent de Paul), students, and seminarians to look after the sick and lonely. The goal was not to replace their current family and neighborhood support system but to augment and support them. She was also keen on maintaining care in the home, where the patient felt at ease in their familiar surroundings. She made all efforts to keep patients from being institutionalized. Having developed the idea, she turned to Father Karol Wojtyla, later bishop of Krakow (and the future Pope St. John Paul II), for advice. He in turn pointed her to Father Machay from the Basilica of the Blessed Virgin Mary, in the old town square in Krakow, who gave his full approval of her plan for Parish Nursing to be implemented in his parish.[1]

She helped the house-bound individuals rediscover the joys of life and gave them strength to bear their daily crosses. When few people had cars, phones, wheelchairs etc., she instituted retreats for the handicapped and housebound at the Salvatorian Retreat Center, ul Glowackiego 3, 32-540, Trzebinia. She coordinated for the Holy Sacrifice of the Mass to be offered in the home for those who could not leave their home. She developed a Code of Conduct for parish nursing with colleagues and Bishop Bronislaw Dabrowski. In 1960, during Lent, she invited Bishop Karol Wojtyla to accompany her on her visits to 35 chronically ill patients in their homes. Under her influence, Karol Cardinal Wojtyla made February 11th (Feast day of Our Lady of Lourdes), an Archdiocesan day of prayer for the sick and those who look after them. As Pope St. John Paul II, he made the Feast of Our Lady of Lourdes the International Day of Prayer for the Sick to be celebrated by the universal church.

In 1960 she published the textbook of "Community Nursing," the fourth edition of which was published posthumously

280

in 1973. In 1965, Pope Paul VI decorated Hanna with the order of *Pro Ecclesia et Pontifice*, in recognition of her work with the chronically ill and house-bound in the Krakow Diocese. The next year, in 1966, she was diagnosed with advanced gynecological cancer. This did not stop her work. She was appointed Deputy Spokesperson for Health Care Workers at the request of the Ministry of Health. She continued to be an active member of the Polish Nurses' Association (PNA), now a "socialist" organization, to which she brought Christian principles. In 1971 she received from Karol Cardinal Wojtyla, an official letter nominating her the coordinator and director of services of the handicapped and chronically ill within the charities commission of the Krakow Archdiocese. She gradually came to realize that in caring for the sick and those who suffered, she was serving Jesus Christ Himself.

On February 14, 1973, two months prior to her death, she delivered a talk on Parish Nursing titled, *"Lay Apostolate and Care of the Sick"* at the annual conference of the Polish Bishops Committee on Pastoral Care. A full transcript of this talk is available in Dr. Gosia Brykczynska, PhD, RN's book *"Blessed Hanna Chrzanowska, RN: A Nurse of Mercy."*[3] In April 1973, Cardinal Wojtyla visited her flat and helped position the dying Hanna Chrzanowska in bed, "his last act of love and human kindness towards her."

Hanna Chrzanowska died on April 29, 1973 on the Feast of St. Catherine of Siena (1347-1380), at her home on Lobzowska Street from cancer. Archbishop Cardinal of Krakow, Karol Wojtyla presided at the Holy Sacrifice

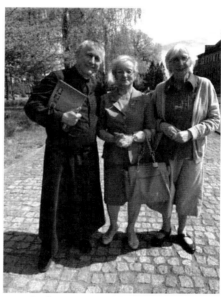

Helena Matoga, RN, MA and Gosia Brykczynska, PhD, RN, OCV with the Rector at the Salvatorian Retreat Center in Trzebinia, Poland

of the Mass and funeral services and accompanied her coffin to the

Rakowicki Cemetery in Krakow. Attendance at the funeral overflowed into the streets with colleagues, friends and patients attending.

The Canonization Process:

Helena Matoga, RN, the Vice Postulator for the Cause of the Canonization of Hanna Chrzanowska described the process:[4]

In 1993, during the meeting commemorating the 20th anniversary of Hanna Chrzanowska's death, Zofia Szlendak–Cholewińska put forward a motion to open her canonization process. After the Holy Mass in the Franciscan Basilica, a meeting of nurses, nuns and the sick was held, during
which they remembered Hanna. It was then when I heard them refer to her as "Auntie" for the first time.

I attended this meeting with my school friend, also Hanna's student, Maryla Cherian, who additionally had a degree in law. After a short discussion, we concluded that opening a canonization process was a very difficult task, so it was necessary to choose people who would find all the information about where to start.

Alina Rumun, a retired nurse and Hanna's oldest student and closest long-time collaborator, and Zofia Szlendak-Cholewińska, also Hanna's student and a teacher of nurses, were able to provide a considerable number of their written and spoken memories of Hanna.

When Alina asked "Who will take care of it?" (i.e. the preparation of the opening of the canonization process), my friend, Maryla Cherian, who was both a lawyer and a nurse, volunteered and asked me to help her. Irena Iżycka, M.A., a distinguished nurse older than us, also Hanna's student, volunteered to help.

At that time (i.e. in 1993) the Catholic Association of Polish Nurses and Midwives (KSPiPP) did not yet exist. We were part of the Pastoral Ministry for Nurses (Duszpasterstwo Pielęgniarek), under the patronage of Cardinal Franciszek Macharski[9], who was Cardinal Karol Wojtyła's successor in this

---

[9]At the request of the nursing community, the Pastoral Ministry for Nurses and Midwives was established by the Primate Cardinal Stefan Wyszyński (now a saint – he was canonised in 2021) in 1957 during his second pilgrimage to Jasna Góra in Czestochowa in Poland. After returning from this pilgrimage, Hanna Chrzanowska and Fr. Wojtyła

282

position. He also celebrated Holy Mass in his chapel for us on the last Sunday of each month, after which we attended a meeting in his representative hall to listen to a lecture or watch a film, depending on what our pastoral minister organised. The Lenten retreats, initiated by Hanna Chrzanowska in the 1960's and held in the Dominican Sisters' monastery, were one of the regular events within our Pastoral Ministry. The retreats have been continuing to this day. Cardinal Wojtyła always attended the closing ceremony of the retreats. I have been taking part in them every year since 1985. This tradition originated from the idea to commemorate the first headmistress of the Vocational Nursing School, Maria Epstein, who was a Dominican nun and is a Servant of God, and under whose supervision Hanna Chrzanowska worked as a young teacher in the years 1926-1929. Maria [Epstein] and her life probably helped in shaping Hanna's Catholic attitude.

Since 1991 I was in charge of a large nursing team in an open health care centre and I presented Chrzanowska as an example to my team. I remembered a phrase that Hanna used to repeat to clergymen, seminarians, students, doctors and to us: "God's Word hardly or not at all reaches the sick who are unwashed and hungry". In the same year I was approached by the newly appointed chaplain of nurses and midwives, Father Kazimierz Kubik, who was a medical doctor, whom I "infected" with Hanna. We have been working together to this day. He defended his doctoral thesis on the social evaluation of Hanna Chrzanowska's heroic life and nursing activity.

In 1995, during another pilgrimage to Jasna Góra in Częstochowa, the Catholic Association of Polish Nurses and Midwives was established. Zofia Żmigrodzka, the Kraków delegate who attended this pilgrimage, informed us about it. We, (i.e. a group of 11 Catholic nurses) formed the Kraków Branch of this Association. Izabela Ćwiertnia, M.Sc, was elected the first president, and with interruptions in her term of office, continues to hold the position to this day[10].

Our meetings were held in a small parish hall at the youth café at St. Nicholas Church on Kopernika Street in Kraków. At that time Fr. Kazimierz Kubik began his priestly ministry there. In this parish Hanna developed parish care for the sick. This parish was the first to implement the celebration of Holy Mass in the homes of

---

organised Pastoral Ministry for Nurses at the Metropolitan Curia in Kraków.
[10] At present there are 42 members of our branch.

283

the sick. During Cardinal Macharski's parish visitation, Izabela Ćwiertnia, the president of our branch, together with Fr. Antoni Sołtysik, the parson of the parish, handed Cardinal Macharski request to initiate the process of canonization of nurse Hanna Chrzanowska.[11] The Cardinal expressed his oral support, but made it dependent on the decision of the Episcopal Conference, which met in Warsaw under the leadership of Józef Glemp, who was then the Primate of Poland.

Having obtained the Episcopate's consent, Cardinal Macharski issued a statement on the commencement of the trial of the Servant of God Hanna Chrzanowska and appointed the Historical Commission for the preparation of documentation and the Tribunal presided over by Rev. Prof. Stefan Ryłko. Several priests, Maria Cherian and I were appointed. We all took the oath on the Gospel in the presence of Cardinal Macharski.

Maria Cherian[12] was appointed a notary in the proceedings. The parson of the parish of St. Nicolas, Fr. Antoni Sołtysik, was appointed a postulator, and I was appointed a vice-postulator. My duties included: running the office of the postulation, handling of the correspondence, searching for witnesses, coordinating and scheduling their hearings, formal work in the cemetery administration related to the exhumation of Hanna's, Servant of God, mortal remains[13]. I also conducted a six-month query in the State Archives in Kraków, where I found many unknown documents related to Hanna's activity during World War II.

The collected documents, together with protocols of hearings of 70 witnesses, amounting to 3000 pages, were delivered to the Congregation for the Causes of Saints in the Vatican. They were the basis for preparing the *Positio*, an important document which assessed the holiness of life and heroic virtues of the Servant of God Hanna Chrzanowska. Rev. Mieczysław Niepsuj, a Vatican prelate, was appointed the Roman postulator. All the documentation gathered in Kraków were entrusted to him. The

---

[11] Fr.Macharski administered to Hanna the Sacrament of Anointing of the Sick before her death.
[12] Maria Cherian +(who died in 2012) participated in the examination of witnesses. She used her seal and signature to approve the procedural documents together with Rev. Prof. S. Ryłko, who conducted the proceedings
[13] This required legal proceedings due to the ownership rights to the grave

parson of the parish, Fr. Antoni Sołtysik and Rev. Kazimierz Kubik delivered it to him personally. They managed to obtain a private papal audience. They informed His Holiness Pope John Paul II about the completion of the work at the diocesan level. The Pope said only: "Tend to this matter, it is very important!"

In summary, the nurses discussed opening the cause of Hanna's canonization in 1993. They formally made the request in 1995. It was approved by the Archbishop of Krakow following agreement of the Episcopal conference under the leadership of the Primate of Poland. The diocesan inquiry began on November 3, 1998 and concluded on January 16, 2002. An intercessory healing attributed to Hanna had occurred in 2001 and was under investigation.

Miracle #1 - 2001

The miracle accepted for Hanna's beatification was the intercessory healing of a fellow nursing instructor who was her former student, Zofia Szlendak-Cholewińska, who was 60 years old at the time and suffered an inoperable brain aneurysm in 2001. Zofia was the same nurse, who in 1993, had made the motion to open the cause for Hanna's canonization.

In the early 1960's, Zofia was a member of a secret Catholic organization, Instutut Świecki [the Secular Institute][14]. The animator was the Abbot of the Benedictine Monastery in Tyniec, Father Piotr Rostworowski[15]. After some time Zofia decided that "this was not her way": *But in leaving the Institute, I also left God.*

Fr. Piotr believed in her return to Him. Zofia valued her friendship with Fr. Peter, they wrote letters to each other. She was arrested during a case against Fr. Peter, although a search of her flat revealed nothing. She was released after two days. She was

---

[14] A young priest, Franciszek Macharski, later to become a cardinal, was also its member

[15] He was arrested and persecuted by the authorities. He spent 4 years in prison. Later he became a Camadolese hermit. Pope St. John Paul II appointed him the Consultor of the Congregation for Monastic Affairs. He took the oath from Chrzanowska, an oblate entering the Third Benedictine

kept under surveillance for several years, and it turned out that the secret informer who 'monitored' her was a nurse from the gynaecological ward, where Zofia underwent surgery for an ovarian cyst (of which the secret services in Poland knew). They also knew that Archbishop Wojtyla (who was very heavily spied on) visited her in hospital. From the secret files to which I gained access, I learned that the Archbishop brought her flowers (5 carnations), lemons and a picture. This was the time of communist terror.[4]

While crossing the tram tracks, Zofia fell almost right under an oncoming tram. She most probably had an epileptic seizure. Zofia was evaluated and a CT scan of her head showed an inoperable brain hemangioma. According to Zofia's own testimony,[16] *"She thanked the doctor for the information. And he said, are you crazy, do you not know what an inoperable aneurysm in the brain is? I replied that I knew, what's more I won't have to pay a fine next time I get under a tram.[17]"*

Going to the Rakowicki Cemetery to visit her husband's grave, Zofia stopped at Hanna's and began to pray the Lords Prayer. She was horrified when she realized that she had forgotten the words. Either this time or at a subsequent visit to the cemetery, Zofia stated in her testimony, *"I went to Auntie's grave and started shouting there, loudly. Auntie do something so that I can reconcile with God..."*

Some time later, in the middle of the night, the aneurysm ruptured and Zofia was taken to the hospital with a massive hemorrhage in the temporal part of the brain. Complicating matters, she also suffered a heart attack in the supracondylar part of the heart. She suffered paralysis of both upper and lower limbs but was able to breath on her own. She was not on a ventilator. Over the next six weeks, Zofia's condition did not improve. The physicians thought there was no real hope for survival. Since an operation was out of the question, she was discharged from the Intensive Care Ward of

---

[16] A long interview with Zofia was published by the Pauline Fathers in Krakow in their jubilee bulletin of 10 May 2009 to mark the 700th anniversary of the Order.
[17] Zofia paid a 100 zloty (PLN) fine, because angry passengers treated her like a suicide.

286

the Neurosurgery Clinic and transferred to the non-invasive treatment ward. Her limbs were paralyzed and muscles constricted.

The news of her illness reached the nurses and others who prayed every month in St. Nicholas Church (ul Kopernika 9) in Krakow for the beatification of Hanna Chrzanowska and for the intentions of those who entrusted their concerns to her. A member of the Krakow Branch of the Catholic Association of Nurses and Midwives initiated a novena "for Zofia's recovery through the intercession of Servant of God Hanna."[4]

At some point, Zofia became aware of her disability and, heartbroken, she again called on Auntie in her dream, who assured her that everything would be all right. And then in the morning, when Zofia awoke, her motor functions began to return. She told her dream to everybody in the ward she had contact with. In her statements Zofia shared,

- *"God made me wait. (I know... it was probably two or three years. Indeed, God did his work. He knocked me down. He literally knocked me down...). I was unconscious for six weeks. There were two worlds then. One here with the body, and the other one that I was experiencing (....).*
- *(....) I was unconscious for six weeks. None of the doctors believed I had any chances of surviving (...)*
- *(...) In fact, I wasted my life and the graces that the Lord gave me (...). The most difficult thing is to forgive oneself. For 37 years, I was far from God. It's no wonder I ended up forgetting the words of 'Our Father' (...)."*

Zofia, after the healing, stated, *"(...) I experienced that God is great love. I felt as if I was surrounded by one great love and I felt very well (...)."*

Not only did Zofia recover without mental or physical deficit, her other symptoms and ailments (i.e. epilepsy, etc.) were gone. Her brain scan showed only a small scar that remained. She was in a better condition than before she had the aneurysm. Perhaps more miraculous is that she returned to the faith.

The head of the clinic, a neurosurgeon and professor wrote, *"With these severe neurological and cardiac problems, from my medical experience, I cannot explain such a rapid improvement of the patient's health."* A similar statement was submitted by the head of the neurology department.

When Helena Matoga, RN, MA, the vice postulator for the

cause of Hanna Chrzanowska's canonization, visited Zofia in the hospital in June, Zofia invited her to her house on July 3rd. Helena did not believe she would leave the hospital that soon. However, Zofia kept her word. "Having confirmed by phone that she was indeed home already, Helena paid her a visit. Zofia opened the door supporting herself with a cane. She was happy."[4] Helena Matoga shared:[4]

> When Zofia returned home, she continued living alone on the third floor in a block of flats without a lift. Someone helped her with cleaning and shopping. She received visitors. She lived for almost 10 more years, spreading the cult of Hanna. The last six months before she died, she was in hospital in the internal medicine ward. She was diagnosed with lymphoma. Her stay in hospital was short. Zofia declared that she wanted to die in her flat "in Auntie's company", whose portrait she had by her bed. And so it happened. The caregiver found her dead in the morning. The death official death certificate read: undiagnosed.

The lack of a diagnosis on Zofia's death certificate was problematic for the Vice Postulator for the cause of Servant of God Hanna Chrzanowska's canonization. Helena Matoga described her dilemma:

> It was necessary to complete the process documents, the cause of death being the most important. This is where my problem began. Fr. Prof. Ryłko died, Fr. Postulator Sołtysik[18] suffered a stroke. I did not have the family's authorization to access her medical history. The authorization was held by her stepson, who lived in Portugal. With difficulty, I was able to find the doctor who visited and treated Zofia. Fortunately, it turned out that she had visited Zofia a few days before her death. Knowing the diagnosis, she advised Zofia to undergo palliative treatment, but she refused. I obtained the necessary document on the cause of death from her.

The diocesan inquiry on the miracle for beatification opened on October 18, 2002 and closed on April 3, 2003. The decree on validity of the diocesan inquiry was issued January 11, 2008. The

---

[18]He described the grace experienced through Hannah's intercession in the book *Dama Miłosierdzia (Lady of Mercy)* on page 166 – 167.

decree on the validity of the diocesan inquiry on the miracle was issued May 21, 2010. The *Positio* was published in 2011. The Vatican particular congress of theological consultors reviewed the cause on November 27, 2012. And the ordinary session of cardinals and bishops reviewed the cause on September 29, 2015. The decree of heroic virtue was promulgated by His Holiness Pope Francis on September 30, 2015. Hanna was now known as Venerable Servant of God Hanna Chrzanowska or just Venerable Hanna Chrzanowska.

Helena Matoga described the next step:

The day of exhumation came in April 2016. I invited Izabela Ćwiertnia and Tadeusz Wadas, a male nurse, who was the president of the Małopolska Chamber of Nurses and Midwives (MOIPiP), to participate in the preparation of the mortal remains excavated from the grave for their later placement in the sarcophagus. Fathers J. Gubala and K. Kubik and the delegates of the Metropolitan Curia were participating in it. The examination and detailed description was done by forensic specialists.

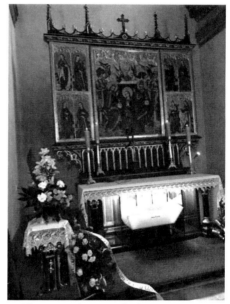

Servant of God Hanna Chrzanowska's remains were re-interred in an alabaster sarcophagus in the southern nave of the Church of St. Nicholas (aka "The Nurses' Church), under the altar depicting the coronation of Our Lady (ul Kopernika 9, Krakow, Poland). The sarcophagus was furnished from donations of the

The sarcophagus of Bl. Hanna at St. Nicholas Church (the Nurses' Church), ul Kopernika 9, Krakow, Poland

Catholic nurses throughout the country of Poland.

289

The Vatican appointed Medical Board reviewed the miracle later that year on November 24, 2016. The particular congress of theological consultors followed by the ordinary session of cardinal and bishop conducted their review on February 21, 2017 and July 7, 2017 respectively. The promulgation of the decree on miracle was issued on July 7, 2017. The steps had been taken to set the date for the beatification of Servant of God Hanna Chrzanowska, RN which would occur on April 28, 2018.

From the motion made by the nurses in 1993 to move forward the cause for canonization of Hanna Chrzanowska, RN to her beatification, 25 years had passed. The canonization delegate of the Metropolitan Curia in Kraków, Fr. Andrzej Scąber, PhD[2] commented on the efforts of the nurses and the unique and generous contribution of Cardinal Dziwisz:

> During one of the meetings preceding the ceremony in Łagiewniki, Fr. Scąber explained that the nurses from Kraków, who were not frightened by the enormity of the formalities, were the initiators of the beatification process: "For the sake of completeness, had it not been for the initiative of these nurses, unprepared for this task in any way, their zeal, their conviction of the holiness of their teacher's life, the cause would not have happened. The beatification will be a celebration of nurses and the sick whom the future Blessed served all her life". Then he also reminded us of the role Cardinal Dziwisz played in H. Chrzanowska's process, who not only appointed the Roman postulator of the case (Prelate Mieczysław Niepsuj) in 2006 but also provided money for the continuation of the process. "I mentioned the financing of the process. I want to say that this burden was taken on personally by Cardinal Dziwisz. I emphasize the word 'personally'", Fr. Scber said.

In addition to conducting the interviews and accumulating the documents required for Blessed Hanna's beatification, the nurses and other organizations have held many conferences and events focused on Hanna Chrzanowska, RN's life and work:

- Symposium on Hanna Chrzanowska's 25th anniversary of her death - May 1998. About 300 people attended it, including the sick who remembered "Auntie" Hanna Chrzanowska
- A trip to Wiązowna in 1999–the place where Hanna was baptised in the Church of St. Adalbert. Organized by: the Catholic Association and

Warsaw nursing community.

- Scientific conference on the 100th anniversary of her birth - 2002. Organised by the Catholic Association and the Jagiellonian University.
- Conference on the 40th anniversary of her death in April 2013.
- Scientific conference (2018) organized before the beatification ceremony by the Pontifical University of John Paul II in Kraków, with the active participation of Fr. K. Kubik, PhD and H. Matoga.
- Press conference at the Polish Episcopate in Warsaw with the participation of Archbishop M. Jędraszewski, Rev. Prof. Robert Tyrała and Helena Matoga.
- Several films, radio and TV programmes dedicated to the Servant of God.
- Ten schools of nursing in Poland have chosen Hanna as their Patroness. Many scientific works have been written about her.
- The relics of the Blessed are being sent to chapels and temples in many countries all over the world. "As of April 2022, Fr. Gubala, the Curator, has issued about 300 relics of Blessed Hanna to chapels, churches, hospices and hospitals. A constant stream of requests and thanksgiving for graces received is coming."
- This year, 2022, thanks to the joint efforts of our community, the Kraków City Council honoured one of the city squares – near Hanna's place of residence and the Carmelite Sisters' Church on Łobzowska Street – with the name of the Blessed.

The Beatification ceremony was organized by the Metropolitan Curia in Krakow and headed by Archbishop Marek Jedraszewski. Three nurses: Izabela Ćwiertnia , Helena Matoga, Tadeusz Wadas and Fathers K. Kubik and J. Gubala were part of the organizing committee.

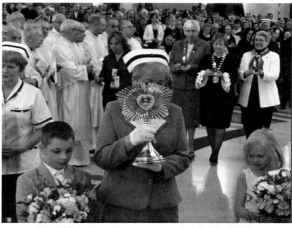

Beatification Ceremony - April 28, 2018
Nurses: Helena Matoga (Poland) carrying relics of Bl. Hanna accompanied by children. Gosia Brykczynska (England), Geraldine McSweeney (Ireland) and Marie Romagnano, (USA) carrying lamps

Servant of God Hanna Chrzanowska, RN was beatified at the Sanctuary of Divine Mercy, in Krakow-Lagiewniki, Poland on April 28, 2018, within 45 years of her death. Helena Matoga, RN, vice postulator for the cause of Blessed Hanna's canonization, now in her 80's, was present and, accompanied by children, brought the relics of the Blessed into the Basilica. Geraldine McSweeney, the International President of International Catholic Committee of Nurses and Medico-Social Assistants — Comité International Catholique des Infirmières et Assistantes Médico-Sociales (CICIAMS) from Ireland, Dr. Gosia Brykczynska, PhD, RN, OCV from the United Kingdom and Marie Romagnano, MSN, RN, CCM from the United States of America carried lamps in the procession. The papal delegate, Archbishop Angelo Amato, handed Pope Francis' five original decrees of beatification to: Marek Jedraszewski, Metropolitan Archbishop of Krakow (2), and one each to the Roman postulator; Fr. Franciszek Slusarczyk, the Custodian of the Shrine of the Divine Mercy; and Helena Matoga, MA, RN, as a representative of the nursing community (1). Izabela Ćwiertnia , and Tadeusz Wadas read the Lessons during the Holy Sacrifice of the Mass. Nurses, from all over Poland, smartly dressed in their nursing uniforms, participated in this joyous occasion.

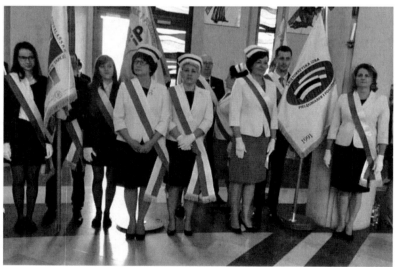

Polish Nurses and Midwives (red strip on cap) from across Poland.
Beatification Ceremony for Bl. Hanna Chrzanowska, RN
April 28, 2018

Blessed Hanna Chrzanowska, RN's feast day is the 28th of April because the 29th, the day she died, was already the important feast of St. Catherine of Siena, one of the patrons of Europe and also a lay Catholic nurse. It was thought better to place Blessed Hanna's feast on the next closest day.(Memorial: April 28).[5]

"God's Word hardly or not at all reaches the sick
who are unwashed and hungry".

"What dignity belongs to our profession!
Christ in us serves Christ in the other person."

Intercessory Prayer
God, who in a special way called your servant Hanna Chrzanowska
to the service of the sick, poor and abandoned,
grant that she who answered your call with all her heart,
should be counted among the saints while encouraging us with her
example to bring help to our neighbours.
Through her intercession grant us the grace… for which we pray
in faith and hope. Through Jesus Christ our Lord. Amen.
Our Father… Hail Mary… Glory be…

Report any graces obtained through the intercession of Blessed Hanna Chrzanowska to the Postulator's Office: Parafia Sw Mikolaja, Kopernika 9, 31-034 Krakow, Poland.
Email: kancelaria@parafiamikolaj-krakow.pl

References:
1) Krakow Catholic Nurses (KSPiPP). Blessed Hanna Chrzanowska. Accessed 14 May 2022. https://hannachrzanowska.pl/en/sample-page/

2) Milosz Kluba Bogdan Gancarz (26Apr2018). Sister of our God. Gosc Media Institute. Accessed 4 June 2022. https://krakow.gosc.pl/doc/4664685

3) Gosia Brykczynska (2019). Blessed Hanna Chrzanowska, RN: A Nurse of Mercy. Marian Press, Stockbridge, MA.
https://shopmercy.org/catalogsearch/result/?q=Blessed+Hanna

4) Personal Communication with Helena Matoga, RN, Vice Postulator for the Cause of the Canonization of Blessed Hanna Chrzanowska, RN, May 3, 2022.

5) Personal Communication with English Biographer for Blessed Hanna, Gosia Brykczynska, PhD, RN, OCV, April 14, 2022.

6) Gosia Brykczynska (2014). Colours of Fire: Biography of Hanna Chrzanowska - a wise and compassionate nurse. William R. Parks: WparksPublishing@aol.com.

Bl. Maria Euthymia Uffing (Germany) (1914-1955)

Graduated with distinction from nursing program on 3 September 1939.
World War II cared for prisoners of war and
foreign workers with infectious diseases.[1]

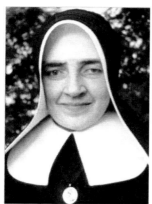

Bl. M. Euthymia Uffing
www.clemensschwestern.de/e
uthymia/biografie/

Emma Uffing[2] was born on April 8, 1914 in Halverde, Germany to August Uffing and his second wife, Maria Schnitt. She was baptized on that same day. Emma was the fifth of seven children. Her parents were farmers. in a small German town. When she was 18 months old she contracted rickets, the effects of which would impact her the rest of her life.

Emma attended elementary school in Halverde and found learning difficult. However, her grades were consistently good. She helped in the kitchen and on the family farm always stating, "I can do that, I can do that." At the age of 14 she expressed a desire to be a nun to her mother who stated that she was too young to make this decision. In November 1931 at the age of 17 she went to work at St. Anna Hospital in Hopsten in the house and on the poultry farm. For a year she worked a cook. There she met the matron, Sister Euthymia Linnenkemper, a Clemens sister who became her role model.

On July 23, 1934 she entered the Sisters of the Congregation of the Sisters of Charity (Sisters of St. Clemens) in Munster together with 46 other women and took the name, Sister Euthymia after the Hopsten supervisor. She was the 2,638[th] women to enter the order taking the vows of poverty, chastity and obedience. Forty people from her home town attended her clothing ceremony, a sign of their appreciation of her.

Sister Euthymia made her temporary vows on October 11, 1936. She was assigned to work at St. Vincent's Hospital in Dinslaken, Germany in October 1936 on the Lower Rhine. She subsequently began nursing training at the School of Nursing at the Raphaelsklink in Münster founded in 1909 and directed by the Clemens Sisters.[3] She found that learning the extensive specialist knowledge was difficult for her, but through perseverance she

295

managed to be successful. She initially worked in the women's ward and then after a year took over the isolation ward. The isolation ward consisted of a wooden barracks with 50 beds. She provided much love and brings happiness to the patients, especially the many children who were without their mothers. On September 3, 1939, Sister Euthymia passed the state-approved nurse exam[3] with the grade of "very good." On September 15, 1940 she made her final vows at the motherhouse in Munster and she thereby committed herself to the order of the Sisters of Clemens for her entire life..

During World War II (1938-1945), Sister Euthymia cared for the contagiously ill prisoners of war and forced laborers. Conditions included: scabies, erythema, typhus, venereal diseases, pulmonary tuberculosis. They usually arrived dirty and infested with lice. She was not repulsed by pus, blood, sputum or feces. She lovingly cared for over 70 patients housed in the St. Barbara barracks. The patients called her the "Angel of Love." On March 23, 1945 when 85% of Dinslaken was destroyed in an American bombing raid, including St. Vincent's Hospital, she helped transport the patients to the surrounding villages until late at night. The next day she collapsed with a high fever.

After the hospital was rebuilt she was assigned to work in the laundry room. Desiring to remain in direct nursing care she was saddened by this decision of her supervisors but quickly recovered with an attitude to be "ready for anything." On January 14, 1948 she was transferred to Munster and took over the management of the laundry in the motherhouse and the Raphael Clinic. She was responsible to clean not only the dirty laundry for the clinic but also the parent company and its affiliated facilities. It was hard and monotonous work. However, she still took time to assist the other sisters with their duties.

She collapsed in the wash house on July 8, 1955 and was taken to the infirmary. Taken to surgery, it is found she had advanced incurable cancer. The doctors were shocked at the stamina of this "laundress." Her pain had to be severe considering the extent of disease. In August 1955, she developed a fever and asked for the Sacrament of the Anointing of the Sick. One nurse recalled, "It was hard to see how much she was suffering."[2] On September 9, 1955 at 6:00 a.m., Sister Maria Euthymia received Viaticum. At 7:30 a.m. she died at the age of only 41. At the same moment the sun shined through the window and illuminated her face – then the weather remained cloudy the rest of the day. Crowds of the sick, nurses, students, employees and visitors flocked to the mortuary chapel where Sister Euthymia was laid out. She was not only prayed for but people immediately began asking for her intercession. Before she died, she had promised others that she would pray to God for them.

On September 10, 1955 a miracle attributed to her intercession occurred. A sister, Sister M. Avelline, who suffered severe burns and bruises when her hand got caught between the rollers of an ironing machine asked for the intercession of Sister Maria Euthymia at her open coffin. The sister's hand was healed within a very short time. The doctors found this medically unexplainable.

The beatification process was begun at the end of 1959 by the Bishop of Munster, Dr. Michael Keller, four years after her death. Blessed Maria Euthymia Uffing was declared venerable with the promulgation of the decree of heroic virtue on September 1, 1988. In March of 2000 Rome accepted the miraculous cure of Sister M. Avelline. Sister Maria Euthymia Uffing was beatified on October 7, 2001[4] both by Pope St. John Paul II.(Memorial - September 9).

References:

1) "Blessed Maria Euthymia Üffing". CatholicSaints.Info. 9 September 2017. Web. 8 December 2021.
<https://catholicsaints.info/blessed-maria-euthymia-uffing/>

2) Clemens Sisters. Biography Sr. M. Euthymia. Accessed 14 April 2022.
https://www.clemensschwestern.de/euthymia/biografie/

3) Personal Communication with Sister Elisabethis Lenfers, Euthymia Center, Munster, Germany. 17 June 2022.

4) Hagiography Circle: An Online Resource on Contemporary Hagiography. 1941. 24) Elisa Angela Meneguzzi (Liduina). Accessed 12 April 2022.
http://newsaints.faithweb.com/year/1941.htm

Bl. Zdenka Cecilia Schelingova (Slovakia) (1916-1955), Martyr

Studied nursing and radiology. Nurse at a hospital in Humenne and then in Bratislava where she worked in radiology.[1]

Cecilia Schelingová, Holy Cross nun, was born on December 24, 1916 in Kriva in Orava, Zilinsky kraj, Slovakia to Pavol Schelingova and Zuzana Panikova. One of ten children, from an early age she along with her brothers and sisters acquired a sense of responsibility, sacrifice and a deep faith from their parents.

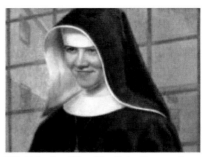

Bl. Zdenka (Cecilia Schelingova).
Source: https://sestrysvkriza.sk/

The Congregation of the Sisters of Charity of the Holy Cross came to the local parish in 1929 while Cecilia was attending the local elementary school. Through observing their presence, she felt the call of God to religious life. In 1931 at the age of 15 she requested admission to the order at the congregations' motherhouse in Podunajské Biskupice, accompanied by her mother. Prior to entrance, she was sent to nursing school and then took a specialized course in radiology. Cecilia Schelingova made her first vows on January 30, 1937 taking the name Sister Zdenka. The Vatican News Service biography records that,

> Sr Zdenka was remembered by her Sisters as a person who lived continually in God's presence, both in prayer and work. She once wrote: "I want to do God's will without paying attention to myself, my comfort or my rest". She demonstrated love and compassion to everyone and was always ready to serve, especially sick hospital patients."

Her first nursing experience was in the hospital in Humenné, near Ukraine. In 1942 she was transferred to the hospital in Bratislava, where she continued work in the radiology department.

In 1948, while Sr Zdenka was in Bratislava, the totalitarian Communist regime began. As a result and until 1953, the Catholic Church was deprived of all rights and her members persecuted. During this period, prisoners were sent to the hospital to receive care, priests among them. One day, Sister Zdenka understood that one of the priests, accused of being a Vatican spy and of betrayal, was going to be shipped to Siberia where death would be awaiting him, and so she acted at the risk of her own life: she slipped sleeping pills into the guard's tea, allowing the priest to escape. After he was free, Sr Zdenka went into the chapel and prayed: "Jesus, I offer my life for his. Save him!".

Some days later, however, on 29 February 1952, when she tried to help three priests and three seminarians escape, her plan backfired and she was arrested. She was interrogated and suffered many humiliations, including being brutally tortured by the police. She finally received a sentence of 12 years in prison and 10 years of civil rights' deprivation. The torture that she underwent left her body mutilated and her right breast torn apart from the continual kicks by the police.

From 1952 until 1955 Sr Zdenka was transferred from one prison to another. She accepted torture and mistreatment with great humility; most difficult of all for her, however, was being deprived of the Holy Sacraments for the three years of her imprisonment.

On 16 April 1955, Sr Zdenka was released from prison by the President of the Republic so she would not die there (she had a malignant tumor in her right breast). When she returned to her congregation's motherhouse in Bratislava, she was not accepted because of the general situation of fear that existed at the time as well as the constant police surveillance; nor was she received in the hospital of Bratislava. Instead, a friend from Trnava took her in. Sister Zdenka was eventually accepted into the hospital of Trnava. On 31 July 1955, after receiving the Sacraments, Sr Zdenka died. She was 38 years old and is remembered as a true martyr of the faith.

One final note: On 6 April 1970, the regional court of Bratislava declared that Sr Zdenka was innocent, having received a "false and artificial accusation... issued [with a] sentence of high betrayal... based on facts manipulated by the state police themselves".[2]

Blessed Cecilia Schelingova (Sister Zdenka) suffered a 12-year sentence for helping detained priests during which she was denied the sacraments and mutilated by torture.[3] She was beatified 48 years following her death. She was declared venerable with the promulgation of the decree of martyrdom on July 7, 2003 and beatified on September 14, 2003[4] at Bratislava, Slovak Republic both by Pope St. John Paul II. www.sestrysvkriza.sk. (Memorial - July 31)

References:

1) "Blessed Cecilia Schelingová". CatholicSaints.Info. 6 September 2017. Web. 8 December 2021. <https://catholicsaints.info/blessed-cecilia-schelingov/>

2) Vatican News Service. Zdenka Cecilia Schelingova (1916-1955). Accessed 7 April 2022. https://www.vatican.va/news_services/liturgy/saints/ns_lit_doc_20030914_s chelingova_en.html

3) Jonathan Luxmoore (7Nov2019). 30 years after Berlin Wall fell, Catholic seek to recognize heroic Eastern European sisters. Accessed 7 April 2022. https://www.globalsistersreport.org/news/world/ministry/news/30-years-afte r-berlin-wall-fell-catholics-seek-recognize-heroic-eastern

4) Hagiography Circle: An Online Resource on Contemporary Hagiography. 1955. 7) Cecilia Schelingova (Zdenka). Accessed 7 April 2022. http://newsaints.faithweb.com/year/1955.htm

Nurses Martyred in the Spanish Civil War - 1936

Bl. Josep Tarrats Comaposada (Spain) (1878-1936), Martyr
Infirmarian at Jesuit Infirmary[1]
Assisted elderly at nursing home run by Little Sister of the Poor [2]

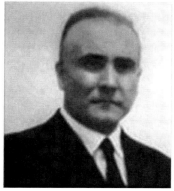

Blessed Jose Tarrats Comaposada
Source: jesuits.global

Josep Tarrats Comaposada, Jesuit Brother, was born on August 29, 1878 in Manresa, Barcelona, Spain. He entered the Society of Jesus (Jesuits) in 1895 and worked first as a tailor before serving as an infirmarian at the Jesuit residence in Valencia in 1910.

In 1932 the Jesuit order was suppressed in Spain and all its properties confiscated. Many Jesuit brothers and priests fled to Rome, Holland, Portugal and Belgium.[3] However, several remained at risk to their lives. One of these was Brother Josep Tarrats Comaposada. He, along with eleven fellow Jesuits were martyred in Gandia and Valencia Spain between August 19 and December 29, 1936 at the start of the Spanish Civil War (1936-1939).

While helping elderly Jesuits at the Jesuit infirmary and other elderly people at the nursing home run by the Little Sisters of the Poor in Barcelona, he was arrested and promptly executed on that same day on September 28, 1936.

Brother Josep Tarrats Comaposada was declared venerable with the promulgation of the decree of martyrdom on December 20, 1999 and beatified on March 11, 2001 both by Pope St. John Paul II.[4] (Memorial - September 28).

References:

1) "Blessed Josep Tarrats Comaposada". CatholicSaints.Info. 24 January 2018. Web. 8 December 2021.
<https://catholicsaints.info/blessed-josep-tarrats-comaposada/>

2) Tom Rochford, SJ. Blessed Jose Tarrats Comaposada. Accessed 5Apr2022.
https://www.jesuits.global/saint-blessed/blessed-jose-tarrats-comaposada/

3) The New York Times. 31Jan1932. Jesuit Expulsion Blow to Vatican. Accessed 5 April 2022.
https://www.nytimes.com/1932/01/31/archives/jesuit-expulsion-blow-to-vati can-spains-action-not-unexpected-but.html

4) Hagiography Circle: An Online Resource on Contemporary Hagiography. 1934, 1936-1939. Martyrs of the Religious Persecution during the Spanish Civil War. Accessed 5 April 2022.
www.newsaints.faithweb.com/martyrs/MSPC30.htm.

Bl. Francisca Pons Sarda (Sr. Gabriella of St. John of the Cross) (Spain/Argentina) (1880-1936), Martyr

28 years religious life spent working in hospitals, nursing homes and care homes for the disabled in Spain and Argentina[1]

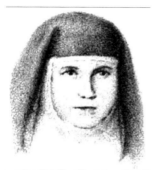

Sr. Gabriella de San
Giovanni della Croce
Source: santiebeati.it

Francisca Pons Sarda was born on July 18, 1880 in Espluga de Francoli, Tarragona, Spain to Jose Pons and Antonia Sarda. She was baptized at birth. She had a strong fiery and determined nature. "She demonstrated it, for example, when she set the antireligious books of a neighbor on fire, without fear of the owner's reaction, when she was just fifteen" years old.[2]

Francisca entered the novitiate of the Carmelite Missionaries in Barcelona, Spain, on May 5, 1907, at the age of 26, taking the name Sister Gabriella of San Giovanni della Croce (Sister Gabriella of St. John of the Cross). She made her solemn profession on October 17, 1913.

Her father was convinced that the religious vocation was not for his daughter. She was exuberant, liked boys and having fun. During the "Tragic Week" in Barcelona in 1909, in which the population experienced public unrest due to the proclamation of the second Spanish republic, he sent word inviting her to come home. When the Spanish Civil War began in 1936, he again sent messengers to invite her to return home. She refused each time and let him know that if the convent was on fire, she would be the last to leave. She believed that God would give her the grace necessary to suffer martyrdom if it was to occur.[2]

Sister Gabriella de San Giovanni della Croce worked at the hospital in Tarrega, the hospice for the blind in Santa Lucia in Barcelona, in Santa Coloma de Queralt and at the diocesan seminary of Barcelona in Las Corts. She was sent to Argentina for a few years and then returned to the Mother House in Gracia, Spain. There Sister Gabriella, along with Sister Daniela di San Barnaba (Vicenta Achurra Gogenola) cared for a sick person in their family home. They traveled by tram, Monday through Saturday, even after the

303

outbreak of the Spanish Civil War on July 18, 1936.

On July 31, 1936, the family of the sick person told the sisters that it was too dangerous to return to the convent in Gracia. A niece of Sister Gabriella, who worked at a local pharmacy of Messrs. Boque, offered a hiding place in her apartment. They tried to disguise themselves as they scurried to the apartment but were recognized as religious by a patrol of militiamen. "The concierge of the Boque house, who was waiting for them, saw that they were captured, insulted and pushed into a pickup truck. Monsieur Boque had an employee of the pharmacy chase the vehicle, but all was in vain. Shortly thereafter the nuns were shot outside the city, on the L'Arrabassada highway in Barcelona, Spain."[2] Sister Gabriella was 56 years old and had been a Carmelite sister for 28 years. They, along with the bodies of two other sisters from their congregation who had been shot and killed were buried in a mass grave.

The four Carmelite Missionaries were included in the cause for canonization that included 64 alleged martyrs: in addition to the 4 Carmelites, 44 Brothers of the Christian Schools, 14 Discalced Carmelites, 1 Carmelite Sister of Charity and a seminarian. All were declared venerable by decree of martyrdom promulgated on June 22, 2004 by His Holiness Pope St. John Paul II. She was beatified on October 28, 2007[3] by His Holiness Pope Benedict XVI. (Memorial - July 31)

References:

1) "Blessed Francisca Pons Sarda". CatholicSaints.Info. 25 January 2022. Web. 6 June 2022.
<https://catholicsaints.info/blessed-francisca-pons-sarda/>

2) Santi Beati. Blessed Gabriella of St. John of the Cross (Francisca Pons Sarda) Virgin and Martyr. Accessed 6 June 2022.
http://www.santiebeati.it/dettaglio/97177

3) Hagiography Circle: Martyrs of the Religious Persecution during the Spanish Civil War (1934, 1936-1939). Accessed 6 June 2022. http

Bl. Benito Solana Ruiz (Spain) (1882-1936), Martyr
Worked as a nurse and tailor in Zaragoza, Spain[1]

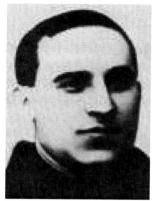

Bl. Benito Solana Ruiz
http://newsaints.faithweb.com/martyrs/MSPC26.htm

Benito Solana Ruiz of the Virgin of Villar, professed religious, Passionists, was born on February 17, 1882 in Cintruenigo, Navarra, Spain, the son of the village carpenter.

His parents were not supportive of his desire to enter the Religious life. However, in 1913, at the age of 31, he entered the Passionist Order in Daimiel, Spain. He was not a very good student and had difficulty with seminary studies. He became a brother taking the religious name Benito of the Virgin of Villar.

He served in may capacities. He worked as a cook and tailor in the Passionist house in Daimiel, Spain. In 1919 he moved to the house in Santa Clara, Cuba where he worked as both a tailor and porter. In 1922 he was assigned to the part of Mexico City called Tacubaya. While assigned in Mexico the anti-Catholic persecution began and the Cristero War began. He was, therefore, recalled to Daimiel, Spain where he worked briefly before moving to Zaragoza.

In Zaragoza, Spain Benito began nursing the sick. *[Note: Located in Zaragoza is the Church of Our Lady of the Pilar - where tradition reports the Blessed Virgin Mary was translocated by angels to give encouragement to Saint James the Great as he preached the Gospel message in Spain].* As a Passionist Brother, Benito was known for his humility, charity and patience especially when nursing sick patients.[2] He, himself, suffered from rheumatism.[1]

Blessed Benito Solana Ruiz was shot to death on July 25, 1936 in Urda, Toledo, Spain at the beginning of the Spanish Civil War (1936-1939). Twenty-five fellow Passionists were also killed.. He was beatified by Pope St. John Paul II on October 1, 1989. (Memorial - July 25).[3]

305

References:

1 "Blessed Benito Solana Ruiz". CatholicSaints.Info. 4 April 2018. Web. 8 December 2021. <https://catholicsaints.info/blessed-benito-solana-ruiz/>

2) Mission Priest (July 23, 2021). Bl. Benito Solana Ruiz: A Jack-of-all-trades. Accessed 5Apr2022. https://missionpriest.com/bl-benito-solana-ruiz-a-jack-of-all-trades/

3) Hagiography Circle: An Online Resource on Contemporary Hagiography. 1934, 1936-1939. Martyrs of the Religious Persecution during the Spanish Civil War. 15. Benito Solana Ruiz. Accessed 5 April 2022. www.newsaints.faithweb.com/martyrs/MSPC30.htm.

Bl. Juan Bautista Egozcuezabal Aldaz (Spain) (1882-1936), Martyr

During the Spanish Civil War, he was seized as he was leaving the hospital where he worked as a nurse caring for crippled children and killed when he would not renounce Christianity.[1]

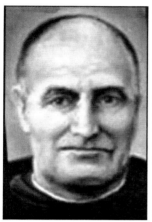

Bl. Juan Bautista Egozcuezabal Aldaz. Source: catholicsaints.info

Juan Bautista Egozcuezabal Aldaz was born on March 13, 1882 in Nuin, Navarra, Spain. He initially entered a Carmelite Order on January 31, 1911. A year later, in 1912 he joined the Hospitallers of Saint John of God. He worked in an asylum hospital. While leaving a hospital where he worked as a nurse with crippled children, he was ordered to blaspheme and renounce Christianity. He refused.

Blessed Juan Bautista Egozcuezabal Aldaz was shot to death on July 29, 1936 in Barcelona and his body was dumped in a field in Esplugas de Liobregat, near Barcelona, in Spain at the beginning of the Spanish Civil War (1936-1939).[1]

He was declared venerable with the promulgation of the decree of martyrdom on May 4, 1991 and beatified on October 25, 1992 both by Pope St. John Paul II.[2] (Memorial 29 July; 30 July as one of the Martyred Hospitallers of Spain).

References:
1) "Blessed Juan Bautista Egozcuezábal Aldaz". CatholicSaints.Info. 2 September 2017. Web. 8 December 2021.
<https://catholicsaints.info/blessed-juan-bautista-egozcuezabal-aldaz/>

2) Braulio Maria Corres Diaz de Cerio, Federico Rubio Alvarez, and 69 Companion martyrs from the Hospitallers of Saint John of God. (Juan Bautista Egozcuezabal Aldaz). Accessed 5April 2022.
http://newsaints.faithweb.com/martyrs/MSPC07.htm

3) Congregazione delle Cause dei Santi. 122 Spanish martyrs (1936). Accessed 4 June 2022.
http://www.causesanti.va/it/santi-e-beati/122-martiri-spagnoli.html

Bl. Juan Agustin Codera Marques (Spain) (1883-1936), Martyr
Worked as a nurse. Murdered on his way to visit the sick during in the Spanish Civil War.[1]

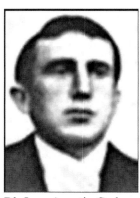

Bl. Juan Agustin Codera Marques.
catholicsaints.info

Blessed Juan Agustin Codera Marques, religious, Salesian of Don Bosco, was born on May 25, 1883 in Barbastro, Huesca, Spain. She was baptized the next day on May 6, 1883.

Juan Agustin Codera Marques entered the Salesians of Don Bosco taking his vows on July 24, 1919 in Carabanchel Alto, Madrid, Spain.

He was arrested several times in the persecutions of Catholics during the Spanish Civil War (1936-1939). Finally he was grabbed while on his way to visit the sick and shot on September 25, 1936 in Madrid, Spain.

Juan Agustin Codera Marques is listed amongst the martyrs of the Religious Persecution during the Spanish Civil War (1934, 1936-1939) with Enrique Saiz Aparicio and 62 companion martyrs from the Salesians of Don Bosco and the Clergy and lay faithful of the Dioceses of Madrid, Cordoba and Seville

He was declared venerable with the promulgation of the decree of martyrdom on June 26, 2006 and beatified on October 28, 2007 both by Pope Benedict XVI.[2] (Memorial 25 September).

References:

1) "Blessed Juan Agustín Codera Marqués". CatholicSaints.Info. 21 September 2015. Web. 8 December 2021.
<https://catholicsaints.info/blessed-juan-agustin-codera-marques/>

2) Hagiography Circle. Martyrs of the Religious Persecution during the Spanish Civil War (1934, 1936-1939). 34. Juan Agustin Codera Marques. Accessed 5 April 2022. http://newsaints.faithweb.com/martyrs/MSPC15.htm

3) Congregazione delle Cause dei Santi. 122 Spanish martyrs (1936). Accessed 4 June 2022.
http://www.causesanti.va/it/santi-e-beati/122-martiri-spagnoli.html

Bl. María Isabel López García (Sr. Mary of Peace) (Spain)
(1885-1936), Martyr
Sister of the Christian Doctrine
Served as a cook and nurse[1]

Maria Isabel Lopez Garcia (Sister Mary of Peace)[2] was born on August 12, 1885 in Turis, Valencia, Spain to Pietro Lopez and Maria Garcia. She was educated in a boarding school by religious sisters from the Congregation of the Sisters of the Christian Doctrine, a religious order founded in 1880 by Mother Micaela Grau for the catechetical instruction and education of children. Maria Isabel joined the congregation in 1911 at the age of 26. Though most of the sister were teachers, Isabel, who took the religious name, Sister Mary of Peace, served as a nurse and a cook.

At the beginning of the Spanish Civil War (1936-1939), many religious communities were dispersed due to great animosity towards religion. Mother Angeles of San Jose, the superior general of the Sisters of the Congregation of the Christian Doctrine gathered into an apartment all those who had no family or friends to host them.[3] There were 15 religious sisters living in semi-clandestine conditions and spending time in prayer and a small apostolate. They actually spent their last months sewing garments for those who would end their lives. The sister lived in fraternal charity and discovered how persecution, poverty and suffering are also ways that lead to God.

Often the militiamen would come to look for them. On the evening of November 19, 1936, a van came to pick them up for their last trip. They left the house praying, encouraging and forgiving each other. They were driven to the Paterna riding school, about six kilometers from Valencia. There, at one in the morning on November 20, 1936, they were shot while uttering words of forgiveness. The last to be killed was Mother Mary Suffrage, crying, "Long live Christ the King!" on behalf of the others.

And so, the nurse, Sister Mary of Peace was shot and killed for her faith on November 20, 1936 in Picadero de Paterna, Valencia, Spain along with 14 other sisters.

A total of 17 sisters from the congregation were shot and killed. They are:[2]

Killed on the night between September 26-27, 1936 near Barranco de los Perros, near Llosa de Ranes (Valencia)
1) Mother Maria del Rifugio (Teresa Rosat Balasch)
2) Sister Maria del Calvario (Josefa Romero Clariana)

Killed on November 20, 1936 at 1 a.m. at the Paterna riding school in Picadero de Paterna, Valencia, Spain
3) Superior General Mother Angela di San Giuseppe (Francisca Desamparados Honorata Lloret Marti)
4) Mother Maria Del Suffragio (Maria Antoniadel Sufragio Orts Baldo)
5) Mother Mary of Montserrat (Maria Dolores Llimona Planas)
6) Sister Teresa of Saint Joseph (Ascension Duart y Roig)
7) Mother Isabel Ferrer Sabria
8) Sister Maria of the Assumption (Josefa Mongoche Homs)
9) Sister Maria della Concezione (Emilia Marti Lacal)
10) Sister Maria Grazia (Paula de San Antonio)
11) Sister Maria of the Sacred Heart (Maria Purificacion Gomes Vives)
12) Sister Maria del Soccorso (Teresa Jimenez Baldovi)
13) Sister Maria de los Dolores (Gertrudis Suris Brusola)
14) Sr. Ignazia of the Blessed Sacrament (Josefa Pascual Pallardo)
15) Sister Maria del Rosario (Catalina Calpe Ibanez)
16) Sister Mary of Peace (Isabel Lopez Garcia)
17) Sister Marcella of St. Thomas (Aurea Navarro)

The diocesan information gathering process began on July 5, 1965 in the Diocese of Valencia and ended on June 1, 1969. Towards the end of this process, on December 12, 1968, the remains of Sister Mary of Peace and the fourteen other sisters were exhumed and placed in a funeral monument in the church of the Mother House. It was not until 1983 that the remains of the first two sisters killed was located.

The sisters were declared venerable by the decree martyrdom promulgated by Pope St. John Paul II on July 6, 1993. The 17 Sisters of the Christian Doctrine were beatified by His Holiness Pope St. John Paul II on October 1, 1995[4], in a group of 45 martyrs who died during the Spanish Civil War (1936-1939), together with 64 victims of the French Revolution (1789-1799) and the Piarist Father Pietro Casani. (Memorial - November 20).

"Lord, make me worthy to be a martyr for Your sake."

References:
1) "Blessed María Isabel López García". CatholicSaints.Info. 1 May 2022. Web. 6 June 2022.
<https://catholicsaints.info/blessed-maria-isabel-lopez-garcia/>

2) Blessed Angela of San Giuseppe (Francesca Onorata Lloret Marti) and 14 companions, Virgins and martyrs. Accessed 6 June 2022.
http://santiebeati.it/dettaglio/78590

3) Congregazione delle Cause dei Santi. Angeles de San Jose and 16 companions. Accessed 6 June 2022.
http://www.causesanti.va/it/santi-e-beati/angeles-de-san-jose-e-16-compagn e.html

4) Hagiography Circle: Martyrs of the Religious Persecution during the Spanish Civil War (1934, 1936-1939). Accessed 6 June 2022.
http://newsaints.faithweb.com/martyrs/MSPC02.htm

311

Bl. Vicenta Achurra Gogenola (Sr. Daniela of San Barnaba) (Spain) (1890-1936), Martyr

Worked at the Las Corts mental hospital,
Badalona asylum,
the Amparo de Santa Lucia house for the blind
and provided home care for the sick[1]

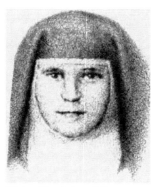

Sister Daniela of San Barnaba
Source: santiebeati.it

Vicenta Achurra Gogenola was born on April 4, 1890 in Berriatua in Biscay, Spain. She was the last of six children born in a poor and deeply religious family. She was baptized in the parish Church of St. Peter on April 5, 1890.

When Vicenta was twenty five, she chose to consecrate herself to God as a Carmelite Missionary Sister. Her novitiate began in 1915 at the Mother House in Gracia, Barcelona, Spain. She made her first profession on October 16, 1916 taking the name Sister Daniela of San Barnaba. She made her final profession on October 17, 1921.

She was first assigned to minister in the communities of Las Corts, the diocesan seminary, and the asylum of Badalona in Barcelona. She also cared for the blind people at the Hospice of Santa Lucia in Barcelona. Just prior to the Spanish Civil War, she returned to the Mother House in Gracia to give care to a sick person in their home along with Sister Gabriella.

Sister Daniela was known to be happy, industrious, friendly and particularly devoted to the Sacred Heart of Jesus and Our Lady of Mount Carmel. She had a great sense of humor but was also know to react abruptly when anxious, for which she always apologized. Her patients were particularly fond of her. One in particular initially refused her care. However, after a week, he refused to have anyone replace her.

In January 1935, Sister Daniela returned to Berriatua to care for her dying mother. She was subsequently tasked to accompany nine young postulants on a long journey from Zaragoza to Barcelona. On the way they prayed, she taught them some religious songs and addressed their fears due to the complicated political

312

situation in Spain and Barcelona, stating, "Even if we are martyrs, it doesn't matter." This mission completed, Sister Daniela returned to the Mother House where she resided while she provided care to the blind at Hospice of Santa Lucia and home care for the sick.

For a few months, Sister Daniela and Sister Gabriella of San Giovanni della Croce took turns caring for the same sick person in Pedralbes.
They traveled by tram, Monday through Saturday, even after the outbreak of the Spanish Civil War on July 18, 1936.

On July 31, 1936, the family of the sick person told the sisters that it was too dangerous to return to the convent in Gracia. A niece of Sister Gabriella, who worked at a local pharmacy of Messrs. Boque, offered a hiding place in her apartment. They tried to disguise themselves as they scurried to the apartment but were recognized as religious by a patrol of militiamen.

> "The concierge of the Boque house, who was waiting for them, saw that they were captured, insulted and pushed into a pickup truck. Monsieur Boque had an employee of the pharmacy chase the vehicle, but all was in vain. Shortly thereafter the nuns were shot outside the city, on the L'Arrabassada highway in Barcelona, Spain."2

Sister Daniela was 46 years old and had been a Carmelite missionary for 20 years. They, along with the bodies of two other sisters from their congregation, Sister Speranza della Croce and Sister Maria Rifugio di Sant' Angel, who had also been shot and killed, were buried in a mass grave.

The four Carmelite Missionaries were included in the cause for canonization that included 64 alleged martyrs: in addition to the 4 Carmelites, 44 Brothers of the Christian Schools, 14 Discalced Carmelites, 1 Carmelite Sister of Charity and a seminarian. All were declared venerable by decree of martyrdom promulgated on June 22, 2004 by His Holiness Pope St. John Paul II. She was beatified on October 28, 2007[3] by His Holiness Pope Benedict XVI. (Memorial - July 31)

Even if we are martyrs, it doesn't matter.

313

References:

1) "Blessed Vicenta Achurra Gogenola". CatholicSaints.Info. 31 July 2016. Web. 6 June 2022.
<https://catholicsaints.info/blessed-vicenta-achurra-gogenola/>

2) Santi Beati. Blessed Daniela of San Barnaba (Vicenta Achurra Gogenola, Virgin and Martyr. Accessed 6 June 2022.
http://www.santiebeati.it/dettaglio/95705

3) Hagiography Circle: Martyrs of the Religious Persecution during the Spanish Civil War (1934, 1936-1939) [22]. Accessed 6 June 2022.
http://newsaints.faithweb.com/martyrs/MSPC22.htm

Three Red Cross nurses killed in the Spanish Civil War
"The Martyr Nurses of Astorga

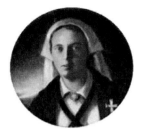
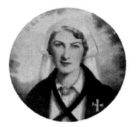
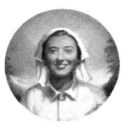

Olga P. Monteserin   Pilar Gullon   Octavia Iglesias
Source: CatholicHerald.com

Bl. Octavia Iglesias Blanco (Spain) (1894-1936), Martyr
Lay woman. Red Cross Nurse.
Raped & murdered in the Spanish Civil War.[1]

Octavia Iglesias Blanco was born on November 30, 1894 in
Astorga, Leon, Spain. She was baptized on December 9, 1894 in the
parish of San Julian. Her family was pious and committed to
virtuous living and charitable works. They assisted in founding the
Convent of the Congregation of the Most Holy Redeemer
(Redemptorists) of Astorga where Octavia's sister consecrated
herself as a nun.

Octavia cared for her elderly and sick father and then her
widowed mother. She was a member of Catholic Action and the
associations of the Daughters of Mary and of the Sacred Heart. She
worked as a Red Cross nurse during the Spanish Civil War (1936-
1939).

On October 27, 1936, at age 41, she was imprisoned,
abused, raped and ordered to renounce Christianity by the anti-
Catholic militia. She refused. After a harrowing night of torture, she
was executed at noon the next day by female militiamen who
volunteered to kill her and her two companions: Maria del Pilar
Gullon Yturriag and Olga Perez-Monteserin Nunez. (continued
below)...

Bl. Maria Pilar Gullon Yturriaga (Spain) (1911-1936), Martyr
Lay woman. Cared for the sick in their homes. Trained and served as a Red Cross nurse at the front in the Spanish Civil War.[2]

Maria Pilar Gullon Yturriaga was born on May 29, 1911 in Madrid, Spain to Manuel Gullon and Pilar Yturriaga. She was the eldest of four children born to their union. She was baptized in the parish church of San Genesio on June 28, 1911 in Arles with the names of Maria del Pilar Peregrina Matea Maximina.[3] She made her First Holy Communion at the Blanca de Castilla school in Madrid. Maria Pilar's father worked as a lawyer and was a member of the Liberal Party in the National Parliament for the constituency of Astorga.

Pilar remained single and cared for her parents, particularly her father who was ill. On July 16, 1936, the family returned to Astorga. There Maria Pilar was a member of Catholic Action and the Daughters of Mary in the Diocese of Astorga, Spain. She also taught catechism to children and cared for ill and infirmed in their homes. She trained as a nurse and served as a Red Cross nurse at the front during the Spanish Civil War (1936-2939).

On October 27, 1936, she was imprisoned, abused, raped and ordered to renounce Christianity by the anti-Catholic militia. She refused. When she was given one last chance to renounce her fait she responded, "Long live Spain, love live Christ the King."[2] At the age of 25, she was executed by shooting at noon on October 28, 1936 by female militiamen who volunteered to kill her and fellow nurses: Octavia Iglesias Blanco and Olga Perez Monteserin Nunez. (continued below)...

Bl. Olga Perez-Monteserin Nunez (France/Spain) (1913-1936), Martyr
Lay woman. Red Cross nurse.
Raped and murdered in the Spanish Civil War. Martyr.[4]

Olga Perez Monteserin Nunez was born on March 16, 1913 in Paris, France, the second of three children born to parents from Astorga. She was baptized on July 5, 1913 in the parish of St. Francis Xavier in Paris. She remained single and dedicated herself to family life and artistic work, particularly painting. Her father was a

316

very famous painter from Leon. He moved his family to Astorga, Spain, in 1920. There Olga was engaged in domestic work along with plastic arts and painting. She also trained as a nurse and served as a Red Cross nurse at the front during the Spanish Civil War (1936-1939).

On October 27, 1936, at age 23, she was imprisoned, abused, raped and ordered to renounce Christianity by the anti-Catholic militia. She refused. After a harrowing night of torture, she was executed at noon the next day, on October 28, 1936, by female militiamen who volunteered to kill her and fellow nurses: Octavia Iglesias Blanco and Maria del Pilar Gullon Yturriag.

...(Continuation) **Martyrdom:** On October 8, 1936 the women arrive at the hospital in Puerto de Somiedo (Pola de Somiedo-Asturias) to serve for eight days. Their time completed, they remained at the hospital in the midst of a very harsh anti-religious atmosphere prevalent during the Spanish Civil War (1936-1939).

At dawn on Tuesday, October 27, 1936 attacks intensified on the front where the small hospital was located. They could have fled but Pilar, Octavia and Olga decided not to abandon the wounded. They placed their own lives in danger as they continued to assist the wounded. When the hospital was overtaken, the wounded were shot and the medical personnel arrested. The three nurses were taken, after a long march, to Pola de Somiedo with other prisoners which included the commander, chaplain and doctor who were killed. Although the women were Red Cross nurses and should have had immunity in combat per the Geneva Conventions, they were handed over to the local War Committee and then to the militiamen who demanded they renounce their faith. When they refused to renounce their faith, the nurses were abused and raped throughout the night. Naked, they were taken to a meadow near Pola de Somiedo, Asturias, Spain at noon on October 28, 1936 and shot while acclaiming "Christ the King." After killing them, the militia women shared the clothes of the three nurses. Their bodies were degraded and left in a common grave dug by some men from the town who were forced to do so by the militiamen.

This was one of the first murders of Red Cross nurses since usually nurses and other health professionals were given immunity. All three declared themselves openly to be Catholic and that they belonged to the Daughters of Mary, the Conference of St. Vincent de

317

Paul and Catholic Action. According to an account of Maria Pilar's nephew Manuel Gullon,

> the Red Cross volunteer nurses rotated every fortnight, and they had the opportunity to return to Astorga and take turns with other young women to care for the wounded from the [Spanish] Civil War at the Hospital de Sangre de Pola de somiedo, they asked to stay on the second shift as well. That was when the Republican militiamen attacked... They were taken handcuffed and tied to the town. The leader of the expedition, nicknamed 'El Patas' offered to set them free and return to Astorga if they renounced their faith and joined his party. When they refused, they locked them in a house in Pola, which still exists, and 'El Patas" told the militiamen to do with them what they wanted during the night. They raped them and their boss even drove a bullock cart through the village so that the screeching of its axles made it more difficult to hear the screams of the three nurses. The next day, on October 28, 1936, at noon, they were shot naked."[5]

The three are known as the martyr nurses of Astorga.[5] Their fame spread immediately in the ecclesial community. On January 30, 1938, the remains were interred in the Cathedral of Astorga, Spain. On June 28, 1948, at the request of the National Assembly of the Red Cross, they were transferred to a new mausoleum in the chapel of St. John the Baptist in the Cathedral.[5]

During his interview Manuel Gullon explained that he was not aware of any miracle specifically attributed to the three nurses. However, his father, Pilar Gullon's brother, composed a prayer for the nurses to intercede for the health of his mother. Nine days after his father prayed the prayer, his mother recovered completely.

Octavia Iglesias Blanco and companions were declared venerable with the promulgation of the decree of martyrdom on June 11, 2019 and beatified on May 29, 2021 both by Pope Francis.[7] (Memorial - November 6)

According to the Catholic News Agency, the Spanish Civil War was fought from 1936-1939 between National forces, led by Francisco Franco, and the Republican faction. During the war, Republicans martyred thousands of clerics, religious, and laity; of these 11 have been canonized, and more than 1,900 beatified.[8]

318

References:

1) "Blessed Octavia Iglesias Blanco". CatholicSaints.Info. 1 November 2021. Web. 8 December 2021.
<https://catholicsaints.info/blessed-octavia-iglesias-blanco/>

2) "Blessed María Pilar Gullón Yturriaga". CatholicSaints.Info. 1 November 2021. Web. 8 December 2021.
<https://catholicsaints.info/blessed-maria-pilar-gullon-yturriaga/>

3) Santi Beati. Maria Pilar Gullon Yturriaga. Accessed 4 June 2022.
http://santiebeati.org/dettaglio/99181

4) "Blessed Olga Pérez-Monteserín Núñez". CatholicSaints.Info. 1 November 2021. Web. 8 December 2021.
<https://catholicsaints.info/blessed-olga-perez-monteserin-nunez/>

5) Aciprensa. (12Jun2019). This is the story of the three nurses whose martyrdom the Pope recognized. Accessed 10 April 2022.
https://www.aciprensa.com/noticias/esta-es-la-historia-de-las-tres-enfermeras-de-las-que-el-papa-reconocio-el-martirio-75899

6) Aciprensa. (15Oct2020). The three lay martyrs of Astorga will be beatified on this date. Accessed 10 April 2022.
https://www.aciprensa.com/noticias/las-tres-martires-laicas-de-astorga-seran-beatificadas-en-esta-fecha-97177

7) Hagiography Circle: An Online Resource on Contemporary Hagiography. Martyrs of the Religious Persecution during the Spanish Civil War (1934, 1936-1939). [199] Maria del Pilar Gullon Yturriaga and 2 compansions from the Lay Faithful of the Diocese of Astorga. Accessed 10 April 2022.
http://newsaints.faithweb.com/martyrs/MSPC55.htm

8) Catholic News Agency. (1Jun2021). Spanish Civil War Martyrs of Astorga 'didn't let themselves be overcome by fear.' Accessed 18 May 2022.
https://www.catholicnewsagency.com/news/247857/spanish-civil-war-martyrs-of-astorga-didnt-let-themselves-be-overcome-by-fear

9) Congregazione delle Cause dei Santi. Maria Colon Gullon Yturriaga and 2 Companions (1936). Accessed 4 June 2022.
http://www.causesanti.va/it/santi-e-beati/maria-colon-gullon-yturriaga-e-2-compagne.html

Bl. Leonella Sgorbati (Italy/Kenya/Somalia) (1940-2006),
Martyr
Assigned at hospitals in Nyeri and Kiambu, Kenya in 1970's.
Midwife and Instructor.
Started Hermann Gmeiner School of Registered Community Nursing attached to the SOS Children's Village hospital in Mogadishu, Somalia.[1]

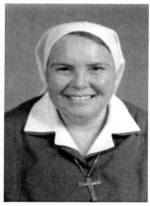

Bl. Leonella Sgorbati
Source: consolatasisters.org

Rosa Maria Sgorbati was born on December 9, 1940 in Rezzanello di Gazzola, Piacenza, Italy to Carlo Sgorbati and Giovannina Teresa Vigilini. She was the youngest of three children. Her father was a farmer and her mother was a homemaker. Rosa was baptized on the day of her birth at the parish church of San Savio.

Immediately following World War II (1938-1945), her father changed occupations from farming to wholesale fruit and vegetable reseller in Sesto San Giovanni, Milan. Thus, when Rosa was 9 years old, On October 9, 1950, the family moved to that Milanese suburb. Her father died a year later on July 16, 1951.

Rosa was sent to a boarding school of Sisters. She had a singular experience at the school one day after the director gave her a book and said, "Take this little book and try to read it." The book was the Gospels. "Sitting in the small chapel of the college, in front of the picture of the crucifixion that was above the altar, she began an increasingly intense dialogue with the Lord..." "...In contact with the Word of Jesus, something great happened to her..." In her diary she wrote, *"I felt INHABITED on that distant day - April 1952 - ... and you kept me in You, my Lord, or You remained in me.. Never again alone... INHABITED...."*[2] Her family even noticed a difference when she returned home. In her teens she expressed a desire to become a missionary but complied with her mother's request to wait until she was older.

When Rosa was 23 years old, on May 5, 1963, she joined the Institute of the Missionary Sisters of the Consolata and was welcomed by Mother Nazarena Fissore, the Superior General. Her

321

six month postulancy began on May 20, 1963 in Sanfre, Cueno, Italy. She then received the habit taking the name Sister Leonella. She studied in the novitiate under Sister Paolina Emiliani beginning on November 21, 1963 in Nepi, Viterbo, Italy. Sister Leonella made her first vows the following day on November 22, 1965.[3] She then traveled to England and studied nursing and midwifery. She

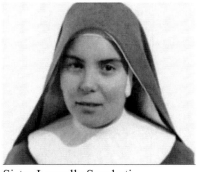

Sister Leonella Sgorbati
leonella.missionairedellaconsolata.org

graduated from the State Enrolled Nursing Program in 1969 and completed the first part of the midwifery course in 1970.[4] The program was intense alternating between training, study and hospital internships. Since the program was fifty kilometers from her community of sisters, she was only able to return to the community on days of rest. Sister Leonella was noted for her brilliant and lively mind and formidable memory.

In September 1970, Sister Leonella was sent to Kenya where she worked at the Consolata Hospital Mathari in Nyeri and the Nazareth Hospital in Kiambu for 13 years from 1970-1983. During this time her duties included serving as a midwife. Also during this time, Sister Leonella made her final religious profession in November 1972. After additional training, in 1985, she began teaching in a school for nurses adjoining the Nkubu Hospital in

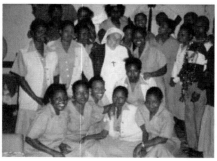

Meru, Kenya focusing on the 100 bed maternity ward. She was very solicitous of the young trainees and also took extra time to give lessons to high school graduates.

In 1993 she was chosen by the sisters to represent them at the VII General Chapter of their Institute. She had been working in the African mission for over twenty years and would help plan for the institute's next six years. After the Chapter, from November 1993 to 1999, she then served as the Regional superior of the Consolata Missionary Sisters in Kenya.

At the conclusion of two consecutive three-year periods as Regional Superior, Sister Leonella was asked to be part of the Sabbatical team for the sisters of the African continent. She cared for the house and the sisters who passed by for their rest time from 2000-2005. She was always on the move with her apron on and sleeves rolled up. "All were amazed by her generosity and attentiveness.[5]

After serving 31 years as a missionary in Kenya, in 2001, Sister Leonella traveled to Somalia to investigate the prospects of opening a nursing school in the hospital run by the organization SOS Children's Village. It was the only health facility in all of Mogadishu providing pediatric care free of charge. During this time Somalia was unstable and dangerous but the sisters were enthusiastic about running the Center, teaching and preparing future nurses. It was the SOS that had asked the Consolata Missionaries to teach in their school of nursing. Nurses and doctors had not been trained in Somalia for ten years.

Sister Leonella had to find common elements between Christianity and Islam. It was necessary to prove that the scientific notions taught were not against the Koran. Also Muslim authorities had to be assured that she did not proselytize. Sister Leonella did not proselytize, instead, she valued interreligious dialogue.[6] Some fundamentalists were not convinced. This created an exhausting environment in which to work. The sisters' activities were restricted to the sisters' house, SOS hospital and crossing the street that divided the two with an escort.

In 2002, the Hermann Gmeiner School of Registered Community Nursing attached to the SOS Children's Village hospital opened in Mogadishu, Somalia. Sister Leonella was the director and also an instructor. "Sister Leonella fought a long bureaucratic battle to obtain internationally recognized diplomas for her students; she succeeded and the World Health Organization (WHO) issued internationally recognized diplomas to her students."[7]

> Following this, Sister Leonella returned to Kenya with three of her students, whom she enrolled at the Medical Training College. Her aim was to have these three students form the nucleus of the future tutors at the school. Getting these students into Kenya, and sorting out the registration and financial difficulties in enrolling them into the college was another struggle, but as soon as Sister saw it through, she headed off to Uganda to scout for hospitals willing to

323

train her other students in operating theater work."[7] They graduated their first class in 2006.

Sister Leonella briefly returned to Italy in 2006 on sabbatical. There, in a television interview, Sister Leonella stated, "I know there is a bullet with my name on it. I don't know when it will arrive, but as long as it does not arrive, I will stay [in Somalia]." Sister Leonella had difficulty returning to Mogadishu because Islamic courts had taken control of the area. She managed to return to her work at the hospital on September 13, 2006. Reportedly some fundamentalist thought that the nursing students were being indoctrinated into the Christian religion.[7]

One morning Sister Leonella arose very early to pray and told the sisters they needed to offer many prayers for His Holiness Pope Benedict XVI and for the Church. She had heard on the radio that the Muslim world was in great agitation because of a speech the Holy Father gave in Regensburg, Germany on September 12, 2006.[8] Some were stirring up violence against the Church. Four days after her return to Somalia, Sister Leonella, along with her bodyguard/driver, were killed:

> "On the fateful day of the 17th of September [Sunday], Sister Leonella crossed the road that separates the hospital from the accommodation of the Consolata Sisters. Hiding behind vehicles and kiosks that are found along this road, two gunmen attacked the Sister. The first shot hit her in the thigh, her bodyguard, Mohamed Osman Mahamud, [a Muslim father of four], opened fire on the to gunmen. They fired back killing him and hitting Sister Leonella twice. One of these bullets entered her back and severed an artery causing a severe hemorrhage. Sister Leonella was rushed into the nearby hospital...[7]

The Consolata sisters relate:[9]

> "Shortly after, someone excitedly knocked on the door, just enough time to hear the name "Leonella" and Sister Gianna Irene Peano with Sister Marzia rushed to the hospital. Where she had been transported; Sister Leonella was very pale and suffering. There they found a feverish bustle of nurses and doctors who tried in every possible way to save her with oxygen and transfusions, while the students offered their blood. They approached Sister Leonella, she was wet with sweat, but conscious.

324

She moved her livid lips and whispered, "I can hardly breathe." Meanwhile, people flocked to the hospital entrance, the tension and pain were strong and almost palpable. The guards managed to make an opening for Sister Annalisa Costardi, who entered the building. Sister Leonella asleep, but conscious. She with the other sisters hastened to communicate the incident to the superior in Italy and Kenya.

Meanwhile, the surgeon called the Flying Doctor's plane, hoping to be able to transport her to Nairobi [Kenya]. In the midst of all this movement, Sister Leonella lay there, suffering, with too little oxygen for her lungs. She took in the air enough to call Sister Gianna Irene, only a whisper came out, but her sister heard and immediately noticed her and brought her face close to Leonella's. Sister Gianna Irene recalls: "There was no sign of fear or tension, not even anxiety, but you could see a great peace that meant something important that was close to her heart and with a faint voice she said: "Forgiveness, forgiveness, forgiveness."

The United Nations helped move Sister Leonella's body and evacuate the other Consolata sisters from Somalia to Kenya. Sister Leonella's funeral was conducted at the Consolata Chapel in Nairobi, Kenya where she was buried. Her body was exhumed on September 30, 2017 and is now kept in the Flora Hostel Chapel in Nairobi.

On September 23, 2006, 6 days following her martyrdom, His Holiness Pope Benedict XVI, in an address to the Bishops taking part in the formation update meeting organized by the Congregation for the Evangelization of Peoples in the Hall of the Swiss at Castel Gandolfo stated,

> *"How can we forget the many priests, men and women religious and lay people in mission lands who have sealed with blood their fidelity to Christ and to the Church, in past centuries and in our times? In the last few days, the oblation of Sr. Leonella Sgorbati, a Consolata Missionary barbarically killed in Moga-dishu, Somalia, has been added to the number of these heroic Gospel witnesses. This martyrology, in the past and in our day, adorns the history of the Church. Even in suffering and apprehension, it keeps alive in our souls trust in the glorious flourishing of Christian faith, for as Tertullian says, "The blood of martyrs is the seed of Christians".*[10]

Sister Leonella Sgorbati was declared venerable with the promulgation of the decree of martyrdom on November 8, 2017 and beatified on May 26, 2018[11] both by Pope Francis. Her beatification was celebrated at the Cathedral of Santa Maria Assunta and Santa Giustina in Piacenza, Italy. Blessed Leonella Sgorbati is the second Italian Consolata Missionary sister working in Africa to be beatified. The first, Blessed Sister Irene Stefani who was beatified on May 23, 2015, was also a nurse. (Memorial - September 17). Website: https://missionariedellaconsolata.org/i-nostri-santi-2/

One must have so much charity to give one's life.
We missionaries are voted to give our lives for the mission [5]

Prayer for the Intercession of Blessed Leonella Sgorbati:[12]
Eternal Father, who through your Holy Spirit,
work in the midst of all peoples, regardless of their culture and their
religion, look with mercy at humankind, often without peace and
reluctant to forgive.
Through the intercession of
the Blessed Sr. Leonella Sgorbati, "faithful and joyful disciple of the
Gospel" who bore witness with her blood to her love for you and for
those mostly in need,
grant us the favour we are asking and
give us the joy to see her recognized as a martyr for the faith.
We ask this through Jesus Christ Our Lord,
model and origin of every martyrdom. Amen.

References:
1) "Blessed Leonella Sgorbati". CatholicSaints.Info. 21 July 2021. Web. 8 December 2021. <https://catholicsaints.info/blessed-leonella-sgorbati/>

2) Suore Missionaire della Consolata. Beata Leonella Sgorbati. Accessed 4 June 2002. https://leonella.missionariedellaconsolata.org/anni-giovanili/

3) Suore Missionaire della Consolata. Beata Leonella Sgorbati. Accessed 4 June 2002. https://leonella.missionariedellaconsolata.org/primi-passi/

4) Consolata Missionaries. Our Saints. Accessed 18 April 2022. https://missionariedellaconsolata.org/i-nostri-santi-2/

5) Suore Missionaire della Consolata. Beata Leonella Sgorbati. Accessed 4 June 2002. https://leonella.missionariedellaconsolata.org/missione/

6) Suore Missionaire della Consolata. Beata Leonella Sgorbati. Accessed 4 June 2002.
https://leonella.missionariedellaconsolata.org/missione-in-somalia/

7) Roman Catholic Mission Somalia. (3Jul2014). Missionaries Murdered in Somalia: Sister Leonella Sgorbati Consolata Missionary Sister. Accessed 18 April 2022.
https://rcmsomalia.blogspot.com/2014/07/missionaries-murdered-in-somalia-sister.html

8) Pope Benedict XVI. (12Sep2006). Lecture of the Holy Father: Faith, Reason and the University-Memories and Reflections. Apostolic Journey to Munchen, Altotting and Regensburg. Accessed 4 June 2022.
https://www.vatican.va/content/benedict-xvi/en/speeches/2006/september/documents/hf_ben-xvi_spe_20060912_university-regensburg.html

9) Suore Missionaire della Consolata. Beata Leonella Sgorbati. Accessed 4 June 2002. https://leonella.missionariedellaconsolata.org/martirio/

10) Pope Benedict XVI. (23Sep2006). Address of His Holiness Benedict XVI to the Bishops taking part in the formation update meeting organized by the Congregation for the Evangelization of Peoples. Accessed 18 April 2022.
https://www.vatican.va/content/benedict-xvi/en/speeches/2006/september/documents/hf_ben-xvi_spe_20060923_corso-evang.html

11) Hagiography Circle: An Online Resource on Contemporary Hagiography.2006. Rosa Maria Sgorbati (Leonella). Accessed 16 April 2022. http://newsaints.faithweb.com/year/2006.htm#Sgorbati

12) Sr. Leonella Sgorbati. Accessed 16 April 2022.
http://consolatasisters.org/sr-leonella-sgorbati/

13) Institute of the Missionary Sisters of the Consolata. (26Oct2019). The Writings of Blessed Leonella Sgorbati. As of 4June2022 only available in Italian, though English version has been requested.
https://leonella.missionariedellaconsolata.org/nuova-pubblicazione-gli-scritti-della-beata-leonella-sgorbati-martire/

14) Congregazione delle Cause dei Santi. Leonella Sgorbati.
http://www.causesanti.va/it/santi-e-beati/leonella-sgorbati.html

Nurses Martyred
by Soviet Communists - 1945

Martyrs-Congregation of St. Elizabeth-Soviet Occupation-1945
Nurses martyred for their faith under
Soviet Communist Regimes in Eastern Europe

The following are religious sisters from the Congregation of Saint Elizabeth, founded in the mid-19th century Silesia by Blessed Maria Luiza Merkert to nurse cholera and typhus patients. In addition to the evangelical counsels of poverty, chastity and obedience, the Sisters take a fourth vow to assist the sick and most needy The sisters of St. Elizabeth were from one of many religious orders which faced brutality during the 1944-1945 Soviet sweep through Poland. These ten (10) professed religious Sisters of St. Elizabeth were chosen for beatification, from among more than 100 murdered sisters from the Congregation of Saint Elizabeth, based upon the availability of documentation and witnesses, 76 years after they were killed.

The women ranged in age from 29 to 70. They were killed while resisting rape and facing other atrocities by Soviet soldiers in the final months of World War II. This mass beatification highlights a little known historical period and recalls the terrible sufferings faced by religious orders during the Soviet's presence in Poland.

"Contemporary opinion still has trouble grasping the parallel criminality of Nazis and communists, and isn't much interested in martyr stories," stated Jan Zaryn, director of Poland's Roman Dmowski and Ignacy Jan Paderewski Institute for the Legacy of National Thought.[1] He further stated, "Poles experienced both totalitarian systems, and remember how Soviets brought terror, rape, arson and captivity with them, arresting and murdering priests and nuns in a bid to prove only lunatics believed in God." Polish cities and towns had been "treated as conquered territory to be plundered and destroyed," with Catholic churches torched and priests and nuns "raped, murdered and driven out." Harsh anti-church measures continued in Poland as the Soviet-backed communist regime took power after World War II, viewing religious orders as secretive organizations threatening its absolute power. In the western region,

323 convents were closed in August 1954 under a campaign code-named "Operation X2," with more than 1,300 nuns rounded up by armed militia and bused to labor camps with no electricity and where tuberculosis was rife. In Czechoslovakia up to 700 Catholic convents were seized in a coordinated action in 1950, leaving an estimated 10,000 nuns incarcerated in prison and detention centers.[2]

A congregation statement said that these 10 religious sisters of St. Elizabeth had been recognized as martyrs from the time of their deaths, as recorded in a 1946 letter by their superior general, Mother Mathildis Kuttner. A statement from the congregation revealed that, "Many girls, women and nuns were raped despite heroically resisting until reduced to a defenseless state by beating. A gunshot often silenced such victims forever." "For many years, we were not permitted even to mention their Christian heroism. But today their names belong to history, revealing these unbroken witnesses of faith to contemporary humanity.[3]

The ten Sister of Saint Elizabeth martyred in *odium fidei* under Communist Regime in Eastern Europe were declared venerable with the promulgation of the decree of martyrdom on June 19, 2021 and their beatification was approved both by His Holiness Pope Francis.[4] The ceremony occurred on June 11, 2022, in Wrocław, officiated by Marcello Cardinal Semeraro, Prefect of the Dicastery for the Causes of Saints (Memorial - May 11).[6]

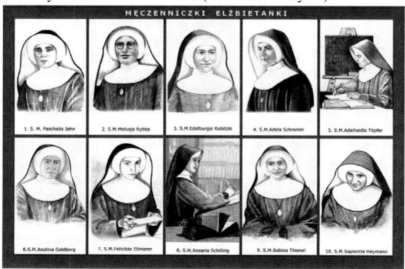

Bl. Maria Magdalena Jahn (Sr. M. Paschalis) (Silesia, Poland) (1898-1945), was born on September 7, 1898 in Gorna Wies, Nysa, Poland. In 1938, she joined the Congregation of Saint Elizabeth founded by St. Mother Maria Merkert and made her temporary profession on October 19, 1939. She was first sent to Kluczbork and Glubczyce as a nurse for the care of children and the elderly. In 1942 she was transferred to Nysa and assigned to cooking and assisting elderly nuns. When the Soviet Red Army entered into the city on March 22, 1945, out of obedience to the Superior, she left Nysa and took refuge in Sobotin (Czech Republic). When Soviet forces occupied the area, she sought safety with another nun in a parish schoolhouse, but was spotted by a Soviet soldier. On May 11, 1945, 47 year old Sister Maria Paschalis was shot when she rebuffed his advances. She died on May 11, 1945 in Sobotin (aka Zoptau), Sumperk, Czech Republic.

"I belong to Jesus, he is my husband"
the last words of Sister Paschalis

Bl. Marta Rybka (Sr. M. Melusja Rybka) (Poland) (1905-1945), was born June 11, 1905 in Pawlow Skabimierz, Brzeg, Poland. She entered the Congregation of the Sisters of Saint Elizabeth and took the name Sister Maria Melusja. Towards the end of World War II, she was shot trying to protect a local girl from a Soviet trooper at Nysa. She died March 24, 1945 in Nysa (aka Neisse Oberneuland), Poland.

Bl. Juliana Kubitzki (Sr. M. Edelburgis) (Poland) (1905-1945), was born on February 9, 1905 in Dabrowska Dolna, Pokoj, Namyslow, Poland. She entered the Congregation of the Sisters of Saint Elizabeth and made her first profession on April 28, 1931 and perpetual vows on June 29, 1936 taking the name Sister Maria Edelburgis. *She worked as an ambulance nurse.* Towards the end of World War II when Soviet Forces occupied the area she hid with other nuns in the presbytery chapel at Zary. She was found, beaten and shot during a struggle when Soviet troops entered the building in February 1945. She died on February 20, 1945 in Zary, Poland at the age of 40.

331

Bl. Klara Schramm (Sr. M. Adela) (Poland) (1885-1945), was born on June 3, 1885 in Laczna, Klodzko, Poland. She entered the Congregation of the Sisters of St. Elizabeth making her first profession on August 16, 1915 and perpetual vows on June 29, 1924, taking the name Sister Maria Adela. At the end of World War II, she was a convent superior in Godzieszów. She was seized by Soviet soldiers while seeking refuge at a nearby farm. She was buried in a bomb crater after being shot with her hosts and others. She died on February 25, 1945 in Godzieszow (aka Gunthersdorf, Boleslawiec, Poland.)

Bl. Jadwiga Topfer (Sr. M. Adelheidis) (Poland) (1887-1945), was born August 26, 1887 in Nysa, Poland. She entered the Congregation of the Sisters of Saint Elizabeth making her first profession on June 15, 1920 and perpetual vows on July 28, 1919, taking the name Sister Maria Adelheidis. Towards the end of World War II, she was killed in Nysa by Soviet soldiers at Nysa. She died March 24, 1945 in Nysa (aka Neisse Oberneuland), Poland.

Bl. Helena Goldberg (Sr. M. Acutina) (Poland) (1882-1945) was born on July 6, 1882 in Dluzek, Nowy Targ, Poland. She entered the Congregation of the Sisters of Saint Elizabeth making her first first profession on June 15, 1908 and perpetual vows on July 25, 1917. She taught war orphans. Towards the end of World War II, she escaped from the village of Lubiaz with a group of girls, only to be apprehended by drunken soldiers. She was shot trying to protect the girls from rape by the soldiers. She died on May 2, 1945 in Krzydlina Wielka, Wolow, Poland.

Bl. Anna Ellmerer (Sr. M. Felicitas) (Germany/Poland) (1889-1945), was born May 12, 1889 in Grafing bei Munchen, Ebersberg, Germany. She entered the Congregation of the Sisters of Saint Elizabeth making her first profession on June 16, 1914 and perpetual vows on July 5, 1923 taking the name Sister Maria Felicitas. Towards the end of World War II, she was killed by Soviet soldiers at Nysa in an attempt to defend younger nuns from the violence of Soviet soldiers.. She died March 24, 1945 in Nysa (aka Neisse Oberneuland), Poland.

332

Bl. Elfrieda Schilling (Sr. M. Rosaria) (Poland) (1908-1945), was born on May 5, 1908 in Wroclaw, Poland. She converted to the Catholic faith from Protestantism and entered the Congregation of the Sisters of Saint Elizabeth making her first profession on April 12, 1930 and perpetual vows on July 29, 1935, taking the name Sister Maria Rosaria. Near the end of World War II, 37-year old Sister Maria Rosaria decided to stay with the sick and elderly who had not been able to escape as the Soviet Red Army approached the city. With them and other nuns she hid in an air raid shelter but was dragged out and raped by a group of 30 Soviet soldiers and shot a day later. She died on February 23, 1945 in Nowogrodziec (aka Naumburg am Queis), Boleslawiec, Poland.

Bl. Anna Thienel (Sr. M. Sabina) (Poland) (1909-1945), was born on September 24, 1909 in Rudzicka, Prudnik, Opole, Poland. She entered the Congregation of the Sisters of St. Elizabeth making her temporary profession on October 24, 1934 and perpetual vows on July 31, 1940, taking the name Sister Maria Sabina. She was killed on March 1, 1945 in Luban, Poland.

Bl. Luczja Heymann (Sr. M. Sapientia/Lucia Emmanuela) (Poland) (1875-1945) was born on April 19, 1875 in Lubiesz, Tuczno, Walcz, Poland. She entered the Sister of Saint Elizabeth in 1894 and made her first profession on July 26, 1897 and perpetual vows on July 2, 1906, taking the name Sister Maria Sapientia. *She served as a nurse in Hamburg-Eppendorf, Germany and Nysa, Poland.*

Near the end of World War II, 70-year-old Sister Maria Sapientia was shot by soldiers of the Soviet Red Army while trying to defend a younger nun from a soldier intent on raping the young religious sister. Sister Maria Sapientia died on March 24, 1946 at the monastery of the Sister of Saint Elizabeth in Nysa (Neisse Oberneuland), Poland. Blessed Luczja Heymann is buried in the garden of the Sisters' house.

Prayer for the favors that are needed and for the canonization of Sister M. Paschalis and IX companions:[7]
Lord Jesus Christ, Crucified and Risen, You strengthened Sister M. Paschalis and her companions to sacrifice their lives. For the price of the blood that was shed, they kept their virgin faithfulness,

333

defended the female dignity of others, and performed acts of mercy.
Let your Church raise them to the glory of the altars and show them
their testimony to the faithful today. May this example encourage us
to be generous in serving others and to be zealous in fulfilling Your
commandments. If it is in accordance with Your will, grant me the
grace through their intercession ... for which I am asking you with
confidence, who live and reign for ever and ever. Amen.

Our Father ... Hail Mary ... Glory be ...

References:
1) The Catholic Sun. (21Jul2021). Polish nuns killed by Soviet army as World War II ended showed courage. Accessed 6 April 2022. https://www.catholicsun.org/2021/07/21/polish-nuns-killed-by-soviet-army-as-world-war-ii-ended-showed-courage/

2) Jonathan Luxmoore. 30 years after Berlin Wall fell, Catholics seek to recognize heroic Eastern European sisters (7Nov2019). https://www.globalsistersreport.org/news/world/ministry/news/30-years-after-berlin-wall-fell-catholics-seek-recognize-heroic-eastern. Acc. 7Apr2022

3) Jonathan Luxmoore (22Jul2021). Polish nuns killed by Soviet army as World War II ended showed courage. Catholic News Service. http://sticna.org/news/polish-nuns-killed-by-soviet-army-as-world-war-ii-ended-showed-courage?uid=166435. Accessed 7 April 2022.

4) Hagiography Circle: Martyrs Killed in odium fidei under Communist Regimes in Eastern Europe. [16] Maria Paschalis Jahn and 9 Companions from the Sisters of Saint Elizabeth. Accessed 5 April 2022. http://newsaints.faithweb.com/martyrs/East09.htm.

5) Congregazione delle Cause dei Santi. Venerable Servants of God - Paschalina Jahn and 9 Companions. Accessed 4 June 2022. http://www.causesanti.va/it/santi-e-beati/paschalina-jahn-e-9-compagne.html

6) 10 Aleteia (27Jun2022). Beatified nuns killed by Red Army represent 100 others who suffered same fate. Accessed 27 June 2022. https://aleteia.org/2022/06/12/10-beatified-nuns-killed-by-red-army-represent-100-others-who-suffered-same-fate/

7) Zgromadzenie Siostr SW. Elzbiety. Martyr Sisters. Accessed 27Jun2022.. https://selzbietanki.com/na-oltarzach/siostry-meczenniczki/

Nurse Martrys of the 19 Martyrs of Algeria (1994-1996)

The following are three nurses who were martyred in Algeria between May 8, 1994 and August 1, 1996. In total 19 Martyrs of Algeria were beatified. They were men and women from 8 different congregations. Through their martyrdom, they witnessed to the universal love of Christ.[1]

The 19 martyred are: Sister Paul-Helene Saint-Raymond, Brother Henri Vergès, Sister Esther Paniagua Alonso, Sister Caridad Álvarez Martín, Fr. Jean Chevillard, Fr. Alain Dieulangard, Fr. Charles Deckers, Fr. Christian Chessel, Sister Angèle-Marie Littlejohn, Sister Bibiane Leclercq, and Sister Odette Prévost; The seven Trappist monks of Tibhrine, who were kidnapped on March 1996 and killed in May 1996: Brother Luc Dochier, Brother Christian de Chergé, Brother Christophe Lebreton, Brother Michel Fleury, Brother Bruno Lemarchand, Brother Célestin Ringeard, and Brother Paul Favre-Miville. Their story was dramatized in the 2010 French film *Of Gods and Men*. The last of the 19 to be martyred was Bishop Pierre Claverie, a French Algerian, the Bishop of Oran from 1981, who was killed on August 1, 1996.[2]

Bl. Paul-Helene Saint Raymond (France/Algeria) (1927-1994), Martyr

Worked as a nurse in poor, working class neighborhoods in Rouen, France. In 1964 worked as a nurse and social worker in Algeria for 30 years. Murdered by Muslim fundamentalists. Martyr.[3]

Helene-Saint Raymond was born on January 24, 1927 in Paris France. She was the eighth of ten children born into a pious family.

Helene initially studied at Sainte-Marie college in Neuilly and then graduated from the Sorbonne in Paris, France with a degree in physical sciences and chemistry. At the Sorbonne she participated in the center for Catholic students created by Abbot Charles (Center Richelieu) and also served as President, following a future Little Sister of the Assumption who invited her to take the habit in 1949. It was here at the Sorbonne that she met the Little Sisters of the Assumption. Following graduation, Helene worked two years as an engineer in the French Petroleum Institute in Rueil-Malmaison. Before entering religious life she also did an internship in a cardboard factory in Bagnolet to experience the harsh working conditions.

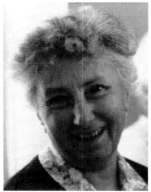

Sister Paul-Helene Saint Raymond.
www.paris.catholique.fr/

Helene entered the Little Sisters of the Assumption in 1952 and on July 29, 1954 she made her first vows taking the name Sister Paul-Helene. She was sent to Creil (1954-1957) where she worked as a family social worker and nurse. She formally studied nursing in 1957 and, initially, worked as a nurse in the poor working class neighborhoods in Rouen, France. She made her final vows in 1960.

In 1963, Sister Paul-Helene left for Algiers, Algeria where she ran the Medico-Social Center in Belcourt serving as the head nurse. "She was a whirlwind of activity so that she would exhaust fellow sisters and had to be told to go easy on them. She became so skilled she could perform minor surgery."[4] In 1974 she was sent to Tunis, Tunisia for a year and then to Casablanca (1975-1984), where she was responsible for caring for premature babies with an entirely Moroccan team. She also cared for those who had to live in hiding.

In 1984 she returned to Algeria working in Boukhari, a town 180 kilometers south of Algiers she reported in a letter, "It's important, interesting and obscure work. There is no nursery, no kindergarten, no family workers. Until now, the big family was enough for everything, but times are changing." This experience was difficult.

In 1988 she was again sent to the Belcourt community in Algiers. She retired from nursing and in September 1988 began working at the library of the Kasbah run by the Marist Brothers. She was obliged to change her route to work each day as tension arose in the country. In October 1990, they suffered an earthquake which caused many homes to collapse. In a 1993, Sister Paul Helene shared in a letter to her congregation:[5]

> I hasten to tell you that we normally continue to go to work, do our shopping, pray, while having suppressed for a long time: walks

336

outside and outings in the evening. Pray for us and for those around us... At the Kasbah library where I have been working for five years, there are still so many young people. We are continuing to develop the collection in Arabic which is essential to them. The relationship between the young people and our team is unchanged. Likewise in our house in the Casbah, two sisters welcome around a hundred young girls, women and children every week for sewing, knitting and tutoring. The "center" is growing. Where you have to be careful is where you are not known. We choose the places to do the shopping and in the evening we do not exceed 7 p. m. / 8 p.m. return. We have obviously given up on any walk — country, sea or mountain. Because of the small number of Christians, we know each other and the relations are very fraternal. The bishops these days in particular, visit the small communities, to realize the particular situations.

Reflecting on the violence that then reigned, she wrote that "one must start oneself to fight against one's own violence." When Bishop of Algiers, Mgr. Teissier warned her of the dangers that they all were facing and gave her the choice of leaving or staying, she responded, *"Father, our lives are already given anyway."* Sister Paul-Helene wrote a last letter before Easter in 1994:[5]

> The situation continues to worsen. If last summer we spoke of hidden war, we must now say: we are in full "civil war." The marquis *[a Salafist movement of Sunni Muslims, now renamed al Qaida in Maghreb, which advocates a return to the traditions of "pious predecessors."]* in the mountainous regions control the villages and make their ruthless and ferocious law reign – in the cities: assassinations, rockets, sabotages multiply and strike anywhere, anytime, anyone. As for everyday life, refueling is so difficult and expensive that the worry of knowing what we are going to put in the pot and how we are going to complete the month, including for those who are lucky enough to have a salary and that it is paid regularly — this concern occupies the minds and in a certain way creates a diversion! And yet in the midst of despair and anguish, life goes on: people help each other, take their lives into their own hands, reflect. The victory of life over death at Easter morning was hardly apparent...

On May 8, 1994 at the beginning of the afternoon, three men appeared at the library saying, "Police" and asked to see the chief. As Sister Paul-Helene directed them to Brother Verges' office, they

337

shot her in the back of the neck. Then they shot Brother Verges in the face. They were the first two victims of the 19 Martyrs of Algeria.[4]

Sister Paul-Helene Saint Raymond died on May 8, 1994 at the age of 67 at the Archdiocesan library on Ben Cheneb Street in the Kasbah in Algiers. Her funeral mass was celebrated at the Basilica of Our Lady of Africa. She was declared venerable with the promulgation of the decree of martyrdom on January 26, 2018 and beatified on December 8, 2018[6] both by Pope Francis. The beatification ceremony for the 19 Martyrs of Algeria was held at the Shrine of Our Lady of the Holy Cross in Oran. (Memorial - May 8)

References:
1) Congregazione delle Cause dei Santi. 19 Martyrs of Algeria (1994-2002). Accessed 4 June 2022.
http://www.causesanti.va/it/santi-e-beati/19-martiri-d-algeria.html

2) Catholic News Agency (14Sep2018). Algerian martyrs to be beatified in December. Accessed 16 April 2022.
https://www.catholicnewsagency.com/news/39384/algerian-martyrs-to-be-beatified-in-December

3) "Blessed Paul-Hélène Saint Raymond". CatholicSaints.Info. 16 October 2019. Web. 11 April 2022.
<https://catholicsaints.info/blessed-paul-helene-saint-raymond/>

4) Catholic Saints Guy (13 February 2018). Accessed 16 April 2022.
https://catholicsaintsguy.wordpress.com/2018/02/13/algerian-martyr-sister-paul-helene-saint-raymond/

5) Sister Madeleine Remond. (13Dec2018). Paul-Helene Saint-Raymond, first of the nineteen Martyrs of Algeria. Petites Soeurs de l'Assumption. Accessed 16 April 2022.
https://assomption-psa.org/paul-helene-saint-raymond-premiere-des-dix-neuf-martyrs-dalgerie-2/

6) Hagiography Circle: An Online Resource on Contemporary Hagiography. Martyrs of Algeria (1994-1996). Helene Saint Raymond (Paul-Helene of Gethsemani). Accessed 16 April 2022.
http://newsaints.faithweb.com/martyrs/Algeria.htm

Bl. Denise Leclerc (Sr. Bibiane) (France/Algeria) (1930-1995),
Martyr
Assigned to a maternity ward in Algeria
working with infants and new mothers.[1]

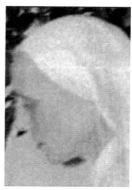

Sister Bibiane
catholicsaints.info

Denise Leclerc was born on January 8, 1930 in Gazeran, Yvelines, France near Paris. She was the eldest of eight children in a peasant family. From an early age, she helped her mother with the household. The family moved to Roye in the department of Somme. Denise attended the Jeanne d'Arc school of home economics. She kept busy with school, farm work and helping with her brothers and sisters. Though she wanted to be a religious sister, she delayed entry until her brother and then a sister, Odile, could finish their studies.

At the age of 29, Denise joined the Missionary Sisters of Our Lady of the Apostles (OLA) on March 4, 1959 in the Mother House of Venissieux, near Lyon. Denise took the religious habit on March 8, 1961 taking the name Sister Bibiane, in honor of Saint Bibiana, virgin and martyr of the 4th century. At the end of her novitiate, she was sent to Constantine, Algeria located in the north-east where she joined a community of sixteen religious sisters and worked on a maternity ward caring for infants and new mothers.

In 1964 Sister Bibiane was assigned to teach sewing and embroidery to young people in the Belcourt district of Algiers, the capital of Algeria at a home economics center for poor girls. On March 8, 1967 in Algeria, Sister Bibiane professed perpetual vows.[2] In 1970 she earned a professional diploma in sewing followed by one in embroidery, each conferred by the academic inspectorate of the city of Algiers. In addition to instructing, she encouraged the girls. With her additional degrees and leadership skills, she was appointed the Director of the School of Industrial and Decorative Arts in Algiers. Amongst the sisters with whom she worked was a OLA Sister, Angele-Marie, who was from Tunis. Sister Angele-Marie (Jeanne Littlejohn) had initially worked at an orphanage and boarding school for young girls in Bouzarea, Algeria and was later assigned to Algiers. She would be martyred with Sister Bibiane.

339

In 1980, Sister Bibiane was appointed to a small community composed of two other sisters. She stood firm in her faith when one day an Islamist disturbed her lessons attempting to force her to teach the Koran. In 1994, as threats to foreigners became more frequent, the superior general of the Missionary Sisters of Our Lady of the Apostles consulted the sister in Algeria to determine if they wanted to leave or stay. After dedicating over thirty years of her life to the mission in Algeria, and now at the height of the Algerian Civil War, Sister Bibiane responded:

> It was the people themselves who asked for Sisters. Now they're asking us to stay. I am very grieved, I feel helpless in the face of so much suffering, but I know, God loves these people and I have great confidence in Our Lady of Africa. Jesus said, 'The father will give you everything you ask for in my name.' His light helps me to discover wonders that are hidden, amazing solidarity, generosity, superhuman courage, the spirit is at work in their heart. The Word of God helps me to stay tuned - to be a glimmer of hope: I choose to stay.[3]

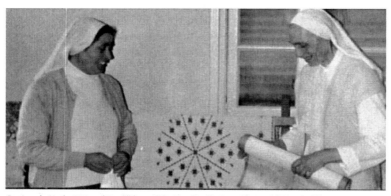

Sr. Angele Marie OLA and Sr. Bibiane OLA, Algerian Martyrs. Photo: (c) OLA Archives

On Sunday, September 3, 1995, Sister Bibiane and Sister Angele-Marie Littlejohn went to the Holy Sacrifice of the Mass with the Salesian sisters. At 7:15 p.m. they left the nun's chapel and walked home. They lived at number 105 Benlouzaid. When they arrived a number 92, they were hit by a hail of bullets, martyred by Islamic forces. Though they had taken the necessary precautions, it appeared that someone had been stalking them.[2] Both had been missionaries in Algeria for over thirty years. Sister Bibiane (65) and Sister Angele-Marie (62) died on September 3, 1995 in the Belcourt area of the capital of Algeria.

340

Both were declared venerable with the promulgation of the decree of martyrdom on January 26, 2018 and beatified on December 8, 2018[4] both by Pope Francis. The beatification ceremony for the 19 Martyrs of Algeria was held at the Shrine of Our Lady of the Holy Cross in Oran. (Memorial - May 8).

References:
1) "Blessed Dénise Leclerc". CatholicSaints.Info. 16 September 2018. Web. 8 December 2021. <https://catholicsaints.info/blessed-denise-leclerc/>

2) Emilia Flocchini (4Dec2018). Blessed Bibiane (Denise) Leclercq, Virgin and Martyr. Accessed 16 April 2022. http://www.santiebeati.it/dettaglio/97813

3) Society of African Missions. (20Nov2019). During 'Week of Witness' we remember two OLA Beatified Martyrs. Accessed 16 April 2022. https://sma.ie/two-ola-sisters-beatified-in-algeria/

4) Hagiography Circle: An Online Resource on Contemporary Hagiography. Martyrs of Algeria (1994-1996). Denise Leclerc (Bibiane). Accessed 16 April 2022. http://newsaints.faithweb.com/martyrs/Algeria.htm

5) Congregazione delle Cause dei Santi. 19 Martyrs of Algeria. Accessed 4 June 2022. http://www.causesanti.va/it/santi-e-beati/19-martiri-d-algeria.html

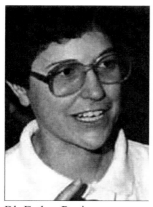

Bl. Esther Paniagua Alonso
Source:catholicsaints.mobi

Bl. Esther Paniagua Alonso (Spain/Algeria) (1949-1994), Martyr
Trained as a nurse and assigned to a hospital in Algeria where she cared for handicapped children.[1]

Esther Paniagua Alonso was born on June 7, 1949 in Izagre, Leon, Spain to Dolores Alonso and Nicasio Paniagua. At age 18, Esther joined the Augustinian Missionary Congregation. She made her perpetual vows in August 1970. She was trained as a nurse.

Sister Esther was assigned to a hospital in the Bab El Oued neighborhood

341

of Algiers, Algeria where she was especially drawn to handicapped children. When asked about the situation in the country she answered, *"No one can take our lives because they have already been given..."*[2]

The wave of violence that broke out in the 1990 in Algeria, and which mainly affected religious missionaries, was so extreme that the bishop of Algiers, Henri Teissier, recommended that the religious communities consider leaving. Sister Maria Jesus Rodriguez, then provincial superior of the Augustinian Missionaries traveled to Algeria to discern with the community about their future. After a few days of reflection, the three members of the community freely decided to continue in Algeria *"out of fidelity to the Gospel, out of love for the Algerian people who had welcomed them, because they were sharing faith and life with the people and did not want to flee but to run their same fate,"* explains Sister Maria Jesus who directly experienced the martyrdom of Sister Caridad and Sister Esther. On the afternoon of October 23, they planned to attend the Holy Sacrifice of the Mass in the chapel of the Little Sisters of Foucauld, a few meters from the house of the Augustinian Missionaries. They traveled in pairs, as the embassy had recommended. Caridad and Esther went ahead and behind them the provincial superior and Lourdes, the third sister of the community, *"Caridad and Esther turned the street and we lost sight of them. At that moment two shots rang out. Moments later, people began to run and a lady took us into her house. We heard crying and learned that a Christian had died. We went up to the roof of the house, from where the chapel of the Sisters of Foucauld could be seen, and we saw the bodies of Carl and Esther lying on the ground."*[3]

On October 23, 1994, Sister Esther was shot three times in the head by *Armed Islamic Group* while walking to the Holy Sacrifice of the Mass on Sunday in Bab-el-Oued neighborhood of Algiers, Algeria. She was 45 years old. Also martyred with her was the Augustine Missionary, Sister Caridad Alvarez Martin (1933-1994) who had served in Algeria for more than 30 years caring for the elderly and poor.[3]

Sister Esther was declared venerable with the promulgation of the decree of martyrdom on January 26, 2018 and beatified on December 8, 2018[4] by Pope Francis. The beatification ceremony for the 19 Martyrs of Algeria was held at the Shrine of Our Lady of the Holy Cross in Oran. (Memorial - May 8)

References:

1) "Blessed Esther Paniagua Alonso". CatholicSaints.Info. 15 September 2018. Web. 8 December 2021.
<https://catholicsaints.info/blessed-esther-paniagua-alonso/>

2) SSVM. (2Jan2019). "I choose to stay"" Starting 2019 with the Newly Beatified Martyrs of Algeria.Accessed 18 April 2022.
https://ssvmusa.org/index.php/2019/01/02/i-choose-to-stay-starting-2019-with-the-newly-beatified-martyrs-of-algeria

3) Theresa Garcia. (6Dec2018). ArchidiocesisBurgos. The Burgos nun Caridad Alvarez, assassinated in Algiers in 1994, will be beatified on Saturday. Accessed 18 April 2022.
https://www.archiburgos.es/2018/12/06/la-religiosa-burgalesa-caridad-alvarez-asesinada-en-argel-en-1994-sera-beatificada-el-sabado/

4) Hagiography Circle: An Online Resource on Contemporary Hagiography. Martyrs of Algeria (1994-1996). Esther Paniagua Alonso. Accessed 16 April 2022. http://newsaints.faithweb.com/martyrs/Algeria.htm

343

VENERABLE

Ven. Rozalia Celakowna (Poland) (1901-1944)

Worked at St. Lazarus Hospital on skin and venereal disease ward.
Replaced dressings, cleaned rotting and stinking wounds,
Worked on night duty, prayed at bedside for the dying
Loved her patients through her great love for Jesus
Also employed at an outpatient clinic at beginning of WWII where German
doctors worked. Had to learn German

Mission from Jesus: "If you want to save the world, you must enthrone the
Sacred Heart of Jesus in all countries and nations of the world."

Mystic

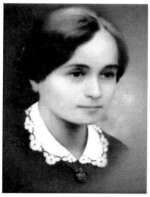

Rozalia Celakowna
Source:przymierzezmaryja.pl

Venerable Rozalia Celakowna[2] (1901-1944) was born on September 19, 1901 in the village of Jachowka, Budzow, Sucha Beskidzka District, Poland to Joanna and Tomasz Celakowna. She as the eldest of eight children and her parents were fervent Catholics.

The family worked hard on their farm and would pray together in the morning, at noon and in the evening, reciting the Rosary and other prayers. They also regularly read the Bible and the Lives of the Saints. They received the Sacrament of Reconciliation every months and celebrated the Holy Sacrifice of the Mass every Sunday and sometimes on weekdays too. Rozalia wrote about her parents, *"From my earliest years, they inculcated into my soul the deep tenets of holy faith and the love of God and neighbor. They watched over my soul to guard it from any corruption. At home, I had never been set a bad example."* In her diary she records, *"The first teacher who taught me to love Jesus was my dear Mother. She instructed me about what Jesus had done for us, what we were to love Him for, how I was to behave so that He would like me, etc. (...) The piety of my parents could be seen above all in the keeping of God's Commandments; it was not some bizarre, warped piety but healthy and reasonable."*

On September 1, 1908, just before she turned 7 years old, Rozalia began elementary school. She was a good student and set an example for other children. Rozalia made her First Holy Communion in 1911 at the age of 10 years old, at which time she declared, *"Dear*

345

Jesus, I want nothing else but love. I want to love You as much as is possible for any creature to love God. You, dear Jesus, nobody else!... I am asking you so ardently for nothing else but to keep me always from offending you with even but a shade of voluntary sin." At this time Rozalia experienced her first mystical experience. The Lord asked her: *"Give yourself to Me, entirely and without reservation, to My exclusive service and you will be very happy. The world can never give you happiness, but I, your God, will make you happy. Love me for the entire world! I will broaden your heart and fill it with love so that you can pay Me with love for love."*

After 6 years, Rozalia finished elementary school in 1914 at the age of 13. The outbreak of World War I (1914-1918) prevented her from continuing her education. She continued to help her parents on the farm and with her younger brothers and sisters. She received the Sacrament of Confirmation in 1917, the same year that the Blessed Virgin Mary was appearing in Fatima, Portugal. Rozalia, herself, continued to have mystical experience. In 1918, she took a private vow of chastity at her parish church.

In 1919 Rozalia experienced spiritual dryness and even darkness lasting six years. She experienced feeling of hopelessness and despair and spiritual attacks. She was very careful, however, never to neglect her prayers. During this time, she visited the Shrine of Our Lady of Czestochowa in Jasna Gora, Poland which houses the picture of the Blessed Virgin Mary and infant Jesus painted by St. Luke. Following this pilgrimage she left the family home and moved to Krakow in 1924.

At the time, the spiritual attacks were at their worst and her confessor was unable to help her because he did not understand her spiritual state. Like the children of Fatima, seven years earlier, in 1917, Rozalia was now given a vision of hell. She described, *"I felt like I was tumbling into the abyss of hell... Before my soul, horrible sins and crimes appeared, and it seemed that I had committed them... I heard a voice: 'You are damned and nothing can save you... I felt hell's fire on me, and it seemed to burn my body. The raring and howling of devils was so piercing that no human mind can imagine."* She understood that, *"When God crucifies a soul in this way and leaves it in darkness, man is then helpless..."* She further stated, *"I saw an open hell, the horror of which I cannot describe."* She reported that the devils experienced satanic joy as they threw huge numbers of souls into the abyss of hell. They competed to see who could being the most souls. They tormented each soul with the sins they had committed. Most were damned for sins against commandment six (Thou shalt not commit adultery) and nine (Thou shalt not covet thy neighbor's wife), followed by the sins of murder and hatred. After this vision, Rosalia's soul was carried to heaven where she received a vision of the love and happiness therein. She "heard" an inner voice say, *"Sainthood is love. The soul will achieve supreme perfection when it comes to love God most passionately."*

Approximately 6 months after her arrival in Krakow, in April 1925, Rozalia began working at St. Lazarus Hospital on the skin and venereal disease ward. The prevalence of syphilis and other venereal diseases testified to a moral decline and the terrible consequences of violating the Sixth Commandment. The Primate Cardinal of Poland, August Hlond, prior to World War II had said that the moral decline of mankind in the 20th century was worse than that of Sodom and Gomorrah. Jesus had told Rozalia, *"There is a need of sacrifice for Poland, for the sinful world. Great harm is done to my Sacred Heart by sins of impurity. I demand expiation."* Rozalia understood that Jesus was calling on her to carry his love and mercy to morally lost people suffering from venereal diseases. Rozalia provided care with great dedication to the patients with venereal disease, many of whom were forgotten by their families. Some were vulgar and exhibited wanton and lewd behavior which pained Rosalia. However, since she knew this was the work Jesus asked of her, she continued to serve the ill for the love of Jesus present in any suffering individual who was in need of her help.

During another mystical encounter, Jesus told Rosalia, *"I Am always with you and support you with My grace and stand by you. Although you cannot see Me now, you are to see Me with your soul's eyes and believe in this; for if I were not at your side, you would not be able to endure on your own under these conditions."*

Two years later at age 26, on December 15, 1927, Rozalia entered the convent of the Poor Clares, a order following the rule of St. Francis. Discovering that this was not her calling, she left the convent a couple months later, on March 1, 1928. She then began working in an eye clinic, a well-paid and prestigious position. However, she experienced another mystical vision in which Jesus was calling her back to the skin and venereal disease ward. While praying she saw Jesus being cruelly whipped by syphilitic female patients. They beat him mercilessly on the face and all over His body. Then, Jesus said to Rozalia: *"My dear child, look, what terrible suffering is inflicted upon Me by sins of impurity. Here, my child, I want to have you, to compensate Me for those horrible sins that harm My Heart so much... You, my child, will suffer a lot in your life in order to console Me, to become like Me, and to save souls... Today, I uncover before you and let you know the mystery and value of suffering. Suffering offers so great a grace that it is hardly comprehensible. It is a greater grace than the gift of working miracles. I shall give you a love of suffering so that you will be able to suffer like Me."* In this mystical vision, Jesus took Rozalia to the edge of a *"huge pit, full of rot and abomination."* Rozalia stated, *"He indicated to me that it was a human heart soiled with a sin of impurity. Jesus told me to work there for the intention of those fallen souls, so that they might mend their ways, and to remember for the rest of my life that my work and life would come to a close there."*

While working at the venereal disease ward, Rozalia had to replace dressings, clean rotting and stinking wounds, work on night duties and accompany the dying. She said that if it had not been for her supernatural love of neighbor and the awareness that she was fulfilling God's Will, she would not have undertaken such a taxing and wretched job for any amount of money.

Rozalia continued to love her patients through her great love for Jesus. She heroically overcame the disgust that rose up in her at the sight and manner of behavior of the syphilitic patients. She provided loving care, kindness and showed the patience of an angel as she cared for their needs. She was tender, modest and firm. She encouraged them to amend their lives and open their souls to Divine Mercy. She would often kneel down at a dying patient's bedside and pray for their reformation and reconciliation with God through confession, right up until they died.

An acquaintance reported one instance they observed,

"Once while on night duty, Rosalia could not persuade a certain middle-aged man to confess and receive Holy Communion before he died. She knelt down at his bed and started to recite the Rosary. After a few minutes, the man asked: 'What are you doing?' *'I'm praying,'* she replied. 'For whom?' *'For you.'* 'For me? I've not asked you to,' he said, then fell asleep. Having woken up, he saw her praying again, and asked: 'Are you still praying for me?' *'Yes!'* At this, he frowned and said: 'But I don't wish you to,' and fell asleep again. When he woke up for the third time and saw Rozalia

348

kneeling, he asked: 'Are you still praying for me despite my unpleasant words?' To this, she replied: *'Yes! Because God's goodness is so great that it embraces you too, in spite of the fact that you hold it in contempt.'* Then, the man asked her to summon a priest; he confessed, received Holy Communion, and was given the Sacrament of the Sick. After two or three hours, he passed away in the early hours of the morning."

Rozalia did everything out of love for Jesus and the Virgin Mary. In addition to her work at the hospital, she continued studying to serve the sick better. She studied evenings and nights for her last exam in nursing, which she passed in 1933. As a registered nurse she received many offers for well-paid work, but continued to be faithful to her calling to care for the people suffering from venereal diseases.

In May 1937, at age 36, Rozalia experienced exceptional mystical encounters with Jesus Christ and a closer union with Him. She wrote, *"Jesus, although invisible, is present in my soul. I feel His presence by having an impression of two persons' souls uniting into one as it were. This coming into contact by Jesus with my soul is far superior to an apparition. Even if I wanted to describe it, I would not be able to because it is far beyond what my mind, so very limited, can comprehend or imagine."*

During a retreat that same year, in September 1937, Rozalia rediscovered what a great gift co-participation in Christ's suffering on the cross was. Accepting the cross of suffering in union with Christ, she desired to learn to love Him even more than any human being had ever loved Him. It was also at that time that Jesus addressed, through her, a call to Poland and all nations to accept Him as the only Lord and to subject all spheres of life to the requirements posed by His love. In the name of the entire nation, this act was to be performed jointly by spiritual and temporal authorities.

In one of her mystical encounters, Rozalia heard, *"If you want to save the world, you must enthrone the Sacred Heart of Jesus in all countries and nations of the world. This is the only hope. Those countries and nations that do not accept it, and do not submit to the reign of Jesus' sweet love, shall perish forever from the face of the earth and shall never rise again... Remember, my child, make certain that so important a matter is not overlooked and forgotten."*

Rozalia proceeded to pray for this intention and offered up all her toils and sufferings for it. The spiritual director of Father Zygmunt Dobrzycki, the Superior-General of the Paulines, Father

Pius Przeidziecki, spoke on several occasions to the Primate of Poland, Cardinal Hlond, about the enthronement of the Sacred Heart of Jesus. Wanting to ensure that Rozalia was reliable, Cardinal Hlond required Rozalia to undergo a medical examination and submit the results to Church authorities. A neurological exam was conducted by Dr. Horodenski, who found that Rozalia was of sound mind.

Rozalia conveyed Jesus and Mary's call to reformation. Poland's failure to reform, in the late 1930's, was to bring about a terrible war, because its main causes were sins of lasciviousness, killing and hatred. Only by enthroning Christ would Poland and the world be protected against a disastrous war. Rozalia greatest wish was to see Poland enthrone Christ and for other nations to follow its example.

During World War II (1938-1945) the Polish people experienced arrest, deportation to concentration camps and mass murder and constant threats to life, Rozalia wrote: *"In spite of all this, I am at peace... If we knew how Jesus loves us, we would not let fear or terror anywhere near our souls for a single moment."* Rozalia cared most to save as many people as possible from eternal damnation.

At the beginning of World War II, Rozalia was employed at an outpatient clinic, where German doctors worked. She learned German. She continued to be greatly upset by the fact that despite a raging war, people would not mend their ways and still kept on offending God with grave sins. She often cried over the fate of her nation. Her pure heart and keen powers of observation allowed her to see the immense moral decline of society. In October 1939, she wrote, *"Such degradation and so many sins have never been found in the Polish nation as recently."* In her prayers, Rozalia incessantly pleaded with God for mercy on sinners. In the spirit of expiation for their sins, she accepted all her sufferings and humiliations with love. Jesus, in return inundated her soul with the indescribable joy of His closeness and love.

In early 1941, Rozalia's health greatly deteriorated, but she did not stop working at the hospital. Until the end, she gave herself entirely to the service of God and her neighbor. She wrote, *"A night duty offers something very important for me... Jesus, the sick and me... This is when Jesus in a special way lowers himself to reach my soul."*

350

Through her work, prayer and suffering, Rozalia did her best to make the day of enthronement arrive as soon as possible, when nations would be given under the reign of Christ the King. She thereby fulfilled Jesus' request: *"I wish to rule absolutely in human hearts. Ask for the hastening of my rule in souls through the enthronement."*

Four years before she died, Rozalia wrote to her confessor, *"I am in the evening of life. I like sunsets so much: then my soul submerges in God, the Sun of Justice, and I think of the Lord, how I am to love Him and please Him, so that my life will end just like the ending of a day, but what follows* (in the next life) *is a bright and fair day."*

In early September 1944, at age 43, Rozalia began to feel very weak. A friend, sick with influenza, asked for her help. During that call, Rozalia caught a bad cold and took to bed. Her health deteriorated day by day. On September 11, 1944 she was taken to the hospital. Never putting aside her Rosary, Rozalia received Holy Communion and the Sacrament of the Sick. Rozalia Celakowna died in her sleep on the night of September 12, 1944.

She was buried at the Rakowice Cemetery in Krakow, Poland. Despite the war, her funeral was attended by many priests, nuns, family members and friends. Soon news spread that through her intercession God had granted people extraordinary graces. (The above are liberal excerpts from the writing of Fr. Mieczystaw Piotrowski, S. Chr.)[2]

Servant of God, Rozalia Celakowna was declared venerable with the promulgation of the decree of heroic virtue on April 9, 2022 by His Holiness Pope Francis.. Vice Postulator is Rev. Pascual Cebollada Silvestre, SJ. Website: www.celakowna.pl.[3]

"If Poland does not revive spiritually and does not abandon her sins, she will perish. Only a complete spiritual revival and surrender to the reign of My Heart may save not only Poland but also other nations from complete doom." - Jesus

"Jesus, grant me love, a love that can love you for the entire world, loving You to distraction, in a way that You have never been loved before on this earth. I can say this because You, Jesus, are able to broaden my little heart to infinity. You are almighty, so You will work this miracle." - Rozalia

References:

1) Rhoslyn Thomas. (29Aug2014) A history of abortion in Poland. Society for the Protection of Unborn Children. Accessed 21 April 2022.
https://www.spuc.org.uk/Article/382473/A-history-of-abortion-in-Poland-Blog-archive

2) Fr. Mieczystaw Piotrowski S. Chr. (1Sep2018). The Servant of God Rozalia Celakowna. Accessed 21 April 2022.
https://www.michaeljournal.org/articles/roman-catholic-church/item/the-servant-of-god-rozalia-celakowna

3) Hagiography Circle. 1944. 22) Rozalia Celek. Accessed 19 April 2022.
www.newsaints.faithweb.com/year/1944.htm.

Ven. Jeanne Mance (France/Canada) (1606-1673)

Lay missionary and immigrant to New France,
landing in Montreal, Quebec in 1642.
Served as the first nurse in New France, working with the sick in her home
and then founding Hotel-Dieu Hospital, the oldest hospital in Montreal in
1645 and directing its operations for 17 years.[1]

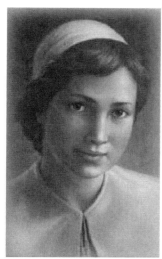

Ven. Jeanne Mance
challengeyouthministry.com

Jeanne Mance, nurse, co-founder of Montreal and founder of Hotel-Dieu hospital. The daughter of an attorney, Jeanne was born in 1606 and baptized on November 12, 1606 in Langres, France. Her mother died prematurely and Jeanne cared for her 11 brothers and sisters. "She is thought to have developed nursing skills working with charitable local societies during the Thirty Years War (1618-1648)."[2] She cared for the victims of the war and the plague in her town.

Once her siblings were older and her father had passed away, Jeanne decided to become a missionary to Quebec. She joined the Societe de Notre-Dame de Montreal which was created in Paris in 1640 to found a colony on the Island of Montreal. "The group had acquired Montreal Island with a view of turning it into a missionary hub for converting indigenous people to Catholicism. Their plan was to push westward past the existing settlement at Quebec and set up a wilderness mission astride the trade routes of the powerful Haudenosaunee (Iroquois)."[2]

On the voyage she provided nursing care to people on board the ship. Once in Quebec, she helped families clear land to build their homes. The Canadian Encyclopedia describes these initial days:

> In May 1642, Jeanne Mance and her companions arrived on Montreal Island. There they pitched tents and began living in woods. Fifty five of them (including 10 women) remained on the Island as winter fell. The next year Mance set up a small hospital within the fort's palisades. The hospital quickly attracted ailing

353

Wendat (Huron), who were allied with the French. They became Christian converts as well as patients. Some beds had to be reserved for French settlers wounded by the Haudenosaune (Iroquois) warriors resisting French encroachment on their trade routes.[2]

Jeanne Mance oversaw the initial construction of Hotel-Dieu Hospital in Montreal whose doors were open to everyone in 1645. In 1649 she returned to France to revive support for the settlement. When the Jesuit mission of Saint Marie des Hurons collapsed in 1649, Montreal became the front-line in the Franco-Iroquois conflict. Greater than one third of the colonist were killed and most moved into the fort in an effort to survive. By mid-1651 only 17 militiamen were left to face 200 Iroquois warriors.

Jeanne Mance convinced co-founder and governor of the colony, Paul de Chomedey de Masionneuve, to return to France and secure the permission of their major benefactor, Madame Angelique de Buillion (widow of a French finance minister) to use the hospital's endowment to recruit colonists. This event, known as the Great Recruitment is believed to have saved the colony. They arrived in 1653.

Among the 177 colonists recruited was Marguerite Bourgeoys who became Maisonneuve's and Jeanne Mance's partner in the administration of the colony. (Canonized on October 31, 1982, St. Marguerite Bourgeoys founded the Sisters of the Congregation of Notre Dame, an uncloistered community, an innovation at the time, which received its civil charter from Louis XIV in 1671 and canonical approbation by decree of the Bishop of Quebec in 1676 with its constitution approved in 1698. They were a teaching order with the apostolate to promote the family, parish and diocesan endeavors).[5] Jeanne Mance was a lay nurse being neither a nun or religious sister. She served as the colony's official treasurer, director of supplies and hospital director.

Jeanne Mance returned to France in 1658, after a fall on the ice that causes her to lose the use of her right arm. The next year she returned to Montreal, her arm miraculously cured. She brought with her the Religious Hospitallers of Saint Joseph who cared for the sick at Hotel-Dieu, the hospital that Jeanne Mance oversaw for the rest of her life. Before she died, in 1672 Jeanne Mance laid one of the first stones of what would become Montreal's Notre Dame cathedral. She

354

ran the hospital for 17 years. Jeanne Mance died of illness in Montreal, New France (current day Canada) on June 18, 1673 when she was 67 year old. In 2014 Pope Francis recognized Jeanne's heroic virtues and declared her venerable. Her tomb is conserved today (2021) in the chapel of the Musee des Hospitalieres de l'Hotel-Dieu on Pine Avenue in Montreal.[6]

"There is nothing in the world that I would refuse to do to accomplish the divine and all-loving will of God. It is the only desire and love of my heart. There in is my passion, all my affections, my only love, and my sole paradise."[7]

Reference:

1) "Venerable Jeanne Mance". CatholicSaints.Info. 13 March 2020. Web. 8 December 2021. <https://catholicsaints.info/venerable-jeanne-mance/>

2) Jan Noel (2021). Jeanne Mance in The Canadian Encyclopedia. https://www.thecanadianencyclopedia.ca/en/article/jeanne-mance. Accessed 13Mar2022.

5) Vatican News Service. Marguerite Bourgeoys (1620-1700) foundress of the Sisters of the Congregation of Notre Dame. https://www.vatican.va/news_services/liturgy/saints/ns_lit_doc_19821031_bourgeoys_en.html (accessed 16Oct2021).

6) Pointe-A-Calliere. Jeanne Mance, co-founder of Montreal. https://pacmusee.qc.ca/en/stories-of-montreal/article/jeanne-mance-co-found er-of-montreal/ (accessed 16Oct2021).

7) Challenge: Catholic Youth Ministry. Saint of the Month: Venerable Jeanne Mance. Accessed 16 October 2021. https://challengeyouthministry.com/saint-of-the-month-venerable-jeanne-ma nce/

Ven. Magdalen of the Sacred Heart (England) (1832-1900)

Volunteer nurse in the Crimean War.
Converted to Catholicism in 1885
Founded the Poor Servants of the Mother of God in 1872.
Set up shelters for prostitutes, homeless women and children.
Founded the Providence Free Hospital in St. Helens, Lancashire, England.
Wrote "Eastern Hospital and English Nurses" exposing the terrible
conditions of soldiers in the Crimea.[1]

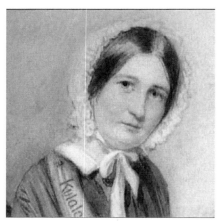

Mother Magdalen
brentfordandchiswicklhs.org.uk

Frances Margaret Taylor (Mother Magdalen of the Sacred Heart) was born on January 20, 1832 in Stoke Rochford, Lincolnshire, England. Her father was an Anglican clergyman.

As a young woman, she nursed casualties in the Crimean War alongside of Florence Nightingale.

She converted to Catholicism in 1855, after she was impressed by the faith of dying Irish soldiers.

In 1872, at age 40, Frances founded the Poor Servants of the Mother of God taking the religious name of Mother Magdalen. With three companions, she set up refuges for prostitutes and homeless women and children. She established the Convent of Our Lady of Pity in 1874 as a base to serve the poor. Mother Magdalen founded the Providence Free Hospital in St. Helens, Lancashire and also took over running the St. Joseph's Asylum in Dublin. By the time of her death in 1900, the Sisters were responsible for over 20 houses and institutions.

Mother Magdalen was a prolific author and journalist often campaigning for the rights of the poor. Her book, *Eastern Hospitals and English Nurses* exposed the neglect of soldiers and the injustice and indignities they suffered. She advocated for better treatment. In addition, she worked to reform the character of paid nurses, whom she often found to be drunk, immoral and insubordinate. The sick and dying deserved much better care.

The Apostleship of Prayer was started in France in 1844 at a Jesuit training college in Vals where the young Jesuits were eager to start their missionary activities abroad. Since they had several years of preparation pending, Fr. Francis Xavier Gautrelet SJ suggested they devote themselves to the mission immediately by simply offering to God everything they were doing in their every day life. This devotion spread quickly. In 1861, Fr. Ramiere SJ published a magazine for the Apostolate, the Messenger of the Sacred Heart of Jesus. By 1941 there were 72 Messengers in 44 different languages. The Apostleship of Prayer. In the late 1800's Mother Magdalen convinced Fr. Dignam, SJ, to change the Messenger of the Sacred Heart from being an expensive literary magazine into a popular penny-worth magazine which quickly circulated freely among the poor. For Dublin, Ireland, she convinced Fr. Cullen SJ to circulate the magazine there. Within a year the Messenger of the Sacred Herat reached a circulation of 73,000 and is still published in Ireland today.

Sister Magdalen of the Sacred Heart died on June 9, 1900 in the Mother House, the Convent of Our Lady of Pity, across from St. Patrick's cathedral adjacent to Soho Square in London, England from natural causes. She was buried in the chapel of the Maryfield Convent in Roehampton, London, England.

In 2014 the Poor Servants of the Mother of God had over 200 sisters working in Kenya, the United States, Venezuela, Italy, Britain and Ireland working among the poor and providing care to the elderly and people with learning disabilities..

Sister Magdalen of the Sacred Heart was declared venerable withe promulgation of the decree of heroic virtue on June 12, 2014.[2]

Say to our dear Lord: "I bear this for love of your dear Heart.
You were worried and harassed on earth for me,
so I will bear it for you."

Prayer for the Beatification of Mother Magdalen:
Heavenly Father you gave to Mother Magdalen Taylor a profound insight into the Mystery of the Incarnation and a great love and compassion for the poor and needy. We pray that her life of deep faith and loving service may continue to inspire us and that, one day, she may be beatified to the glory of your name.
We ask this through Christ Our Lord. Amen.[3]

References:

1) "Venerable Magdalen of the Sacred Heart". CatholicSaints.Info. 10 March 2020. Web. 8 December 2021. <https://catholicsaints.info/venerable-magdalen-of-the-sacred-heart/>

2) Hagiography Circle: An Online Resource on Contemporary Hagiography. Frances Margaret Taylor (Mary Magdalen of the Sacred Heart). Accessed 21April2022. http://newsaints.faithweb.com/year/1900.htm#Taylor

3) Poor Servants of te Mother of God. Beatification. Accessed 21Apr2022. https://www.poorservants.org/our-beginning/beatification/

4) A Lady Volunteer [aka Frances Margaret Taylor]. (1856). Eastern Hospitals and English Nurses; The Narrative of Twelve Months' Experience in the Hospitals of Koulali and Scutari. London: Hurst and Blacket Publishers. Available online at https://archive.org/details/easternhospital01taylgoog/page/n1/mode/2up

Ven. Mary Jane Wilson (India/England/Portugal) (1840-1916)
Worked as a nurse and taught catechism to children.
Founded the Franciscan Sisters of Our Lady of Victory
Cared for children and the sick and
worked with victims of the smallpox epidemic of 1907.[1]

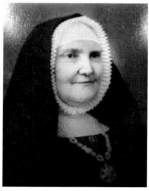

Sister Mary of St. Francis
(Public Domain)

Mary Jane Wilson (Sister Mary of St. Francis) was born on October 3, 1840 in Hurryhur, Mysore, Karnataka, India to English parents who practice the Anglican religion. She was orphaned as a child and raised by an aunt in England.

Mary Jane worked as a nurse and also taught catechism to children. One difficulty she had with the Anglican religion and what drew her to Catholicism was the belief in the true presence of Jesus in the Most Holy Eucharist. This quandary was overcome through the intervention of Our Lady of Victories on April 30, 1873. The following year on May 11, 1874, she received Catholic Baptism in Boulongne-Sur Mer, France at the age of 33.

On May 26, 1881 she moved to the Madeira Island, the largest and most populous of the Portuguese Madeira Archipelago, working as a nurse for an English patient. She settled in Funchal where she catechized children, cared for the sick and established several charitable works: orphanage, dispensary, pharmacy and Colegio de S. Jorge.

After three years, on January 15, 1884, with Amelia Amaro de Sa, she founded the Congregation of the Franciscan Sisters of Our Lady of Victory taking the name Sister Maria de St Francis. The congregation restored the Hospital da Vila de Santa Cruz where the sisters worked. As they did so, their congregation also flourished and expanded to various parts of Madeira Island. They opened schools, promoted literacy and culture, evangelized and helped the poor.

When an epidemic of smallpox ravaged the southern region of Madeira in 1907, the sisters fearlessly helped the sick. King D. Carlos awarded her the "*Torre e Espada*." In 1910, when Portugese Republican Party over threw the centuries-old Portugese monarchy on 5 October 1910, the congregation was extinguished and Sister Maria de St. Francis was arrested and expelled to England. After a

359

year of exile, she returned and while in hiding she gathered together the sisters bringing new life to the congregation she had founded. The congregation received diocesan approval of the statutes on May 8, 1916. On October 18, 1916, as she was laying the foundation for the pre-seminary (novitiate), she died at the age of 76, in Camara de Lobos, Funchal Madeira, Portugal from natural causes.

The foundation she established has foundations also in mainland Portugal and the Azores, Mozambique, England, Italy, Germany, Brazil, South Africa, the Philippines, Angola, India, DR Congo, Timor and Tanzania. An Association of "Friends of Sister Wilson" was founded for the lay faithful. The charity that Sister Maria de St. Francis exhibited earned her the title, "Good Mother."[2]

Sister Maria de St. Francis (Mary Jane Wilson) was declared venerable via the promulgation of th decree of heroic virtue on October 9, 2013. Website: www.cifnsv.com[3]

Along your path, seek to live from this great truth:
"God is our Father, our best and dearest Friend..."
As we pay attention, life appears full of opportunities
to perform acts of love.

References:

1) "Venerable Mary Jane Wilson". CatholicSaints.Info. 3 March 2020. Web. 8 December 2021. <https://catholicsaints.info/venerable-mary-jane-wilson/>

2) Mary Jane Wilson. Accessed 4 June 2022. https://web.archive.org/web/20181111211352/http://www.cifnsv.com/2009/index.php?option=com_content&view=article&id=12&Itemid=34&lang=pt

3) Hagiography Circle: An Online Resource on Contemporary Hagiography. 1916. Mary Jane Wilson (Maria of St. Francis). Accessed 21 April 2022. http://newsaints.faithweb.com/year/1916.htm#Wilson

Ven. Coloma Antonia Marti y Valls (Spain) (1860-1889)
Infirmary nurse

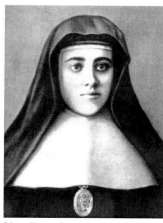

Ven.Francisca de las Llagas de Jesus Marti y Valls
Source: ofm.org

Coloma Antonia Marti & Valls was born on June 26, 1860 in Badalona, in the diocese of Barcelona, Spain, into a deeply religious Christian family.

She felt the call to religious life at age 11. Obedient to the opposition of her father, she awaiting the right moment to enter the Monastery exhibiting great patience.

She joined the Poor Clares of Divine Providence on October 2, 1882 in Badalona, Spain at the age of 22.

She made her first vows in 1883 taking the name Sister Francesca of the Wounds of Jesus. (Francesca delle Piaghe di Gesu). She made her final profession on September 29, 1891 at the age of 31. She subsequently served as a teacher, infirmary nurse, sacristan, choir director and novice mistress. She formed young women in true love for our Lord, true devotion and observance of religious life.

She had a deep devotion of Jesus in his Passion on the Way of the Cross and an equally intense love for the Blessed Virgin Mary. She recited frequently the Rosary, the crown of Our Lady of Sorrows and the chaplet of the twelve stars. She was known for her charity to her sisters and her spirit of penance for the sins of the world and for her deep contemplative prayer life.

Sister Francesca of the Wounds of Jesus died on June 4, 1889 at the age of 39, in the monastery of the Poor Clares in Badalona, Barcelona, Spain of endocarditis, an inflammation of the heart. She was buried at the convent of the Poor Clares of Divine Providence in Badalona.

The fame of her holiness of life spread extensively after her death, to the point that her tomb was left untouched during the destruction of convents during the persecutions of the Spanish Civil War (1936-1939).[3]

361

She was declared venerable by the promulgation of the decree of heroic virtue on May 19, 2018 by His Holiness Pope Francis.[4]

References:

1) "Venerable Coloma Antònia Martí y Valls". CatholicSaints.Info. 25 May 2022. Web. 5 June 2022.
<https://catholicsaints.info/venerable-coloma-antonia-marti-y-valls/>

2) Congregazione delle Cause dei Santi. Venerable Servant of God - Frances of the Wound of Jesus (born: Colomba Antonia Marti y Valls). Accessed 4 June 2022.
http://www.causesanti.va/it/venerabili/francesca-delle-piaghe-di-gesu-al-sec olo-colomba-antonia-marti-y.html

3) OFM. (21May2018) Venerable Francisca de las llagas deJesus Marti y Valls, Professed Nun of the Second Order of St. Francis. Accessed 4 June 2022.
https://ofm.org/blog/venerable-francisca-de-las-llagas-de-jesus-marti-y-valls -professed-nun-of-the-second-order-of-st-francis/

4) Hagiography Circle: News 2018. 12 decrees promulgated - Coloma Antonia Marti Valls. Accessed 4 June 2018.
http://newsaints.faithweb.com/news_archives_2018.htm

Ven. Giovanni Nadiani (Italy) (1885-1940), Incorrupt

Professed lay brother in the Congregation of the Blessed Sacrament.
Served as infirmarian.[1]

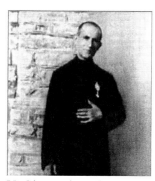

V. Giovanni Nadiani
Source:
blessedsacramentphil.org

Giovanni Nadiani was born on February 20, 1885 in Santa Maria Nuova in Cesena, Province of Forli, Italy to Ercole Gaspare and Annunziata Piazzi. He was the youngest of three, having an older brother and sister, Erminio and Maria.

His father was an anti-clerical republican who ran a grocery store and tavern and married his mother in 1880. When Giovanni was three years old his mother died at the birth of her fourth child, Adolf, who also died immediately after her. In 1892 his father married his first wife's sister to whose union was born Giovanni's half-sister, Annunziata, who died at age 5. Lucia also died and in 1897 Giovanni's father married for the third and final time to the maid, Giovanna Ruffili. His mother and both step-mothers raised him in a Christian manner, educated him in the faith, taught him to pray and ensured he received the sacraments, even though his father was not a practicing Christian.[2]

Vanitti, as he was called, was a fine student. He showed a particular disposition for singing and was a fine soloist. He completed elementary school in 1898, at the age of 13, and briefly entered the seminary in Cesena, Italy.

Discovering this was not his vocation, he returned home after 4 years in 1902 and worked in his father's restaurant. He continued to read religious books and would make the sign of the cross if he heard a bad word. He grazed their horses near the chapel of the Blessed Mother where he would sing and pray. His sister loved to hear his beautiful voice. Vanitti entered the Christian Democratic Circle of Prodezza and served as the secretary.

As he contemplated his future, he thought about being a missionary. He went to work in Switzerland in order to learn French and German. There he worked in a chocolate factory. In 1905, he enlisted for military service in Italy and was transferred to Rome where he worked as a bartender.

363

Once, when visiting the Church of San Claudio, he observed Eucharistic Adoration. Jesus, in the Blessed Sacrament, was solemnly exposed with two priests praying in adoration as the lay faithful came in and out to pray for a long time or just for a few minutes. Kneeling he came to understand this would be his mission. He got to know the Blessed Sacrament Father who welcomed him, not as a candidate for priesthood, because of his age, but as a lay-brother.

When he entered the Congregation of the Blessed Sacrament (formally known as the Congregation of the Presbyters of the Most Holy Sacrament) at Turn on July 2, 1907, Vanitti was 22 years old. On November 14, 1907, he began the novitiate at Castelvecchio di Moncalieri under the direction of Father Carlo Maria Poletti. Here he began writing his *"Spiritual Notes."* He decided to be consecrated in a nuptial communion to Jesus in the Eucharist, through the *"Eymardian Vow of Personality."* His mystical insights, his passion for the Eucharist and the Blessed Mother reached the highest levels. The Vow, initially made by St. Peter-Julian Eymard on March 21, 1865, and the source of its name described by St. Eymard is as follows:

> I made the perpetual vow of my personality to our Lord Jesus Christ through the hands of the Blessed Virgin Mary and Saint Joseph, under the patronage of Saint Benedict: nothing for me and anyone, and asking for the essential grace, nothing by me... Everything through Him, with Him and in Him."[3]

Brother Giovonni was professed in the Congregation of the Blessed Sacrament, as a lay brother, on November 14, 1909. He served as the sacristan and promoted the Blessed Sacrament periodicals and was of humble service wherever he was needed.

During World War I, from January 1917 to the autumn of 1918, he worked on the front near Strassoldo (Udine) as an assistant to a military chaplain. After this, he returned to the community and served in many capacities including the vice-treasurer.

In October 1931 at the age of 46, he was transferred to Ponteranica, where he was made the infirmarian of the community. Though he did not have a diploma in nursing, he learned on the job and undertook his duties with kindness and generosity. He earned the esteem of the doctors, who recognized in him a "really maternal care for the sick." He set down his own thoughts in *"The Spiritual Maternity of the Religious of the Blessed Sacrament."*

Brother Giovanni, in contemplating Jesus in the Blessed Sacrament, would prepared by choosing themes --- then following adoration he would note the spiritual fruits.

When Brother Giovanni was fifty-five years old, the doctors discovered that he had stomach ulcer which they eventually determined was cancer. He thanked the Blessed Virgin Mary for "that little living cross." He continued to work as the infirmarian. On September 9, 1939 he traveled to Bergamo on foot alone to the clinic where he was told the diagnosis. He responded: "Deo gratias." Surgery was performed on December 22, 1939 at the main hospital. He asked others to pray for a miracle but also placed himself in the will of God.

Brother Giovanni died, from cancer of the stomach, on January 6, 1940, the solemnity of the Epiphany of the Lord in Ponteranica, Bergamo, Italy.

Seventeen years after his death, in 1957, the canonization process began. Forty-eight years after he died, his coffin was opened on November 8, 1988, his body was found to be intact.[4] Giovani Nadiani was declared venerable by a decree of heroic virtue on June 11, 2019.

Intercessory Prayer:
"O Most Holy Trinity, we thank you for the gift of the Eucharist, the font and strength of all holiness, and ask you to glorify the Venerable Giovanni Nadiani, who witnessed in humility and service the life of love springing from this Sacrament. Through his intercession grant us the graces that we are asking from you."

Say 3 "Glory be to the Father...," to the Most Holy Trinity.

References:

1) "Venerable Giovanni Nadiani". CatholicSaints.Info. 1 July 2021. Web. 4 June 2022. <https://catholicsaints.info/venerable-giovanni-nadiani/>

2) SSS Congregatio. Accessed 4 June 2022. The Venerable Giovanni Nadiani, Blessed Sacrament Brother. https://www.ssscongregatio.org/en/news/causes-of-saints/item/61-the-venerable-giovanni-nadiani-blessed-sacrament-brother.html

3) Father Francis Mwanza. SSS. (4May2020). The Gift of self in an eymardian perspective. Accessed 24 April 2022. https://www.ssscongregatio.org/en/news/recent-news/item/1407-the-gift-of-self-in-an-eymardian-perspective.html

4) Daniele Bolognini (28Jun2019). Venerable Giovanni Nadiani. http://www.blessedsacramentphil.org/venerable-giovanni-nadiani/ Accessed 4 June 2022.

Ven. Noeme Cinque (Sister Serafina) (Brazil) (1913-1988)

Worked as a teacher and nurse often taking sick men and women and pregnant women off the street providing health care and giving them a place to stay establishing first "The Refuge"
Founded the Divine Providence Home for pregnant women and infants fondly called "The House of Sister Serafina" by many
Tirelessly begged for beds, sheets, furnishings, food and money to care for the poor sick and/or pregnant in her care
Known as, "The Angel of the Transamazonian Road."

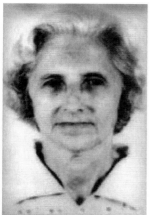

Ven. Noeme Cinque
(Sister Serafina)
Angel of the the
Transamazonian Road

Noeme Cinque was born on January 31, 1913 to Vincent and Sarah Cinque in Boca das Gracas, Urucurituba, Amazonas, Brazil. This was a village on the Amazon River. She was the second of twelve children (Mario, Noeme, Aura, Renato, Miguel, Sylvio, Jose, Humberto, Attilo, Marieta, Nair, Alfredo and Yolanda). Her parents were of Italian heritage. Her father owned a cacao plantation, a store for buying and selling cloth and was a tapper of rubber trees.

Noeme made such great progress in her studies that, at the age of eleven, her father entrusted her to the Dorothean sisters in Manaus to teach and educate her. The Dorothean Sisters prepared Noeme for her First Holy Communion, at which time she felt called to become a religious sister. She wrote:

> On the day that Jesus entered my poor heart for the first time, I felt a great love for Jesus and a great desire to belong entirely to Him. With true fervor I made my own consecration, hoping that one day my desire would be fulfilled.

At the age of 16, Noeme told her parents about her desire to become a religious Sister. Her parents strongly disagreed. Her father purchased a home in Manaus and sent his wife and Noeme and oldest sons to live there and continue their education at te state school, the Institute of Education of Amazonas, where Noeme completed her studies.

Noeme involved herself in the local parish of St. Sebastian administered by an Italian Capuchin priest. He hired her as a catechist. Noeme worked hard as a catechism of children, youth and adults in her parish in Manaus. She took the allowance that her father sent every month and gave it to the sick and the poor whom she encountered.

In 1934, after completing her teacher training courses at the Institute of Education, Noeme was sent to the interior of the state to teach and fulfill the obligatory requirements of new teachers. Noeme worked in the small town of Tabocal, in a school housed in the home of one of the families. She taught Portuguese, mathematics and catechism, preparing the children for baptism. She also taught adult religious education and provided marriage counseling.

In 1936 Noeme returned home to Urucurituba where she taught and prepared people for the sacraments awaiting the priest's periodic visit to the town. Under her leadership, an abandoned chapel that was used as an animal shelter was transformed back to a lovely chapel. There she taught the children catechism and the older people came there to pray the rosary and to receive religious instructions.

The Secretary of Education transferred her to teach in several different schools to include: Benjamin Constant and Saldanha Marinho schools. She was recognized for her zeal as a teacher and catechist.

During World War II (1938-1945), people of German and Italian and Japanese descent were considered enemy foreigners and were shunned by many people. Fellow teachers accused her of being a Nazi or a Fascist and of not teaching correctly. She was forbidden to teach religion and was under constant scrutiny. During this difficult time, Noeme's mother Sarah Cinque died on January 11, 1945. Despite these difficulties, Noeme was very active in the Church. She enrolled in the Pious Union of the Daughters of Mary organized at the cathedral of Manaus. She also joined the Apostolate of Prayer and became one of its leadership. She became a member of Catholic Action. And also took time to join members to visit inmates in a large prison in Manus.

At the request of Archbishop Dom Joas da Matta Andrade e Amoral, Noeme assisted a new Redemptorist priest, to learn Portuguese, establish a new parish, Our Lady of Aparecida, and establish a branch of the Pious Union of the Daughters of Mary there. Her enthusiasm attracted many young people to join.

In order to help the sick poor people, she took a course to become a practice nurses registered in the Health Department of Amazonas. She visited the sick and the elderly in their home.

In 1946, Noeme, made the decision to entered the Congregation of the Adorers of the Blood of Christ, an American congregation from Wichita, Kansas, who had just begun working in mission field of Brazil. On November 7, 1946, accompanied by Sisters Evelyn and Julitta, she travel to Wichita, Kansas where at the provincial motherhouse in early December she would begin her postulancy. Almost immediately she was given a postulant veil and joined fourteen other postulants. She sewed the long white gowns and made the cords for all fourteen postulants' investiture ceremony as they entered the next phase, the novitiate.

Noeme began her novitiate on July 1, 1947 and was given the religious name, Serafina. On July 1, 1948, Sister Serafina professed her vows of poverty, chastity and obedience and became the first Brazilian Adorer of the Blood of Christ. Four months later in November 1948, Sister Serafina began her journey back to Brazil landing in Belem on November 18, 1948. They continued on to Manaus the next day.

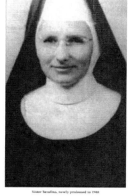

Sister Serafina, - 1948

In Manaus, on government donated land, the sisters built a convent and novitiate. On February 21, 1949, they received the candidates. Sister Serafina now was fulfilling the role of an older sister amongst the young Brazilian candidates.

On March 4, 1949, Sister Julitta assigned Sister Serafina as the Director of the High School at Coari. She departed for Coari the next day. On July 1, 1953, the feast of the Precious Blood of Jesus, Sister Serafina pronounced her perpetual vows. The next year Sister Serafina was sent to Codajas, where she served for three years as local superior and director of Our Lady of Grace School. While assigned there, in June 1955, she was called to Manaus to be with her father during his last illness. She was at his bedside when he died on July 2, 1955. She then transferred, in 1957, to Altamira as the superior of the Adorers there and director of the Institute of Maria De Mattias.

369

There she began the Pedagogical Institute of Altamira in 1958 to train good teacher.

In 1959 she moved to Santarem to be directress of a new high school dedicated to St. Raymond Nonnatus which had been opened two years earlier. This year she was also selected to be a delegate to the General Chapter of the Congregation of Adorers and in July traveled to Italy, the country of her ancestors. After two year she was transferred back to Coari as a teacher in the pedagogical course started six years earlier. She took seriously the importance of providing a sound education for local teachers. In 1963 she was assigned at the Teacher Training School in the town of Manacapuru on the banks of the Amazon River.

By 1965, Congregation of the Adorers of the Precious Blood had 135 professed Adorers serving in twenty communities scattered up and down the Amazon and its tributaries. That year, at the General Chapter of 1965, they decided to form the Vice-Province of Manaus into a Province which caused great joy amongst the adorers.

Sadness engulfed the community following the Second Vatican Council which concluded in late 1965. For many Sisters in Brazil and elsewhere, the poorly understood changes mandated by the Council raised doubt and questioning of the value of their religious vocation. Many young Adorers in Brazil chose to withdraw from the Congregation. This unexpected exodus deeply troubled Sister Serafina. She, herself, was puzzled by some of the changes that were introduced in the province of Manaus. She expressed these concerns in a letter dated May 18, 1971 to members of the General Chapter meeting in Rome that year.

In 1966, Sister Serafina was assigned to the community at Nova Olinda do Norte, in the Borba Prelacy of Amazonas. The North American Franciscan priests of the Third Order invited the Adorers to this area. Already in 1965, the Sisters had opened a parochial school and health clinic. Sister Serafina taught in the school which became Nazareth High School and also worked in the clinic.

Many sick people died because of the shortage of doctors in the interior. Sister Serafina arranged to transfer to Manaus those who needed immediate assistance and were too serious to be handled at the clinic. Transfer was via a tiresome boat ride, where the more critical could be placed in the hospitals for treatment. A former Adorer gave the following statement about Sister Serafina:

As a temporary professed Sister, I was sent to Nova Olinda where I personally witnessed Sister Serafina's dedicated love for the poor and the sick. Hers was the witness of a true saint as she assisted with the births in the maternity ward and with various general services in the clinic. Those who know the difficult circumstance in the interior of Amazonas can understand the major health problems and hazards that pervaded this region.

Sister Serafina's untiring zeal and unlimited service in attending to the sick at any hour, especially to those who came from distant rural communities, was not always understood by some of the Sisters. They were concerned about Sister Serafina's personal physical condition. Some felt that adhering more regularly to a community schedule was fundamental, while Sister Serafina gave greater priority to caring for the needs of the poor at whatever house they presented themselves. There were also those, however, who admired her humble acceptance of the criticisms and even offenses she received from some of the Sisters. Sister Serafina always defended the sick and poor, but at the same time, she also treated each Sister and every person with kindness and gentleness.

Some of the Sisters witnessed to the fact that Sister Serafina seemed to exemplify a new ways of being involved in community and ministry at that particular time of renewal in the Church. In the midst of all her involvements with God's people in need, Sister Serafina did not forget nor neglect the primacy of prayer. She was seen many times in the chapel. Her concern for priests during this difficult Post-Conciliar period was likewise evident. She counseled younger community members to listen to the priests and to pray much for them.[3 p56-57]

One particular instance that demonstrated Sister Serafina's astute nursing care was recognizing a fellow religious Sister, Sister Genoveva's, very critical condition and then being instrumental in getting her to the hospital in Manaus for the treatment she desperately needed for typhus. She had both the nursing skills and the gentle caring love with which she reached out to the poor. When asked which ministry she preferred among: education, nursing, social work, domestic service and vocational work, Sister Serafina chose nursing and added, "In this work I feel fulfilled and I am happy."

Working continuously without a real and prolonged vacation, Sister Serafina contracted tuberculosis and remained in the provincial house all of 1969. During this time she also saw the demise of the petroleum industry in this poor amazon area. Vacant

371

buildings were transformed into schools for children within walking distance. Others went into ruin, a reminder of what could have been. Still in poor health, she was sent to Marituba in 1970 where she served as the secretary for the seminary of the Redemptorists and took up residence with the Sisters there. Soon Sister Serafina regained her health and once again began working with the poor in the Xingu River region.

In 1972, Sister Serafina was sent to Altamira on the Xingu River, to work in the parish health care center to serve the needs of the sick and the poor. She was also to help train teachers by working with other Adorers in their Pedagogical Institute in Altamira. She was recognized by many as caring for the poor pregnant women, who had traveled from the interior for a safe delivery but were dismissed from the hospital because it was not yet time to deliver. The journey to the hospital was exhausting and many were now in a larger city, very pregnant and with no money. Since the hospital would not shelter them, Sister Serafina found them on the streets, exposed, alone and hungry. She initially housed several in her clinic which quickly exceeded capacity. She worked with parishes and government officials to house the pregnant women. Some complained that the pregnant women were too young and should have used contraception. Others criticized her saying that she was "giving fish to these people instead of teaching them to fish." Sister Serafina ignored these accusations, cared for them and many then became assistants in her work.

In 1972, soon after Dom Erwin Krautler was made bishop, he had his Vicar General, Father Frederico Tschol, oversee the construction of a shelter for Sister Serafina's sick which was fondly called, "The Refuge." It had a dining room and dormitory and could accommodate twelve people. With extra blankets, the shelter could house 50 people. According to their condition, Sister Serafina would either take care of them at The Refuge or coordinate their admission at the hospital for treatment. At times she would manage to send critical patients to Belem for admission.

One day when she was at prayer in the community chapel of the Institute of Maria De Mattias, she heard a voice from outside the window call, "Sister Serafina, help me! I'm dying!" She looked and saw a poor man clothed in rags, trembling and unable to walk. He had been discharged from the hospital after a month and told to leave because he would never get well. His family lived 150km away. Sister Serafina took him to The Refuge and gently and expertly bandaged his leg and prepared a meal for him. She borrowed a hammock and sheets from the priests and made the poor man as comfortable as she could.

In 1973 Sister Serafina celebrated her silver jubilee as an Adorer of the Blood of Christ. She was celebrated in the newspapers as "The Angel of the Transamazonian Road." The building of the Transamazonian Road had impoverished many of the locals who had traveled from their homes in the interior to find work on the road which was not available. Sister Serafina's work was compared to that of Mother Teresa of Calcutta and they referred to her as "Mother Teresa of Altamirea." Sister Serafina was intent on doing God's will as an Adorer of the Blood of Christ and reaching out to meet the needs of her "dear neighbor."

Sister Serafina dreamed of a permanent building to care for the many, many pregnant women who kept arriving in Altamira after an often perilous journey, hoping for a safe delivery for their baby. Bishop Erich Krautler became her advocate in this endeavor and on a visit to Europe made her needs known and raised a considerable sum from friend in the parish of Biberach in southern Germany and also from the Governor of Voralberg in Austria. Interestingly one Austrian magazine reported, "Our women no longer want more children. So let us help those who still have the courage to have them!"

The House of Divine Providence, as it was called, was built on Antonio Vieriea Street, 214 Bairro Brasilia with construction begun in 1979 and completed in 1984. The building was spacious with a chapel, rooms for the pregnant women and an area to house the Adorers who staffed it. On the front of the building was a large mosaic of Our Lady of the Most Precious Blood. And also out front to welcome the women was a statue of Our Lady with the infant Jesus. The House of Divine Providence opened on May 13, 1984.

Sister Serafina's work was not done. She tirelessly begged for beds, sheets, furnishings and money. In one encounter a man told them they should make those "witches" work instead of allowing them to "make" children. Another store keeper told Sister Serafina and a mother who had recently delivered and was helping raise funds, "No one should give anything to this old witch who only knows how to beg." Sister Serafina approached the man, thanked him for the 'compliment' and continued quietly on her way.

373

Despite this, many, many people were very generous and at times she would return from her begging trips with a Diocesan truck loaded with sacks of rice, beans, corn, peppers and coffee. The House of Divine Providence was called by many of the local citizens, "The House of Sister Serafina."

In her book on the life of Sister Serafina, Irma Marilia Menezes relates an example of Sister Serafina's trust in God which occurred in 1983:

> Sister Serafina had an unshakeable trust in God's goodness and love believing that since God is good and God's goodness is limitless, God certainly would never abandon those who are the object of God's love. This gave her unshakable confidence in Divine Providence. One day, in great anguish, Sister Serafina asked Sister Rosa to loan her a large sum of money to pay off, with great urgency, a part of the debt of one of the men who was working on the construction of The House of Divine Providence. Sister Rosa withdrew the money from the bank, leaving both the large school and the Adorers' community without any money left in the bank. The money, Sister Serafina gave to the poor workers with a heart overflowing with gratitude to God. Sister Rosa prayed asking God to take care of the situation and the very next day, Father Dario, whom one of the nuns had been teaching Portuguese, arrived with a donation in the exact amount of what had been withdrawn.[3] p89-90

In 1986, Sister Serafina celebrated the fortieth anniversary of her entrance into religious life with a trip to Wichita and reunion with the group with whom she had entered her postulancy. This was a joyous occasion and many celebrations were held. Within two years, however, Sister Serafina would meet that Good God who accompanied her those so many years nursing the poor, sick and abandoned. The sisters observed her becoming weaker and one day she fell on the streets. After she recuperated, a car was donated by friends that she was able to use briefly. She was sent to the Hospital of Our Lady of Guadalupe in Belem where tests revealed that she had a form of cancer called lymphoma. She received chemotherapy which caused great physical pain, terrible itching, a rash all over her body, hair loss and great weakness. Despite this, she assisted Sister Bernitz Marie with household tasks.

Sister Serafina was moved to the provincial house in Manaus to received care in their newly constructed Nazareth

374

Infirmary wing there. She patiently accepted suffering with meekness and gentleness towards the Sisters and everyone else. She continued in prayer with complete surrender to God's will. She tried with faith to understand and to accept the mystery of pain and helplessness, when there was still so much that she had hoped to do. She so much wanted to recover and return to Altamire to serve the sick and the pregnant women there. Here, however, she offered her suffering for the province of Manaus, for the entire Congregation of the Adorers of the Blood of Christ, and for the whole Church.

As her condition deteriorated, she was taken to the public Hospital Getulio Vargas in Manaus. She was unable to speak the last three weeks. Sister Serafina died on October 21, 1988 on the Feast Day of St. Gaspar del Bufalo, founder of the Missionaries of the Precious Blood. Her body was buried in the Cinque family tomb in St. John the Baptist Cemetery in Manaus at the family's request.

Sister Serafina Cinque, ASC was declared venerable with the decree of heroic virtues promulgated on January 27, 2014 by Pope Francis.[2]

Since her death, several people in the city of Altamira and along the Transamazonian Road have reported receiving graces due to the intercession of Sister Serafina. Irma Menezes lists several of these in her text[3 p111-112] Graces received should be reported to the postulator below:

Postulator: Sr. Maria Paniccia, ASC. Irmas Adoradoras do Sangue de Cristo, Av. Constantino Nery, 1667-Sao Geraldo, 69011-970, Manaus - AM, BRAZIL

How good God is.

References:

1) "Venerable Noeme Cinque". CatholicSaints.Info. 21 June 2015. Web. 26 April 2022. <https://catholicsaints.info/venerable-noeme-cinque/>

2) Hagiography Circle: An Online Resource on Contemporary Hagiography. 1988. Noeme Cinque (Serafina). Accessed 25 April 2022. http://newsaints.faithweb.com/year/1988.htm#Cinque

3) Irma Marilia Menezes. (26 Oct 1999). Serafina Cinque: Angel of Altamira. ASC Profiles 12. Accessed 25 April 2022. https://adorers.org/profile-of-serafina-cinque/

4) Nadine McMillan. (2020). Saint of the Month, February, Venerable Serafina Cinque. Challenge: Catholic Youth Ministry. https://challengeyouthministry.com/saint-of-the-month-venerable-serafina-cinque/. Accessed 25 April 2022. (Photo source).

Ven. Enrica Beltrame Quattrocchi (Italy) (1914-2012)
Accompanied the sick to Lourdes and Loreto
Red Cross volunteer from 1939
Served as a nurse in military hospital during the war,
helping the politically persecuted, soldiers and refugees.

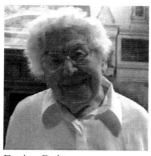

Enrica Beltrame
Quattrocchi
Source: diocesidiroma.it

Enrica Beltrame Quattrocchi was born on April 6, 1914 in Rome, Italy to Luigi Beltrame Quattrocchi and Maria Corsini. She was the youngest of four children. Before the age of 13, between 1924 and 1927, her siblings all left home entering religious life.

In her youth, Enrica was involved with the Daughters of Mary, the Christian Sisters and the Ladies of San Vincenzo. She helped the poor and most needy in the poor areas of Trastevere and Montagnola.

When she was 22, she regularly accompanied the sick to the sanctuary and miraculous healing spring at Lourdes, France, where the Blessed Virgin Mary had appeared to St. Bernadette in 1858. She also accompanied the sick on pilgrimage to Loreto, the location of the home from Nazareth in which the Blessed Virgin Mary was born, received the message from Angel Gabriel and conceived Jesus in her womb. The altar that had been placed in the house in the 1st century was consecrated by St. Peter, the Prince of the Apostles. The house was removed from the Holy Land in 1291, by angels to protect it from Muslims bent on destroying Christian artifacts. It came to its final resting place in Loreto in 1294.[2]

In 1939, as World War II was beginning, she served as a Red Cross volunteer and subsequently graduated from nursing school She worked as a nurse in military hospital during World War II and took care of the politically persecuted, soldiers and refugees. She graduated from the University of Rome with a degree in Modern Literature in 1942. She specialized in art history and began teaching this in 1944.

Enrica considered entering a religious congregation in 1956. However, after consultation with her spiritual advisor, she decided to care for her aging family. Enrica was active in the International Catholic Association of Works for the Protection of Young Women

377

along with her mother. She became the secretary general serving until 1976. Continuing her volunteer activities, she then served as the Superintendent of the Ministry for Cultural and Environmental Heritage beginning in 1976.

On November 15, 2001, at the age of 87, she became a consecrated member of the Witnesses of the Risen movement founded by Don Sabino Palumbieri, SDB. She continued active in volunteer activities welcoming young people, couples, priests, seminarians, religious, bishops and cardinals. Enrica Beltrame Quattrocchi had dedicated her life to the care of her parents, totally disregarding her own aspiration. She was involved in many charitable works including accompanying couples in crisis. As a Lady of San Vincenzo, she cared for those in need.

Her day was shaped by prayer, reading and meditating on the Word of God, daily participation in the Holy Sacrifice of the Mass. She was available to anyone who asked her advice or assistance. Beginning in 2009, her health began to deteriorate, though now 95 years old, she continued to care for the needs of others. In 2010 she adopted Franceso Beltrame, the son of a cousin, thereby allowing the surname Beltrame Quattrocchi to continue. She died two years later on June 16, 2012 in Rome at the age of 98.

Enrica Beltrame Quattrocchi was declared venerable by Pope Francis on August 30, 2021 with the promulgation of the decree of heroic virtue.

References:

1) Congregation for the Causes of Saints. Enrica Beltrame Quattrocchi. http://www.causesanti.va/it/venerabili/enrica-beltrame-quattrocchi.html. Accessed 3 June 2022.

2. Sr. Katherine Marie. (11Jul2005). The Holy House of Loreto. Accessed 3 June 2022. https://catholicism.org/loreto-house.html

Martyrs of Charity - Nurse Victims of the Ebola Epidemic, Democratic Republic of the Congo/Zaire (Italy) - 1995

Died of the Ebola virus contracted while caring for victims of the hemorrhagic fever in Kikwit, Kwilu, Democratic Republic of Congo. Members of the Sisters of the Poor, Palazzolo Institute, composed mostly of experienced nurses, and founded in 1869 in Bergamo, Italy

In 1995 a very aggressive virus that causes a terrible hemorrhagic fever, Ebola, ravaged Zaire taking the life of six nurses, missionary sisters from the Congregation of Sister of the Poor, Palazzolo Institute between April 25 and May 28, 1995. The religious sisters contracted the disease in the hospital wards and operating room while providing nursing care to those infected by the virus. The terrible Ebola virus killed them along with thousands of people in Africa. In Kikwit it affected 220 people and 176 died. The Bishop of Bergamo, Msgr. Francesco Beschi, described these nurses as "martyrs of charity," stating, "There is no greater love than giving one's life like Jesus." They gave their lives to serve the sick and poor in the turbulent country known as the Belgian Congo (1908-1960), Democratic Republic of the Congo (1960-1971), Zaire (1971-1997) and again DRC (1997 to the present).

In May 1995, after caring for victims of Ebola, as they began to succumb to the deadly effects of the virus, the Sisters faxed the Mother General in Bergamo, Italy:

> "We understand your trepidation, but we are totally in God's hands. No evacuation can be done. It is very hard for you and for us to accept this separation from the sisters. Painful events have overwhelmed us but the life of the Congregation must continue: the situation is quite dramatic, especially inside. But it is necessary to remain calm. In Kinshasa there are no outbreaks and all the roads towards the interior are blocked."[1]

The United States of American Center for Disease Control and Prevention recorded the outbreak in a 1998 Emerging Infectious Disease letter.[2]

At the request of the Congregation, on April 28, 2013, Bishop Edouard Mununu, Bishop of Kikwit, initiated the Cause for Canonization of the six religious Sisters by opening the diocesan inquiry to ascertain their heroic virtues. Eight years later, Sister Floralba, Sister Clarangela, and Sister Dinarosa were declared

379

venerable on February 20, 2021. And the next month, on March 17, 2021, Sister Danielangela, Sister Annelvira, and Sister Vitarosa were also declared venerable all with the decree of heroic virtue[3] promulgated by Pope Francis.

The remains of the six nurse, missionary, religious sisters, at the express request of the Bishop of Kikwit Monsignor Edouard Mununu, rest in front of the Cathedral of Kikwit.

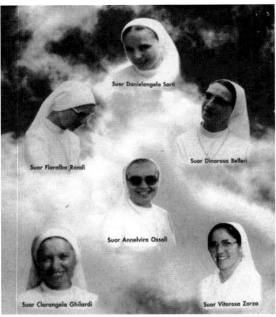

Ven. Luigia Rosina Rondi (Sr. Floralba) (1924-1995) was born on December 10, 1924 in Pedrengo, Bergamo, Italy. At the age of 14, when her mother died giving birth, Luigia took charge of the family, taking care of her father and seven siblings.

In 1944, at the age of 20, she initially entered the Institute of the Sisters of Charity, in Bergamo (aka Maria Bambini). The next year, she met the Sisters ofthe Poor, Palazzolo Institute (Poverelle Sisters) and on April 10, 1946, she entered their novitiate. Two years later, on October 3, 1948, she made her temporary vow as a Poverelle Sister taking the name Sister Floralba.

380

She attended professional nurses training and was then assigned to work in a hospital. After attending a tropical medicine course in Antwerp, Belgium, on April 15, 1952, she departed for the Belgian Congo with four other sisters to begin the order's first mission there. Their first mission was established in Kikwit caring for the sick and poor. It was in Kikwit that Sister Floralba made her perpetual vows as a religious sister on November 11, 1954. She served in Kikwit at the Kikwit Civil Hospital for 25 years. During these years, she faced with faith many difficulties which included an attack of the Soviet backed Simba rebels in 1964. In 1977 she was sent to Kisangani, on the outskirts of Kinshasa, the Congo capital, to work in the poor and populous neighborhood. In 1983 she was transferred to the Mosango Hospital Center located between Kinshasa and Kikwit where she cared for leprosy patients.[4]

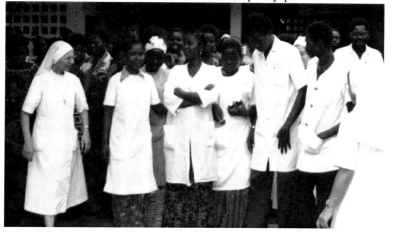

Sister Floralba Rondi, Congo;   Source
ecodibergamo.it

Over a 43 year period, Sister Floralba cared for the poor and sick in the Congo and also often held the office of Superior. Her hope was in our Lord and she relied heavily on Divine Providence not losing her peace and serenity during periods of great difficulty: civil war, hospital management difficulties, shortages of food, doctors and medicines. The Vatican Congregation for the Causes of saints describes her as follows:

> Her life of faith and hope, as well as her dedication to her brothers and sisters, was nourished by the love for God, which transpired in every gesture and in every behavior. He wanted other to love God

too: following him faithfully, if they were priests or religious, regularizing their marriage, if they were cohabiting, trying to assure the seriously ill the anointing of the sick or confession, accompanying the path of conversion of those who had need. For this reason, she often offered sacrifice and continuous prayers with a spirt of sacrifice that affected everyone.

The love she has for the Lord represented for her the constant urge to love her brother and give all of herself for them. She paid particular attention to the poorest and the most sick, to whom she dedicated the most intense care. At the same time, she took care of everyone without making any discrimination based on culture or religious. Her love and availability were also the reason for her death: she took care of the first patients affected by the Ebola virus with her usual dedication and generosity and in turn contracted the infection.[5]

In 1993, two years prior to the Ebola epidemic, Sister Floralba returned to Kikwit to work as a nurse in the Kikwit General Hospital. Her plans were to eventually return to Mosango to work with leprosy patient. On April 15, 1995, as the Ebola epidemic was beginning, she developed symptoms: profuse diarrhea, vomiting, high fever and severe agitation with delirium. She thought she was coming down with typhoid. As symptoms worsened, she was hospitalized at the Mosango General Hospital. She received the sacrament of the Anointing of the Sick around 3pm on April 22nd. Her condition worsened and she developed petechiae, bruises and bleeding at injection sites on hospital day 4, April 23rd. Hemorrhages increased on hospitalization day 5 and her fever remained high. She became comatose and died on April 25, 1995 at 9:45 a.m.

No special nursing precautions had been taken either during the hospitalization or after her death. Her body was transferred to Kikwit for burial.[2] Her funeral was held on April 27, 1995 in Kikwit with an large number of people attending. They remembers her as "mama mbuta" (or "elderly mother"), a name which carried with it great esteem and veneration. She was buried in front of the Kikwit Cathedral.

Sister Floralba was the first of the six Poverelle Sisters to die from Ebola, though as yet, they did not know the cause. Sister Clarangela was the next to become ill. She had taken care of Sister Floralba during the night of April 23rd and according to the CDC report became ill with fever, headache and myalgia on April 30th (see below).

I know in Whom I have placed my hope.

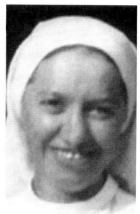

Sister Clarangela
Ghilardi
Source: aciafrica.org

Ven. Alessandra Ghilardi (Sr. Clarangela) (1931-1995) was born on April 21, 1931 in Trescore Balneario, Bergamo, Italy to Michele Ghilardi and Angiolina Oldrati. She was the youngest of four children. Her father worked as a sharecropper. Following elementary school, she was taught the trade of sewing by the local seamstress, Ercolina. She initially worked in a button factory and later moved, with her brother Mario to Milan, to work in the rest home of the Sisters of Poverelle on via Aldini.

She was attracted to the vocation of the Sister to serve the poorest, including the sick and abandoned elderly. Thus, on September 8, 1952, Alessandra Ghilardi entered the Congregation of the Poverelle Sisters. Notably, it was the birthday of the Blessed Mother on which Alessandra took the religious habit and name Sister Clarangela. In 1952, the order had sent five religious sisters to a mission in the Belgian Congo. One day, the Mother General asked for volunteers. Sister Clarangela exclaimed, "If I am asked for obedience, I will go." On March 31, 1955 Sister Clarangela made her Temporary Profession as a Religious Sister in the Mother House church in Bergamo. In the autumn of 1955 she was sent to Rome to attend a boarding school for professional nurses obtaining a diploma in 1957. After she graduated Sister Clarangela, then, was sent to Antwerp, Belgium for a course on tropical disease. She also earned a diploma in obstetrics. She would serve in the Belgian Congo as a nurse midwife..

In 1959 she was assigned to the mission in the Belgian Congo. For the first eleven years, she worked in Kikwit. Here she made her perpetual vows on March 26, 1961. In 1970 she was assigned to Tumikia where she continued to care for pregnant women and the sick poor. From 1983 to 1993 she served at the Mosango Hospital Center. She was described as exuding joy. She could be heard singing softly or whistling as she worked on the maternity ward. She was given a moped to assist her in her work

383

travels and therefore nicknamed, "the Sister of the scooter."

Sister Clarangela returned to Kikwit in 1993 and dedicated herself to many small services including working in the hospital. She continued to have a dedicated prayer life, participated in monthly retreats and annual Spiritual Exercises, having a Trappist monk as her spiritual director. The fruit of one of these retreats she shared with the Mother General in a letter of September 1994 and is written at the conclusion of this summary.

In Easter 1995, the Kikwit health care workers had participated in surgery on a seriously ill patient who died within two weeks. Fellow Poverelle Sister, Sister Floralba Rondi died on April 25, 1995. After taking care of Sister Floralba Rondi, Sister Clarangela fell ill on April 26, 1995, with similar symptoms. Professor Muyembe Tamfum, an expert virologist noticed the red spots on her body and send a blood sample to the Center for Disease Control and Prevention in Atlanta, Georgia, USA on May 5th.

Sister Clarangela said to her sisters, *"Let me go to my Lord."* At another time she prayed, *"I recommend Zaire to you, Lord. I recommend this country to You."* On May 6, 1995 at 135 a.m. Sister Clarangela died in Kikwit, Kwilu, Democratic Republic of the Congo (Zaire). Two days later the definitive diagnosis arrived from the CDC in the United States of America. Both Sister Clarangela and Sister Floralba and several other doctors and nurses had died of the Ebola, a very contagious hemorrhagic fever virus. Four other Poverelle sisters succumbed to the Ebola epidemic of 1995: Sister Danielangela Sorti, Sister Dinarosa Belleri, Sister Annelvira Ossoli, Sister Vitarosa Zorza. Their relics were enshrined in front of the cathedral of Kikwit

Lord, open me entirely to your Fatherly Love,
place me next to my brothers free, welcoming, happy,
poor among the poorest like a drop of water
lost in the immense ocean of your love.

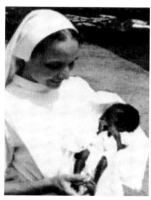

Ven. Anna Maria Sorti (Sr. Danielangela) (1947-1995) was born on June 15, 1947 in Bergamo, Italy. She was the youngest of 13 children, seven of whom survived. Her mother and father died in 1956 and 1957. At age 10 she was left orphaned, grieved and lost her faith becoming a troubled teenager. Through the influence of the Sisters of the Poor (Poverelle Sisters) she reformed her life.

Sister Danielangela Sorti
suoredellepoverelle.it

She desired to enter the order at age 18 but her brothers and sisters opposed. The age of majority was 21. They took her to court but she prevailed due to her strong character and the support of her cousin and guardian Lucia Bacis. At age 19, Anna entered the convent and took the name Sister Danielangela in honor of her parents. She professed temporary vows on September 29, 1968 and perpetual vows in 1974. She was sent to Milan to study for her nursing diploma. There she worked on via Palazzolo caring for the elderly.

Desiring a more contemplative life, she asked this of her superiors. Instead the Superior proposed that she go to Zaire where there was a greater need. On July 4, 1978, Sister Danielangela left for Mosango where she worked at the Hospital Center. She then moved to Kikimi, a suburb of Kinshasa, where she established a maternity ward, so that women no longer gave birth in inhumane conditions. This she did in an area with no electricity or running water! In 1991, she was appointed head of the mission in Tumikia. She was concerned about the suffering of the people under the oppressive Mobutu regime. She did her best to help wherever she was needed.

She was nicknamed by the other sisters, "trappistina" for her contemplative ways. She led community prayers, participated in Eucharistic adoration, wearing her Sunday best to adore Jesus in the Blessed Sacrament. In a letter dated March 23, 1995 she wrote, "Time passes quickly for everyone and we must be prepared because we know neither the hour nor the day when the Lord call us. Stay in joy, because love asks for love."

In order to relieve other sisters already tired from previous vigils caring for Sister Floralba, Sister Danielangela drove to

385

Mosango to look after the gravely ill Sister Floralba on the night of April 24, 1995. In addition to washing blood-soaked bandages, she cut herself on her finger with an injection vial. In the morning she returned to Tumikia. On May 1, she experienced chills, fever. She was hospitalized in Mosango and then transferred to Kikwit when ebola was suspected. Sister Danielangela died on May 11, 1995 in Kikwit, Kwilu, Zaire, one month before her 48th birthday.

Servant of God Sister Danielangela Sorti was declared venerable with the decree of heroic virtue on March 17, 2001 by Pope Francis.

Time passes quickly for everyone, and we must be prepared because we do not know the hour or the day when the Lord can call us."
Stay in joy because love asks for love.

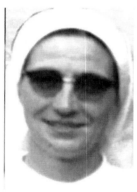

Sr. Dinarosa Belleri
Source: Aciafrica.org

Ven. Teresa Santa Belleri (Sr. Dinarosa) (1936-1995) was born on November 11, 1936 in Cailina di Villa Carcina, Brescia, Italy to Battista Belleri and Maria Riboldi. She was the middle of three children. Her father worked in a workshop and her mother worked in a cotton mill.

She was taught to sew by her mother's cousin Agnesi. She did not enjoy this work and so changed jobs becoming a worker in an iron bolt factory named Bossini located in Lumezzane. She rode her bike each day to the factor and saved the money she made to help pay for her Sister's trousseau. Teresina, as she was called, already knew that she wanted to be a Poverelle Sister.

She entered the Sister of the Poor of the Palazzolo Institute when she was 21 years old, on March 18, 1957, at the Mother House in Bergamo, Italy. She made her first vows on October 3, 1959. The next day she left for Rome for nursing training. After obtaining her diploma, she was assigned to Marine Hospital in Cagliari, Italy which specialized in treating all forms of tuberculosis.

In 1966 she was sent to the Democratic Republic of the Congo (previously known as Belgian Congo). She worked for the

386

next seventeen years in the Mosango Hospital Center. She cared for lepers and other seriously ill patients along with children. During this time she did return to Italy and then was sent for the tropical medicine course in Antwerp, Belgium.

In 1983, at the age of 47, she was transferred to Kikwit cared for lepers, tuberculosis and AIDS victims. In a rare letter, she described the situation, "450 beds for about 1200 sick people, without pipes, without adequate medicines, with food often consisting of insects." She was known to cheer up the other sisters and defuse tension during stressful times. She sang, wore funny wigs and clothes and even and even a dental prosthesis to make them laugh.

Sister Dinarosa remained at her post as the Ebola virus epidemic surged. Sister Floralba had died on April 25th followed by Sister Clarangela on May 6th. The first week in May, Sister Dinarosa began to feel ill and was placed on antimalarials and antibiotics. On the 8th word came back from the CDC that the illness was ebola. Sister Danielangela died on May 11th. On May 14, 1995, around 3 a.m. Sister Dinarosa went into a coma. Sister Vitarosa had been watching over her and realized she was no longer responding. Sister Dinarosa died on May 14, 1995 around 9 a.m. in Kikwit, Kwilu, Democratic Republic of the Congo.

Servant of God Sister Dinarosa Belleri was declared venerable with the decree of heroic virtue on February 20, 2001 by Pope Francis.

When I see them nourished like that [eating insect for their food],
*I feel great compassion and confront our so-called economic crises
with warehouses full of every good thing ...
What a terrible and incomprehensible social justice!"*

"But I am here to serve the poor; the Eternal Father will help me."

387

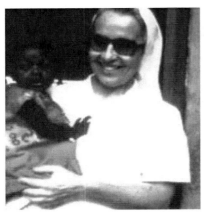

Ven. Celeste Maria Ossoli (Sr. Annelvira) (1937-1995) was born on August 26, 1936 in Orzivecchi, Brescia, Italy to Lodovico Ossoli and Elvira Zerbini. She was one of four children born to their union. Her father worked as a peddler of groceries and her mother in a grocery shop in the village. At a young age, Celeste learned how to knit. She spent her free time with the Poverelle Sisters in the town's oratory.

Venerable Celeste Maria Ossoli (aka Sr. Annelvira)

When Celeste turned 17, her father promised to purchase her a knitting machine. She informed him she did not need one since she planned to be a Poverelle Sister. He over reacted and slapped her so hard that he knocked out a tooth and she fell to the ground. He later repented on his action and gave her permission to depart to the Poverelle Mother House in Bergamo.

Celeste entered the Sister of the Poor on October 5, 1953. Following her postulancy, she took the name Sister Annelvira. She made her first vows at age 20 in 1957. She was then sent to Rome to obtain a diploma as a professional nurse. She completed nursing training and training in nursing administration. In January 1960, she was assigned to the Milan retirement home at via Aldini and worked there for about a year.

Sister Annelvira and was sent to the Democratic Republic of the Congo (previously the Belgian Congo) on November 1, 1961 to work at the Kikwit Civil Hospital. She generously gave herself to her work until she contracted pulmonary tuberculosis. She soon recovered and refused to complete the TB antibiotic regime believing it unfair that those suffering from TB in the hospital did not have access to the same treatment.

She returned to Italy and attended the obstetrics school in Rome graduating in 1969 as a nurse midwife. She returned to the Democratic Republic of the Congo (DRC) and worked in Kingasani, a suburb of the capital Kinshasa. She delivered 30-40 babies a day and was honored with a nickname. "Woman of Life".

In 1977 she served as Superior of the community in Kikwit. She suffered from severe pain in the knees, so much so, that she had to use a wheelchair. She returned to Bergamo. She had surgery and was able to return to Kikwit following her recovery. She work in the mission of Tumikia in 1988 and returned to Kingasani in 1990 as the Superior there. In her letters she expressed concern about the country's political instability.

Sister Annelvira was elected the Provincial Superior in Africa in 1992. She traveled to each of the missionary communities in the Congo, Ivory Coast and Malawi. When Sister Floralba was stricken ill, Sister Annelvira drove 310 miles (500 km) to be with her. After Sister Floralba died on the unknown virus, Sister Annelvira sensed danger and faxed the Mother General in Bergamo, Italy, telling her about the course of their illnesses and her dismay about the deaths.

Sister Annelvira began to feel ill on May 13. She developed a fever and red patches formed on her arms. On May 19 she was quarantined in the little house where the sisters had died along with Sister Vitarosa Zorza. Both received the Sacrament of the Anointing of the Sick that afternoon. Sister Annelvira, Provincial Superior of the Poverelle Sisters in Africa died at age 58, from Ebola on May 23, 1995 in Kikwit, Kwilu, Democratic Republic of the Congo, just a month after the first sister succumbed to the disease.

Servant of God Sister Annelvira Ossoli was declared venerable with the decree of heroic virtue on March 17, 2001 by Pope Francis.

It is Jesus who must be at the center of our life and our apostolate. Then we will do everything with love, finding and discovering, and making known, Who and for Who we are at the service

Ven. Maria Rosa Zorza (Sr. Vitarosa) (1943-1995) was born on October 9, 1943 in Palosco, Italy to Angelo Zorza and Maria Merigo. She was the youngest of seven children. Her mother died when she was two years old. She was raised by her maternal grandmother, Faustina. Her father remarried Maria Calegari and to their union was born two more children.

In 1950, when Maria Rosa was 7 years old, the family moved to Bettole di Cavenago where her father worked as an

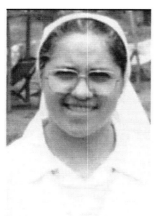

agricultural expert and farmer. Her father was industrious in his work and very religious. Every evening he gathered the whole family to pray the Holy Rosary. At an early age, she felt called to religious life. When she was seventeen, in 1960, the family returned to Palosco. Maria Rosa worked doing house work and also in an umbrella handle making factory.

Maria Rosa began dating a young man named Giuseppe and their relationship lasted two years. Determining that they were not meant to be married, Giuseppe entered religious life and Maria Rosa began in search of her calling.

Maria Rosa met the Poverelle Sisters of the Palazzolo Institute in Palosco. In order to determine if she was called to their mission and charism, she began working in the psychiatric hospital in Varese where the sisters also worked. This experience confirmed her calling to work with the poor and the sick. Maria Rosa entered the Congregation of the Sisters of the Poor on September 1, 1966 at the age of 22. She took the name Sister Vitarosa. She professed temporary vow on March 25, 1969 in the chapel of the Mother House in Bergamo. She was sent to via Palazzolo in Milan where she studied professional nursing specializing in geriatrics. She encountered some fatigue while in her studies and wrote a childhood friend who had also become a Poverelle Sister, "But I want to become a nurse at all costs, to go on a mission to treat sick children."

Sister Vitarosa served the sick elderly at the Milan nursing home, then at Torre Boldone and then the mentally ill in Varese. During her childhood, she had been accustomed to move with her family so she readily adapted to her various assignments. However, she continued to have the desire to serve in the missions and wrote the Mother General expressing her availability three times. In 1981 her request was accepted and she was sent to the tropical disease course and instructed to learn French.

October 20, 1982 at the age of 39, Sister Vitarosa was sent to Kikwit to work in the civil hospital. She tried to bring joy to the malnourished and sick children, mothers, sick people of all ages and conditions and hospital collaborators. In her letters to the Mother General, she expressed concern about the political situation in Zaire: great poverty, injustice, oppression and internal wars. In addition to her work in the hospital, she would bring food and comfort to the inmates in the local jail.

In 1991, at age 48 she returned to Italy for care of an ischemia. She wished to return to Zaire and was therefore sent to Kingasani, the large mission on the outskirts of Kinshasa. She was concerned about the frequent looting and riots but entrusted herself to God.

She was 51 year old when the Ebola epidemic hit. Thinking that they simply had serious diarrhea, with the permission of the Provincial Superior Sister Annelvira, she packed a suitcase full of medicines and drove the 42 kilometers to assist the sisters. Sister Vitarosa assisted the Provincial Superior in the care of the first four deceased sisters. When asked if she was afraid, Sister Vitarosa responded, *"Afraid of what?"* She would then sing along in the Kinshasa language, *"If in the church Jesus Christ calls you, accept to serve Him with all your heart."*

Both sisters contracted ebola and were quarantined in a small house on May 19, 1995. In the afternoon they both received the Sacrament of the Anointing of the Sick. Sister Vitarosa did not seem sick like the others and she took precautions while quarantined. After Sister Annelvira died on May 23, Sister Vitarosa said to the doctor from Atlanta who treated her, "Now it's my turn." She died on the night of May 28, 1995 at the age of 51 in Kikwit, Kwilu, Zaire.

Servant of God Sister Vitarosa Zorza was declared venerable with the decree of heroic virtue on March 17, 2001 by Pope Francis.

"Afraid of what?"
"If in the church Jesus Christ calls you,
accept to serve Him with all your heart"

"I felt that life is a gift from God, that everything that surrounds us is made by Him with love and that every person was also a sign of God's love. I understood that the Lord has a particular project for each person: it is the task of each of us to know this project and carry it out according to the gifts we are filled with. But what was my project?"

391

Reference:

1) FarodiRoma (21Feb2021). Move forward towards the beatification of the nuns killed by Ebola. Accessed 29 April 2022.
https://www.farodiroma.it/passi-avanti-verso-la-beatificazione-delle-suore-uccise-dallebola/

2) Centers for Disease Control and Prevention (Sep 1998). Unrecognized Ebola Hemorrhagic Fever at Mosango Hospital during the 1995 Epidemic in Kikwit, Democratic Republic of the Congo. Accessed 4 June 2022.
https://wwwnc.cdc.gov/eid/article/4/3/98-0349_article

3) Hagiography Circle: Martyrs of Charity. Accessed 28 April 2022.
http://newsaints.faithweb.com/martyrs/Kikwit.htm
http://newsaints.faithweb.com/news_archives_2021.htm

4) Santi Beati. Venerable Floralba (Luigia Rosina) Rondi, Nun of the Poverelle. Accessed 4 June 2022. http://www.santiebeati.it/dettaglio/97446

5) Congregazione delle Cause dei Santi. Venerable Floralba Rondi (born Luigia Rosina). Accessed 29 April 2022.
http://www.causesanti.va/it/venerabili/floralba-rondi-al-secolo-luigia-rosina.html

6) Emilia Flocchini & Sister Linadele Canclini, Postulator General of the Poverelle Sisters. (7April2021). Venerable Clarangela (Alessandra) Ghilardi, Sister of the Poverelle. Santi beati e testimoni. Accessed 28 April 2022. http://www.santiebeati.it/dettaglio/97444

7) Congregazione delle Cause dei Santi. February 20: Clarangela Ghilardi (Alessandra). Accessed 28 April 2022.
http://www.causesanti.va/it/archivio-della-congregazione-cause-santi/promulgazione-di-decreti/decreti-pubblicati-nel-2021.html
http://www.causesanti.va/it/venerabili/clarangela-ghilardi-al-secolo-alessandra.html

8) "Venerable Alessandra Ghilardi". CatholicSaints.Info. 27 June 2021. Web. 28 April 2022.
<https://catholicsaints.info/venerable-alessandra-ghilardi/>

9) Aleteia. Accessed 28 April 2022.
https://aleteia.org/2021/03/23/6-heroic-nuns-who-fought-the-ebola-pandemic-and-are-on-their-way-to-sainthood/

392

10) Santi Beati. Venerable Danielangela (Anna Maria) Sorti, Nun delle Poverelle. Accessed 4 June 2022. http://santiebeati.it/dettaglio/97445

11) "Venerable Anna Maria Sorti".CatholicSaints.Info. 27 June 2021. Web. 5 June 2022. <https://catholicsaints.info/venerable-anna-maria-sorti/>

12) Santi Beati. Venerable Dinarosa (Teresa Santa) Belleri, Sister of the Poverelle. Accessed 4 June 2022. http://www.santiebeati.net/dettaglio/96028

13) "Venerable Celeste Maria Ossoli". CatholicSaints.Info. 26 June 2021. Web. 5 June 2022. <https://catholicsaints.info/venerable-celeste-maria-ossoli/>

14) Santi Beati. Venerable Annelvira (Celeste Maria) Ossoli, Sister of the Poverelle. http://www.santiebeati.eu/dettaglio/96037

15) "Venerable Maria Rosa Zorza". CatholicSaints.Info. 27 June 2021. Web. 5 June 2022. https://catholicsaints.info/venerable-maria-rosa-zorza/

16) Santi Beati. Venerable Vita rosa (Maria Rosa) Zorza, Sister of the Poverelle. Accessed 4 June 2002. http://www.santiebeati.it/dettaglio/96041

393

SERVANT OF GOD

Servant of God Sr. Magdalena Maria Epstein, OP (Poland)
(1875-1947)

Established a small hospital adjacent to the
Daughters of Charity dispensary.
Established the first School of Professional Nurses in Krakow in 1911
Established the modern University School for
Nurses and Hygienists in Krakow

Maria Epstein was born on August 2, 1875 in the Pilica castle near Olkusz to a wealthy family of a convert, Warsaw banker of Jewish descent, Leon Epstein. Her mother, Maria, from the Skarżyńska family, belonged to the class of the Polish landed gentry. In her childhood, Maria's family moved to Krakow. Maria was an only child. She had three half-brothers and a large family to which she was very attached. From her family home she developed a deep sense of patriotism and received a comprehensive education. She knew several foreign languages. From her early childhood days, Maria showed great compassion for the distressed and the suffering. After the deaths of her parents, though she had no professional training, she completely sacrificed her life to help the ailing and the poor.

Before the First World War, she lost all the property inherited from her parents. Not only did she endure it calmly, but she was also able to take care of five elderly people from her former ministry, with whom she shared everything she had for the rest of their lives. She was characterized by a sense of responsibility for

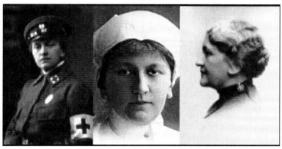

Maria Epstein.   Source: jura-pilica.com

others and a great desire for charity.

Charity work

During the partitions, the only possibility of organized charitable activity was provided by charitable associations. Maria started working in the Association of Women Economists, whose aim was to care for and help the poor. Ladies collected money,

395

materials and clothing, reworked and repaired it, and sewed new ones. They met regularly. After a few years, Maria, despite her young age, became the president of the Association. Her apartment turned into an office and a meeting place. In addition to her activities in the Association, she organized a reading room and simple nourishment for workers.

In 1909, three members of the Association accidentally came into contact with the work of a small dispensary run by the Sisters of Charity. The sisters worked without a doctor providing medical and material assistance. Meals were provided in the same room where they made dressings. Cooperation with the Association of Women Economists brought a change in this situation. With the collected funds, a room intended exclusively for an outpatient clinic was equipped, and medical training for staff in the field of emergency assistance was organized. One initiative gave birth to another. An operating room was organized at the infirmary, and the next stage was the opening of a small eight-bed hospital. Volunteers from the outpatient section were on duty day and night. Over time, they understood that professional nursing preparation was necessary to work with the sick. It was then that Maria Epstein had the idea of organizing a nursing school in Krakow.

With great effort, thanks to contributions and private donations, funds were obtained for the renovation and adaptation of a barn, donated by the Daughters of Charity for the needs of the future school. The opening of the Nursing School took place on November 5, 1911. Since there was no registered nurse who could officially take up the position of the school's director, this position was taken by Dr. Wacław Damski – vice-president of the Krakow Medical Chamber, but in fact it was managed from the beginning by Maria Epstein. Maria and several members of the outpatient section were students of the first class of 14 people. Together they ran the school, at the same time learning in it.

Maria and her colleagues took care to provide a high level of teaching for these future nurses. Maria ensured that their education included a spirit of patriotism and religiosity. She also cared for her own spiritual development and zealously carried out religious practices.

Resourceful director

From 1914-1916 Maria Epstein organised short First Aid/nursing courses which were run by the graduates of the [Krakow] school, and were aimed at Red Cross volunteers. Each group of trained volunteers was to take over the running of a designated military hospital located along the front-line or sometimes deep within the country. The groups were directed to work in Polish units serving in the Austrian Army.

Maria Epstein and her companions directed this action, at the same time working in Prof. Rutkowski's surgical group at the front and in sanitary points at the rest station for soldiers, at the Krakow railway station. Maria was involved in helping the victims of the war through the Ducal-Episcopal War Victims Relief Committee. This committee, under the leadership of Prof. Emil Godlewski, ran infectious hospitals, vaccination points and disinfection stations. Maria Epstein was for some time a supervisor in a hospital in Bielcza near Tarnów, where as a result of the great concentration of evacuated population, epidemics broke out:

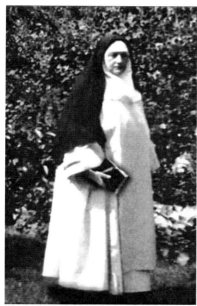

Sister Magdalena Maria Epstein, OP.
Source:
http://www.niepelnosprawni.pl/files/no
we.niepelnosprawni.pl/public/2019/ma
gdalena_maria_epstein.png

dysentery, typhus and typhoid fever. At the same time, she conducted the training of nurses and organized additional medical facilities. She remained in each facility as she launched the works, and then, together with Prof. Godlewski, she carried out inspections of subordinate institutions. Their efforts largely contributed to the extinction of the epidemic.

In 1916, after the resumption of the School of Professional Nurses, Epstein again became its headmistress, struggling with great financial difficulties both at school and in her own home. From 1920 she sought funds to run the school. She received the help of the Rockefeller Foundation and the consent of the Jagiellonian University to launch the University School of Nurses and Hygienists as an auxiliary study of the Faculty of Medicine of the Jagiellonian University. She was appointed headmistress of the same School. In the direct circle of Maria Epstein's collaborators as a director, apart from Anna Rydlówna (her successor, sister of the Young Poland poet Lucjan Rydel), prominent figures of the Krakow circle of professional nursing included: Blessed Hanna Chrzanowska (beatified on April 28, 2018), Teresa Kulczyńska and Maria Starowieyska. Together they formed the first editorial committee of "Pielęgniarka Polska," a monthly professional nursing publication. Thanks to the energy and perseverance of Maria Epstein, the headmistress, the school, despite very difficult conditions, developed successfully.

Fulfillment in God

Despite her success in organizing various works of charity and forms of nursing education, which culminated in the establishment of the University School of Nurses and Hygienists, Maria Epstein felt that she should serve only God, behind the cloister. In shaping her spiritual desires, an important role was played especially by Archbishop Metropolitan of Krakow Prince Adam Stefan Sapieha. The development and formation of Epstein's Dominican vocation was also influenced by her numerous contacts with cloistered sisters of the Order of Preachers in Krakow's Gródek, dating back to 1918. At a mature age, when she was 56 years old, her inner desire to join the community of nuns of St. Dominic, in which she took the name Magdalena, was fulfilled. She enriched the community with her humility, love and zeal in religious life. To the question posed to her as a postulant: "What caused you to enter the monastery?" She replied: "*The desire to strive for a higher perfection and to offer a sacrifice of myself to God, for the Homeland and priestly vocations in Poland.*" After passing the administration of the University School for Nurses and Hygienists into good hands (at the end of 1930), she joined the enclosed Dominican convent in Grodek, Krakow on March 24, 1931. There she spent 16 years setting a good example of humbleness, love, and zeal for the monastic life. At the center of her devotion she placed the Crucified Christ.

During World War II (1939-1945), most of her family members, due to their Jewish origins, died at the hands of the Nazis.

398

She, on the other hand, succumbed to the left-sided paralysis of the body. She endured her sufferings especially for the last five years of her life with submission to God's will and offered them for the intention of the sisters' quick return to the mother convent in Gródek. The sisters had been deported to the convent of the Poor Clare Sisters. During her stay in the monastery, her spiritual director, apart from the Metropolitan Prince Archbishop Adam Stefan Sapieha, was also Blessed Father Michał Czartoryski OP. Sister Magdalena Maria Epstein died in the odour of sanctity on September 6, 1947 and was buried in the Rakowicki Cemetery in Cracow.

On September 30, 2004, Cardinal Franciszek Macharski in the church of the Dominican Sisters in Gródek opened the beatification process of the Servant of God Sister Magdalena Maria Epstein. The diocesan stage was completed on April 20, 2007 and the case file was handed over, through the postulator general of the Dominican Order, to the Congregation for the Causes of Saints in Rome.[1] The decree on validity of diocesan inquiry was issued the next year on November 28, 2008. In 2022, the Positio was being elaborated on.

From the spiritual notes of Sister Magdalena Maria Epstein, OP

"I want to love Jesus for the present and the future time; for all those days when I did not love Him enough."

"To perform all our duties only for love of God and with care about the salvation of souls. To try to be pleasing to God in everything."

"When our thoughts drift apart from God and we forget about his presence, we should often say ardent prayers with our hearts."

"Not to dwell on thinking about our faults in order not to flounder into them, to turn away from them in order to give ourselves to God, who loves us, more fully and with boundless trust."

"Our love for God should be the most beautiful and the purest. The real love for God is indicated by deeds."

"Each deed reacts with our soul. Goodness brings goodness, but one conscious act of evil causes further evil. Let us seek virtues, because each deed shapes our soul."

"To boundlessly trust God and to pray for reaching the level of perfection destined for us by Him."

"In everything that is pleasant, but also in the greatest humiliation, if you, God, wish to send it on me, I want to repeat these words always and everywhere: Fiat Voluntas Tua."

399

Prayer for the beatification & intercession of the Servant of God Sr. Magdalena Maria Epstein OP

Almighty and merciful God, look benevolently on the humbleness, love, and utter devotion to You of Your Servant, Sister Magdalena Maria Epstein and deign to include her among the Blessed. Accord us, with her intercession, the following grace:... for which we implore You through our Lord Jesus Christ. Amen.

Our Father..., Hail Mary..., Glory be to the Father...

Please inform the following of any graces received through the intercession of Servant of God Magdalena Maria Epstein: Dominican nuns, ul Mikolajska 21, 31-027 Krakow. Email: grodek@dominikanie.pl; www.grodesk.mniszki.dominikanie.pl. Servant of God Sr. Magdalena Maria Epstein OP Foundation, www.fundacjadominikanki.pl

References:

1) Apostolstwo Chorych. Nurse and nun - Servant of God Sr. Magdalena Maria Epstein OP. Accessed 6 February 2022. https://www.apchor.pl/temat/2020/04/09/Pielegniarka-i-mniszka-Sluzebnica -Boza-s-Magdalena-Maria-Epstein-OP

2. Hagiography Circle: 1947. 19) Magdalena Maria Epstein. Accessed 5 June 2022. http://newsaints.faithweb.com/year/1947.htm

Servant of God Stanislawa Leszczynska (Poland) (1896-1974)

Polish midwife for 38 years, no child or mother died under her care
Delivered over 3,000 babies in Auschwitz
Known as "Angel in Auschwitz Hell"

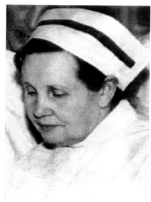

Stanislawa Leszczynska
odkrywamyzakryte.com

Stanislawa Zambrzycki (married lay woman) was born on May 8, 1896 to Henryka and Stanislaw Zambrzycki in Lodz, a portion of the partitioned Poland controlled by the Russians. Stanislawa had seven siblings, five of whom died in infancy. Two younger brothers remained.

At the time of her birth, and since before 1795, Poland had been partitioned between the rulers of Russia, Prussia (Germany) and Austria. As an independent country, Poland disappeared from the map of Europe until 1918. When Stanislawa was five years old, her father was called up to serve in the Russian Army in Turkestan which he did for 5 years. Her mother worked 14 hours per day in Poznanski's Factory in Lodz to provide for the family and Stanislawa took over the care of her two younger brothers and household chores.

Stanislawa began Waclaw Maciejewski's private school, taught in Polish, at age seven as her parents tried to preserve their culture while under foreign rule. In 1908 the family emigrated to Rio de Janeiro, Brazil looking for better living conditions. There Stanislaw attended school and studied in both Portuguese and German. In 1910 they returned to Lodz settling in one of the poorest districts, Bulatach. There her parents ran a shop in which she also worked while continuing her education in a junior high school.

Her father was drafted again for World War I (1914-1918) and support of the family fell upon her mother and now also Stanislawa. Stanislawa still found time for charity work and time to pray. She believed strongly in Divine Providence.

When Stanislawa was 20 years old she married Bronislaw Leszczynski. To their union were born four children: Bronislaw, Sylwia, Stanislaw and Henryk. An important family event was meal times when they met together, talked and shared their day.

When she was 24 years old, from 1920-1922, Stanislawa

401

attended the State School of Obstetrics (Panstwowa Szkola Poloznicza) on the Karowa in Warsaw studying to become a midwife. During the next 38 years that she served as a midwife, no child died, nor did any women who gave birth under Stanislawa's care. She would go to a woman in labor, any time, day or night and make the sign of the cross as she entered the house, over herself and over the woman who was to give birth and finally over the child after he or she was born. If it was a complicated delivery, she petitioned the Mother of Jesus for help.

During WWII, she collected and donated food to Jewish families who were her friends and lived in the ghetto. Her husband and sons took part in the September defensive battles in 1939. Bronislaw and Stanislaw worked as paramedics in a miliary hospital. Her youngest son, Henryk, worked with the firefighting team in Warsaw to extinguish fires following the bombings. Her husband, Bronislaw Leszczynski, had been working as a typesetter in the Kotkowski printing house in Lodz. Her husband and son helped make false documents for Jews to enable them to escape their pursuers.

Arrested by the Gestapo in February 1943, her two sons, Henryk and Stanislaw were sent to the stone quarries of Mauthausen-Gusen concentration camps. Her husband managed to flee the Gestapo but died in the Warsaw Uprising in 1944. Stanislawa and her daughter Sylwia, a medical student, were transported to Auschwitz-Birkenau (Oswiecim) where Stanislawa became prisoner no. 41355. In the concentration camp, she worked as a midwife for two years.

When the German midwife Klara fell ill, Stanislawa asked Dr. Mengele if she could take over her duties. The German woman, Pfani, told Stanislawa that there was an order to treat every born child as dead, to which she did not agree and so was beaten. She still did not listen. The German women, Klara and Pfani, up until May 1943 had drown all children born at Auschwitz. Over 3,000 children were delivered by Stanislaw Leszczynska, and no newborn or mother died at birth. Dr. Mengele could not believe that none died because even in the best university clinics, this was not the case. Stanislawa prayed before each delivery. Many were baptized. She secretly tattooed infants born with blue eyes and fair hair, who were removed from the camp and sent to Naklo to be brought up to become "real Germans, so that after the war they could be

402

recognized. Stanislawa delivered the babies in horribly unsanitary condition surrounded by filth, turmoil, disease, rats, lice, shortage of water, in hunger and cold. Her only supplies were a small pair of scissors like the ones used to remove cuticles, a kidney basin with a solution of potassium permangnate, a very limited amount of cellulose fiber tissue, some bandage to tie the umbilical cord, and a bowl of water to wash the neonate and the mother. After wrapping the infant after delivery, Stanislawa always baptized it with water or a herbal brew, named the newborn and reminded the mother of the first Christian catacombs.

Camp regulations required that Jewish infants were not to have their umbilical cord cut and tied. As soon as they were born, they were to be thrown, placenta and all, in the "shit-bins." Though punishable by death, Stanislawa ignored this rule. She delivered the babies of Jewish prisoners, baptized them too and gave the infants back to the mothers. Most died of starvation because the mothers were forbidden to breast-feed them and even if they could, had little or no milk.

How did Stanislawa survive in the midst of all this misery? She writes in her book, "Midwife's report from Auschwitz:

> this is what made me stronger every day and every night I spent on strenuous work, the toil and sacrifice being just an expression of my love for the little children and their mothers, whose lives I tried to save at all cost. Otherwise, I would not have been able to survive.[1]

Stanislawa was released from Auschwitz in February 1945 and she returned to Lodz and continued to work as a midwife until the mid-1950's. In 1957 she wrote a book titled, *"Report of a midwife from Oswiecim."*[2] In 1970 she met with mothers from Auschwitz and their saved children.

Stanislawa Leszczynska died March 11, 1974 from intestinal cancer. When Pope St. John Paul II visited Lodz in June 1987, he recognized Stanislawa Leszczynska as an example of Christian heroism. On April 9, 1992, the Congregation for the Doctrine of the Faith gave permission (nihil obstat=nothing stands in the way) to initiate the Cause for the Canonization of Stanislawa. On March 3, 1992, the Decree establishing the Tribunal for the Canonization of the Servant of God Stanislawa Leszczynska was issued.[3]

The following is "*A midwife's report from Auschwitz*" written by
Stanislawa Leszczynska (1896-1974) Midwife, Auschwitz-Birkenau
survivor, No. 41335. The paper was originally delivered on 2 March
1957 during a Polish midwives' jubilee held in the health department
of the Baluty district of the City of Lodz:[2]

I spent two out of the thirty-eight years of my professional
life working as a midwife imprisoned in the women's concentration
camp at Auschwitz Birkenau.

There were plenty of pregnant women in the transports of
women brought to this concentration camp. I worked as a midwife
in three blocks which were all alike in terms of structure and
interior furnishings, except for one detail—one of them had a brick
floor. The three blocks were wooden barracks about 40 meters
long, with numerous gaps gnawed in the walls by rats.

The camp was located on a lowland area with clay soil, so
whenever there was heavy rain, water flooded the barracks and
there were up to twenty centimeters of standing water on the floor,
or even more in lower lying barracks.

Three story bunks lined the two long walls inside each
barrack. Each bunk had to accommodate three or even four sick
women on a dirty straw mattress full of the vestiges of dried blood
and excrement. So it was overcrowded; patients had to let their legs
hang down from their bunk or pull their knees up to their chin. The
bunks were hard and uncomfortable, as the straw filling in the
mattresses had long since crumbled into dust, and the sick women
were effectively lying on bare boards, which were not at all
smooth, but parts of old doors or window shutters from demolished
buildings, with "panels" which pressed and cut into their flesh and
bones.

A brickwork stove in the shape of a trough ran lengthwise
along the middle of the barrack. It had a fireplace at either end, but
they were hardly ever used for heating. Instead the "stove" served
as the only place viable for childbed, since no other facility,
however makeshift, had been provided for this purpose. As there
was no heating, the premises were savagely cold, especially in
winter, with long icicles hanging down from the ceiling, or more
precisely from the roof.

The thirty bunks nearest the stove made up what was
known as the "maternity ward."

The block was full of infectious disease and a nasty smell,
and it swarmed with worms of all kinds and rats, which bit off the
noses, ears, fingers, toes, and heels of the women who were so ill

and drained of energy that they could not move.

I did my best to chase off the rats from the patients, taking turns with a woman on Nachtwache (German "night watch duty"). We were helped by convalescing women, taking turns to get a couple of hours of sleep. The rats, which had fattened on human corpses, were as big as huge cats. They were not scared of humans, and if you shooed them away with a stick all they would do would be to duck their heads, dig their paws into a bunk, and get ready for their next attack. They were attracted by the stinking smell of the seriously sick women, for whom we had no water to wash nor a clean change of clothes. When a woman was in labour I had to fetch the water to wash her and the baby myself. It took me about twenty minutes to bring a bucket of water.

The vast numbers of worms of all kinds exploited their biological supremacy over the dwindling vitality of the humans. Not only the sick women but also the newborn babies fell victim to the endless onslaught launched by the rats and vermin. Death came quickly to these human bodies debilitated by hunger and cold, and tormented by their ordeals and diseases. There was a total of 1,000–1,200 patients in the block, and every day 10–20 of them died. Their corpses were taken out in front of the block and were a daily report documenting their tragedy.

The women having to give birth in such conditions were in an appalling situation, and the position of their midwife was extremely difficult. There were no aseptic medical supplies at all, neither dressings nor medications; all the medicine allotted to the entire block was a daily ration of a few tablets of aspirin.

At first I was completely on my own. Whenever there were any complications, such as having to remove the placenta manually, which called for the attention of a specialist physician, I had to manage as best I could. The German doctors in the camp, Rhode, Koenig, and Mengele, could hardly be expected to "tarnish" their medical vocation by attending non Germans, so I had no right to ask them for help. Later, on several occasions I availed myself of the services of a Polish woman doctor, Dr Janina Węgierska, who worked on another ward but was totally dedicated to patients; later still there was another, very generous Polish doctor, Dr Irena Konieczna. When I went down with typhus myself, I was attended by the extremely helpful Dr Irena Białówna, who looked after my patients and me with a lot of diligence and concern.

I won't write about the work of the doctors who were held in Auschwitz as prisoners, because what I observed surpasses my ability to say what I really feel about the tremendous dignity of the physician's vocation and the heroism with which they carried out their duties. The magnificence of these doctors and their dedication was the last thing their poor, agonized patients looked upon but will never be able to say what they saw. These doctors fought to save lives that were doomed, and for those doomed lives gave their own. All they had to treat their patients was a handful of aspirins and their own, great hearts. They were not working for the sake of a grand reputation or blandishment, nor to satisfy their professional ambition; all these incentives had vanished. What was left was just the physician's duty to save lives in all the cases and any circumstances she or he happened to encounter, augmented by the need to show sympathy for their neighbour.

The chief disease decimating the women was dysentery. Often their loose stools would drip down onto the bunks below them. Other serious diseases included typhus and typhoid fever, as well as pemphigus, which covered a patient's body with nasty sores and blisters. The emergence of a few of these pustules, some as big as dinner-plates, spelled death. We did our best to hide cases of typhus from the Lagerarzt (viz. the chief SS physician) by writing in the patient's medical record that she was suffering from "flu" because typhus patients were automatically sent to the crematorium. In practice no one managed not to contract typhus, because there was such a mass of lice in the camp that you just could not avoid getting infected.

It would be no exaggeration to say that about 20% of the putrid, overcooked weeds which made up the patients' staple diet were made up of rat feces.

These are the conditions I worked in day and night for two years, with no one to substitute for me. Sometimes my daughter Sylwia helped me, but the serious illnesses which were her lot, too, made her unavailable most of the time.

Women in labour went on the stove to give birth. I delivered over 3,000 babies. In spite of the appalling filth, the teeming vermin and the rats, in spite of the infectious diseases, the lack of water and other dreadful, indescribable things, something that was most extraordinary went on there.

One day the Lagerarzt told me to present a report on the postpartum infections and mortality rate for the mothers and newborns. I told him that I hadn't had a single death of a mother or neonate. He looked at me in disbelief and said that even the best German university hospitals could not boast of such a success rate. In his eyes I could see anger and hatred. Perhaps the extremely

406

debilitated bodies of my patients were too poor a culture medium for bacteria to thrive on.

A woman about to deliver was compelled to give up her bread ration for some time in advance in order to exchange it for a sheet (or as they used to say, "organize a sheet"), which she could then tear up to make nappies and baby clothes, because, of course, there were no such things in the camp [to see how the conditions described by Leszczyńska compare to the situation in other concentration camps, see, for instance, the 2021 study "Childbirth in Stutthof concentration camp" by Agnieszka Kłys—Editor's note].

The ward had no water, so washing nappies was a big problem, especially as there was a strict prohibition on prisoners leaving the block, and a restriction on moving from place to place on the premises. Mothers dried nappies on their backs or thighs, because hanging them up where they could be seen was strictly prohibited and punishable by death. The rule was that there was no food ration for babies, not even a drop of milk. The babies were only irritated by their mothers' breasts which had been dried out by starvation. Suckling only frustrated them and aggravated their hunger.

Until May 1943 all the children born in Auschwitz were murdered in a most cruel way—drowned in a barrel of water. This was done by two German women, Schwester ("sister") Klara and Schwester Pfani. Sister Klara was a midwife by profession, and she was sent to Auschwitz for infanticide. When I was appointed midwife an injunction was put on her prohibiting her from assisting at deliveries because she was a Berufsverbreherin (viz. she had committed an offence in her professional capacity). She was appointed to perform a job for which she was far better suited. She was also appointed to a management job as Blockälteste (senior block officer). She was given an assistant, Sister Pfani, a ginger freckled streetwalker. Each birth was followed by a loud noise of something gurgling coming from the room of these two, and then the sound of splashing water, sometimes for a fairly long time. Not long afterwards the mother could see her baby's body thrown out in front of the block and being pulled to pieces by rats.

In May 1943 for some children the situation changed. The blue eyed blond ones were taken away from their mothers and sent to Nakło to be Germanised. Whenever a baby transport left the block it was accompanied by the mothers weeping aloud to bid their babies farewell.

407

For as long as the mother had her baby with her the very fact of maternity itself was a ray of hope for her, but parting with the baby was terrible.

To secure a chance of identifying the abducted children at some time in the future and returning them to their mothers, I devised a way of tattooing the babies due for deportation. I did it in a way the SS men did not notice. Many a mother was consoled by the thought that one day she would find her lost child.

Jewish children continued to be drowned. This was done with unrelenting cruelty. There was no chance of concealing a Jewish baby or hiding it among non Jewish children. "Sisters" Klara and Pfani took turns to keep an eye on Jewish women in labour, which made it impossible to keep the birth of a Jewish baby secret. As soon as it was born it was tattooed with the mother's prison number, drowned in the barrel, and thrown out of the block.

The remaining children suffered the worst fate—they died slowly of starvation. Their skin became thin and parchment like, and through it you could see their sinews, veins, arteries, and bones. Soviet babies survived the longest; about 50% of the women were from the Soviet Union [for a detailed discussion on the starvation disease in children in the ghettoes and comparison in respect to the data presented by Leszczyńska, see "Pediatrics in the Warsaw Ghetto," a paper delivered at the 2021 Medical Review Auschwitz conference by Agnieszka Witkowska-Krych—Editor's note].

Out of all the tragedies I saw there is one I remember most vividly: the story of a woman from Vilnius, sent to Auschwitz for aiding resistance fighters.

As soon as she had given birth her number was called (when prisoners were summoned to report they were called by their prison numbers). I went to excuse her, but that didn't help, it only infuriated the SS staff. I realized that she was going to be sent to the crematorium. She wrapped her baby in a dirty sheet of paper and pressed it to her bosom. Her lips moved in silence, perhaps she was trying to sing a lullaby for her baby, as mothers often did to make up for the cold, hunger, and torments their babies had to suffer. The Vilnian had no strength left to sing, only tears came from under her eyelids and fell on the condemned baby's head. It's hard to tell what was the most tragic: the simultaneous death of these two beings who were so dear to each other, or the mother's agony on watching the death of her child, or her dying before the baby and leaving it to its own fate.

Among all these ghastly memories there is one thought

that lingers in my mind. All the babies were born alive. They all wanted to live. Only thirty survived. A few hundred were sent to Nakło for Germanisation. Klara and Pfani drowned over 1,500. Over 1,000 died of cold and hunger. These are approximate figures, but they don't include the period up to the end of April 1943. Contrary to all expectations and in spite of the extremely inauspicious conditions, all the babies born in the concentration camp were born alive and looked healthy at birth. Nature defied hatred and extermination and stubbornly fought for her rights, drawing on an unknown reserve of vitality.

So far I have not had an opportunity to deliver a midwife's report from Auschwitz. I am presenting my account on behalf of the mothers and children—those who could not tell the world about the wrong done them.

References:

1) Stanislawa Leszczynska.. Medical Review Auschwitz. https://www.mp.pl/auschwitz/journal/english/206159,stanislawa-leszczynska Accessed 29 April 2022.

2) A midwife's report from Auschwitz. (2Mar1957) https://www.mp.pl/auschwitz/journal/english/193055,a-midwifes-report-from-auschwitz. Accessed 29 April 2022.

3) Stanislawa Leszczynska - Polozna-Angel in Auschwitz Hell. Accessed 29 April 2022. https://www.odkrywamyzakryte.com/stanislawa-leszczynska/

4) Hagiography Circle: 1974. 6) Stanislawa Leszczynska. Accessed 5 June 2022. http://newsaints.faithweb.com/year/1974.htm

Servant of God Janina Woynarowska (Poland) (1923-1979)
Highly respected nurse in Chrzanow
Helped abandoned and unwanted people, single mothers, their children and
the elderly, organized material and spiritual support
Organized retreats at the Marian Sanctuary in Pioki
Visited poor families in their home
Fortified for the strenuous work of during through daily participation at the
Holy Sacrifice of the Mass and Eucharistic Adoration
Appointed instructor and nurse supervisor, Dept. of Health and Social
Welfare in the Presidium of the County National Council in Chrzanow
Opened a home for unwed mothers
Removed from leadership for stopping at a monastery with a patient
Active participant in the Synod of Pastoral Care
of the Archdiocese of Krakow (1972-1979)
Member of the Secular Institute of Christ the Redeemer of Man

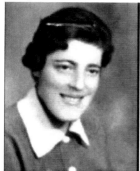

Servant of God Janina
Woynarowska, RN
woynarowska.blogspot.com

Janina Woynarowska was born on May 10, 1923 in Piwniczna-Zroj, Nowy Sacz, Poland. Her mother died in the typhus epidemic and as buried in Istebna. As a child, Janina was adopted by Kazimierz Witold Strzemie-Woynarowski and Maria Jadwiga nee Twarog. Her foster father was a Colonel and physician.

They lived at "white manor house" on Al. Henryka 24 in Chrzanow. The family was wealthy and charitable giving meals, material and medical assistance to the poor. They were a religious and patriotic family. Though Janina suffered from progressive scoliosis, she had a lovely childhood composing poems, playing the piano, visiting with her cousin, Leszek, ice skating, and other activities. Due to her health, she completed the first two years of primary school at home after which she attended primary school No. 3, near her house.

In 1936 she entered Michalina Moscicka, a private school for women, until schooling was interrupted on September 1, 1939 due to the outbreak of World War II. Her parents taught school in their home for a time which also was interrupted due to responsibilities in the home from which they were subsequently ordered to leave.

411

The family moved to an apartment at Krakowska Street and then to Al. Henryka 32. During the occupation Janina was ordered to work digging anti-aircraft ditches. At the end of the war the family returned to their devastated house where on May 21, 1945, her foster father died.

Janina began working at the Obvodows Outpatient Clinic at ul Koniewa 19 (currently Zklad Lecznictwa Ambulatoryinego st ul Skola 19), as a junior hygienist. She was promoted to senior hygienist after 6 months. On June 26, 1946 she took a nursing oath and a year later completed an additional course for employees of the Social Insurance Institution. She was active at St. Nicholas Church and coordinated the Living Rosary.

In 1950 Janina obtained the state certificate as a registered nurse. She was fortified for the strenuous nursing work through full daily participated in the Holy Sacrifice of the Mass and adoration of Jesus Christ on the Cross. She was known to visit the side chapel of St. Stanislaus, the bishop, and lay on the cold floor with a cross and dialogue silently with Christ. In prayers before Jesus in the Blessed Sacrament, she presented matters that awaited her during that day.

She was a highly respected nurse in Chrzanow. She cared for both the sick individual's body and soul. She helped abandoned and unwanted people, single mothers with their children and the elderly. She organized material and spiritual help for those in her care. She kept herself abreast of new development in medicine and implemented these in practice as appropriate. She was always learning so that she could better care for her patients.

With the cooperation of priests, she organized retreats at the Marian Sanctuary in Pioki. She visited poor families in their home bringing advice and help in the form of vouchers (so-called numbers) with which they could obtain basic food in the store. She arranged for tutors for children and if they were not baptized, she often became their godmother. She prayed for the grace of conversion of her patients and several returned to the Church after years of neglect.

The Ministry of Health awarded her "For exemplary work in the health services" on April 8, 1951. Two years later her foster mother died on July 2, 1953. She fainted during the funeral and was taken to the hospital. After she returned home to the empty house, she wrote a beautiful poem in memory of her mother:

She did not give birth, but gave the Love,
which she enveloped a helpless, orphan being for ever.
She invited into her life, she shared her life -
watching day and night with the readiness of tender hands.
The light of serene glances was distracted by the fear
of a child's heart, which ...
sings a ceaseless song - Mateńko[1]

On January 13, 1955, she was awarded with the 10th Anniversary Medal for merits in nursing work by the Minister of Health. Four days later, on January 17, she was awarded the Silver Cross of Merit for exemplary work in the Health Service. On January 1, 1956, she nominated as the Head Nurse of the District Clinic in Chrzanow and the chairman of the Polish Nursing Society.

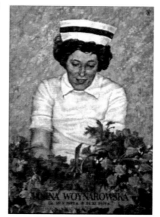

Janina Woynarowski, RN
Source:grafik.rp.pl

In 1961 she took annual vows of chastity, poverty and obedience, becoming a member of the Secular Institute of Christ the Redeemer of Man in Krakow. In 1964 she became the editor of *Ora et Labora*, the institute's bulletin. She was appointed to the position of instructor and nurse supervisor at the Department of Health and Social Welfare in the Presidium of the County National Council in Chrzanow. She worked with Fr. Zbigniew Monko to establish a home for unwed mothers at ul Skola 44. The entire ground floor of this building was donated by the Szurek-Lusinski family for this purpose. At the Adoption Center, she found foster parents for abandoned children. In 1966, she made her perpetual vows with the Secular Institute of Christ the Redeemer of Man in the presence of Karol Cardinal Wojtyla, Archbishop of Krakow and future Pope St. John Paul II, and Fr. Witold Kacz, founder of the Institute.

Unable to afford the upkeep of the family home, the next year, in 1967, she moved into an apartment with her cousin, Elzbieta Twarog-Rawicz at ul Grunwaldzka 13. After several awards and accomplishments noted above, in 1969, she was disciplined and

413

released from her leadership position. She was permitted to work in the clinic treatment room for the next 10 years until her death. What was her offense? She brought, at his request, a man who had a double amputation via ambulance to visit a monastery en route to their final destination. The communist atheist authorities opposed this detour.

Janina's professional accomplishments were many. She wrote articles for the nursing professional magazine: Sluzba Zdrowia i Zdrowie (Nurse and Midwife). She participated in the International Congress of Secular Institutes in Rome. She was an active participant in the Synod of Pastoral Care of the Archdiocese of Krakow (1972-1979) where she met Blessed Hanna Chrzanowska, RN (the first lay Catholic Registered Nurse to be beatified on April 18, 2018 in Krakow). In 1979 she graduated with a master's degree in Psychology and Christian Philosophy. She founded the parish charity team at St. Mikolaja Church. She also worked as a social probation officer, worked at the Adoption Center and provided marital counseling. And she continued throughout her life to write beautiful poems, many of which were the fruit of her pious reflection. Many of her poems were published by her friend Lucyna Szubel in several volumes. She was also an active members of the Gronie Literary Group in Zywiec and was a prolific writer. Some of the most mature and valuable of her writings were: *Our Spirituality* (1971), *Reflections* (1971) and *An outline of the theology of work* (1972)..

Janina Woynarowska died on November 24, 1979 in a car accident. It was a rainy and snowy Saturday. She was driving from Bochinia to Chrzanow with Dr. Emilia Szurek-Lusinska near Krakow's Pasternik. The car skidded off the road and hit a roadside tree. Janina was buried in the parish cemetery in the plot of her adoptive parents in Chrzanow on November 29, 1979. Bishop Jan Pietraszko from Krakow and Fr. prelate Witold Kacz officiated. Fr. Prelate Witold Kacz, Archdiocesan Chaplain of the Sick in Krakow delivered the sermon at the Holy Sacrifice of the Mass funeral.[2]

The canonization process of the Servant of God Janina Woynarowska was opened on June 18, 1999 by Franciszek Cardinal Macharski and the nihil obstat issued by the Vatican on April 26, 1999. The diocesan inquiry began on June 18, 1999 and closed on April 24, 2002. The Positio was published in 2017.

In Chrzanow, the memory of Servant of God Janina Woynarowska, every month on the 24th at 8 a.m. in the church of St. Nicholas, the Holy Sacrifice of the Mass for the elevation of Janina to the Altar is celebrated. Lamps are also lit on her grave and flowers placed there by those who faithfully remember her goodness of heart.[1]

Prayer for beatification

Lord Jesus, Redeemer of man,
Your Servant Janina Woynarowska
has always rushed to help the sick and the poor.
We beg you to help all those who suffer from pain and suffering through her intercession, and to teach us everyday Christian love by her example. Who live and reign with God the Father in the unity of the Holy Spirit, God forever and ever. Amen.[1]

Report any graces received to the vice postulator for the cause of the canonization of Servant of God Janina Woynarowska
Vice-postulajca Sł. B. Janinie Woynarowskiej, ul. Kadłubka, 22 a/4, 32-500 Chrzanów, POLAND; Instytut Świecki Chrystusa Odkupiciela Człowieka, Pl. Mariacki, 5, 31-042 Krakow, POLAND

References:

1) Secular Institute of Christ the Redeemer of Man. Servant of God Janina Woynarowska. Accessed 15 May 2022. https://woynarowska.blogspot.com/

2) Secular Institute of Christ the Redeemer of Man. Sermon of Funeral Mass-Janina Woynarowska. Accessed 30 April 2022. https://woynarowska.blogspot.com/2011/04/zycie-pojea-powaznie.html#more

3) Janina Woynarowska-Biography. Accessed 15 May 2022. https://www.peoplepill.com/people/janina-woynarowska

MARTYRS

Tertio Millennio Adveniente

On November 10, 1994, His Holiness, Pope St. John Paul II promulgated *Tertio Millennio Adveniente* (On the Preparation for the Jubilee of the Year) in which he recommended that the "Consistory, the local Churches should do everything possible to ensure that the memory of those who have suffered martyrdom should be safeguarded, gathering the necessary documentation."[1]

He also stated that,

> "This witness must not be forgotten. The Church of the first centuries, although facing considerable organizational difficulties, took care to write down in special martyrologies the witness of the martyrs. These martyrologies have been constantly updated through the centuries, and the register of the saints and the blessed bears the names not only of those who have shed their blood for Christ but also of teachers of the faith, missionaries, confessors, bishops, priests, virgins, married couples, widows and children."[1]

To facilitate this effort, several nurse martyrs who, as yet, have not had a cause for canonization opened, are included herein.

References:
1 Pope St. John Paul II. (10Nov1994). Tertio Millennio Adveniente (On Preparation for the Jubilee of the Year 2000). Accessed 15 April 2022. https://www.vatican.va/content/john-paul-ii/en/apost_letters/1994/documents/hf_jp-ii_apl_19941110_tertio-millennio-adveniente.html

249-262, Alexandria, Egypt. In Alexandria, Egypt a memorial attests to the fact that many saints --- priests, deacons and laity - died between 249 A.D. and 262 A.D. caring for the plague-stricken victims.[1] Historians conjecture that the cause was either a novel influenza virus or hemorrhagic fever. It spread rapidly and reduced the population of the known world by a third. The equivalent number of death today would be 2.5 billion.[2] (Memorial - 28 February).

The Roman Martyrology records on the twenty-eighth day of February:[3]

> [At Alexandria..]"Likewise the commemoration of the holy priests, deacons, and many others who, in the time of Emperor Valerian, when a most deadly pestilence was raging, willingly faced death while ministering to the sick. The religious faith of the pious is wont to honour them as martyrs.

Martyrs, Who Died in the Great Pestilence in Alexandria (February 28), from the *original* Rev. Alban Butler's (1883) *Lives of Saints*:[4]

> A violent pestilence laid waste the greatest part of the Roman empire during twelve years, from 249 to 263. Five thousand persons died of it in one day in Rome, in 262. St. Dionysius of Alexandria relates, that a cruel sedition and civil war had filled that city with murders and tumults; so that it was safer to travel from the eastern to the western parts of the then known world, than to go from one street of Alexandria to another. The pestilence succeeded this first scourge, and with such violence, that there was not a single house in that great city which entirely escaped it, or which had not some dead to mourn for. All places were filled with groans, and the living appeared almost dead with fear. The noisome exhalations of carcasses, and the very winds, which should have purified the air, loaded with infection and pestilential vapors from the Nile, increased the evil. The fear of death rendered the heathens cruel towards their nearest relations. As soon as any of them had caught the contagion, thought their dearest friends, they avoided and fled from them as their greatest enemies. They threw them half dead into the streets, and abandoned them without succor; they left their bodies without burial, so fearful were they of catching that mortal distemper,

which, however, it was very difficult to avoid, notwithstanding all their precautions. This sickness, which was the greatest of calamities to the pagans, was but an exercise and trial to the Christians, who showed on that occasion, how contrary the spirit of charity is to the interestedness of self-love. During the persecutions of Decius, Callus, and Valerian, they durst not appear, but were obliged to keep their assemblies in solitudes, or in ships tossed on the waves, or in infected prisons, or the like places, which the sanctity of our mysteries made venerable. Yet in the time of this public calamity, most of them, regardless of the danger of their own lives in assisting others, visited, relieved, and attended the sick, and comforted the dying. They closed their eyes, carried them on their shoulders, laid them out, washed their bodies, and decently interred them, and soon after shared the same fate themselves; but those who survived still succeeded to their charitable office, which they paid to the very pagans their persecutors. "Thus," adds St. Dionysius, "the best of our brethren have departed this life; some of the most valuable, both of priests, deacons and laics; and it is thought that this kind of death is in nothing different from martyrdom." And the Roman Martyrology says, the religious faith of pious Christians honors them as martyrs.

In these happy victims of holy charity, we admire how powerfully perfect virtue, and the assured expectation of eternal bliss, raises the true Christian above all earthly views. He who has always before his eyes the incomprehensible happiness of enjoying God in His glory, and seriously considers the infinite advantage, peace, and honor annexed to his divine service; he who is inflamed with an ardent love of God, and zeal for his honor, sets no value on anything but in proportion as it affords him a means of improving his spiritual stock, advancing the divine honor, and more perfectly uniting his soul to God by every heroic virtue: disgraces, dangers, labor, pain, death, loss of goods or friends, and every other sacrifice here becomes his gain and his greatest joy. That by which he most perfectly devotes himself to God, and most speedily and securely attains to the bliss of possessing Him, he regards as his greatest happiness.[3]

References:

1) Ministers of the Infirm: Camillian Religious. The Camillian martyrs to charity. Accessed 15 June 2022.
https://www.camilliani.org/en/the-martyrs-to-charity/

2) Mike Aquilina. (2 June 2020). How the Church survived — and thrived — after a third-century plague. Angelus. Accessed 17 June 2022. https://angelusnews.com/faith/finding-hope-in-the-third-century-churchs-plague-survival-instincts/

3) Canon J.B. O'Connell (1956). *The Roman Martyrology*. Maryland: The Newman Press, 42-43.

4) Reverend Alban Butler (1883). *The Lives of the Saints*. Book II, Vol II-III. Re-published by Loreto Publications: Fitzwilliam, New Hampshire, 2020. (Original texts reproduced with permission), 243-244.

In addition to the vows of poverty, chastity and obedience, the Camillians take a fourth vow of perpetually serving the sick. More than three hundred Ministers of the Sick, as the Camillians are also called, have given their lives in service of the sick. Only a few are known by name.

1589, Palermo, Italy. Father Pasquale and eight other Ministers of the Sick (Camillians) (out of the nine that were there) died in Palermo caring for the sick when the plague broke out in that city.

1625, Genoa, Italy. Father Francesco died, along with his other religious brothers, in Genoa in 1625 caring for members of the Spanish fleet struck by the plague.

1630, Milan, Italy. Brother Olimpo Nofri, along with sixteen sons of Camillus, died in Milan in 1630 when the Asian disease assaulted Milan. This heroic brother, after exhausting his strength in caring for the plague-stricken, noticing that he, too, had the disease, dragged himself after receiving the sacraments, outside Porta Ludovica to the cemetery and there awaited his death --- not wanting to distract his religious brothers from serving other people.

1630, Mantua, Italy. Fr. Antonio Buccelli, who was present when St. Camillus died, was among the fifteen members of the Ministers of the Sick who died in Mantua after caring for citizens, who after being attacked by the Lansquenets, were invaded by the plague. The Camillians were seen running everywhere to give comfort to the dying. (1630).

1630, Bologna, Italy. Seven additional Camillians died in Bologna where they had been called and responded to minister to the sick affected by the plague and hospitalized at the Annunziata e di S. Giuseppe hospital, outside Porta Saragozza. There were thirty thousand victims of the plague in Bologna in 1630.

1630, Piacenza, Italy. Father Marapodio and three other Camillians died in Borgonuovo (Piacenza) caring for victims of the plague. Fr. Marapodio was known for his burning love for Jesus in the Eucharist and for the poor. He dragged himself to the foot of the tabernacle and there, in adoration, he breathed his last.

1630, Monovi, Italy. Father Pizzorno, Father Morelli and Father Lavagna and four others died in Mondovi ministering to the sick in 1630.

1630, Florence & Lucca, Italy. Father Bisogni, in Florence, and Father Domenico De Martino, in Lucca, died caring for the sick struck by the plague in Florence and Lucca respectively. Fr. Domenico had lived for a long time working side by side with St. Camillus de Lellis, the founder.

1630, Rome, Italy. In Rome, almost every day of 1630 saw the death of one of the members of the Ministers of the Sick. The Major Superiors therefore requested to answer the call to assist in Bologna. The Father General, Pieri and the members of the General Consultor, Father Novati, Father Zazio and Father Prandi hurried to Bologna to assist when the plague struck that city. Two of them caught the plague. One of them died there. The others were spared for future labors including that of 'cleaning houses' and disinfecting offices in places where the plague was present.

1630, Rome, Italy. Father Zazio, who was very experienced in cleaning and disinfecting houses with the caustic sprays of Sulphur, bitumen and mixtures of resinous substance and even direct flames, lost his sight and his life was shortened due to the chemical exposure. He was another martyr of charity.

1630, Naples, Italy. When the city state of Naples was attacked by the plague, the number who became martyrs of charity was the greatest. All of the Ministers of the Sick volunteered to serve in the hospital caring for the infected. Of the 100 priests who volunteered, 96 succumbed to the plague. The names of twenty-seven of these are known. Of them are: Prospero Voltabio, Giovanni Battista Crescenzi, Luifi Franco, and Troiano Positani - these four had been

421

trained in the school of the Founder and had previously worked by his side. Of the brothers, the names of only thirteen are known.

1630, Rome, Italy. Father General Albiti died in Rome of the contagion and made there as his last recommendation to persevere "entire service to God in order to always be minister and faithful servants of the poor."

1630, Viterbo, Italy. Two additional Camillians died caring for those infected by the plague in Viterbo.

1630, Genoa, Italy. In Genoa, the loss was only second to that in Naples. The plague killed approximately 64,000 citizens in Genoa. All fifty Sons of St. Camillus who went to care for them came down with the plague. Thirty-seven of these died. Brother Giacomo Giacopetti was one of the victims "who was crowned in such a worthy way a life of hard work and immolation in the apostolate of nursing charity." 1630

Additional Martyrs of Charity: Turin epidemic of 1679; Genoa, 1709; and Rome, 1714 and 1731; Plague in Messina in 1743.wenty-six religious sacrificed themselves caring for victims of the plague which struck that city.

Additional Martyrs of Charity as the Sons of Camillus entered their field of nursing charity in a superabundant fashion: 1835-1911-Cholera; nursing war victims in Europe between 1595 to 1914-1918.

Reference:
1) Ministers of the Infirm: Camillian Religious. The Camillian martyrs to charity. Accessed 15 June 2022.
https://www.camilliani.org/en/the-martyrs-to-charity/

2) M. Vanti (1929). San Camillo de Lellis (1550-1614), Libreria Editrice, Francesco Ferrari, Rome. 681-689.

Anna Sonsalla (Sr. Maria Herais) (Poland) (1867-1945), Martyr
Certified Nurse, Caretaker Sanct Anna Stift Nursing Home
Congregation of Nursing Sisters of the Third Order Regular of Saint
Francis (Hospitaller Franciscan - OSF)
Burned alive by Russian forces with 16 charges including 4 children

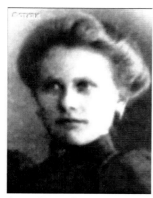

Anna Sonsalla
(Sister Maria Herais)
swzygmunt.knc.pl

Anna Sonsalla was born on October 10, 1867 in Dobrzen Wielki, Opole, Poland. She joined the Congregation of Nursing Sisters of the Third Order Regular of Saint Francis (Hospitaller Franciscan - OSF). She became a certified nurse in the Congregation on April 26, 1916. She made her perpetual vows on October 24, 1924. From 1936-1945 she lived in the religious house in Pokoju near Opole and served as the caretaker and nurse of the "Sanct Anna Stift" nursing home.

During the Russian winter offensive in 1945, when it became clear that the Russians were winning and the front was getting closer, on January 21, 1945, she moved her charges from the old people's home to a wooden barn (or rather a brick house) in the forest. She hid there for over 3 weeks until a group of Russian discovered them in the forest. The Russians surprised, poured gasoline over the walls of the barn and set her on fire. She was burned alive with 16 charges, including 4 children.

Sister Maria Herais died with her charges on February 16, 1945 in Pokoj, Namyslow, Poland.

References:

1) Hagiography Circle: Poland. Anna Sonsalla (Maria Herais). http://newsaints.faithweb.com/new_martyrs/Poland2.htm. Accessed 5 June 2022.

2) St. Zygmunt Roman Catholic Parish. White Book. Martyrdom of the Clergy 1914-1989. Anna Sonsalla (Sister Maria Herais). http://www.swzygmunt.knc.pl/MARTYROLOGIUM/POLISHRELIGIOUS/vPOLISH/HTMs/POLISHRELIGIOUSmartyr2537.htm. Accessed 5 June 2022.religious, Hospital Sisters of Saint Francis

423

Barbora Boenigh (Sr. Florina) (Poland/Slovakia) (1894-1956), Martyr

Serve the sick and poor all her life
Nurse at the hospital in Nitra
Arrested and tortured in prison

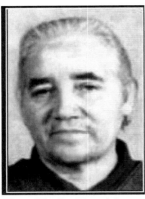

Sister Florina Boenigh
newsaints.faithweb.com

Barbora Boenigh was born December 21, 1894 in Wegajty (aka Wengaithen), Jonkowo, Olsztyn, Poland. She jointed the Society of Daughters of Charity of St. Vincent de Paul on June 27, 1914, at age 17. She served the poor sick all her life. She cared for the children in the Trnava orphanage for 10 years. She was the superior of the hospital communities in Kremnica, Ruzomberok & Levoca

Of Sister Florina, the other sisters would say, *"When I say she was good, that's not enough, she was pre-eminent! Pious, modest, unobtrusive, hardworking. She did the lowest work. In Levoca, she was in charge of supplying the hospital kitchen. She raised pigs and poultry for the hospital, and grew flowers for the chapel. Sometimes she surprised her sister on night duty and brought her some sweets. She took great care to ensure that the sisters were faithful in their vocation and ministry."*

In 1948 she worked as a nurse at the hospital in Nitra. She was arrested at the hospital by communist "State Security Service" on November 22, 1951, at age 57, for: 1) sheltering Fr. Stefan Kristin CM who escaped from concentration monastery in Hronsky Benadik and 2) helping Lazarist theologians continue their seminary studies, locating private homes, provided food, clothes, and finances.

Sister Florina was beaten and exposed to hunger and cold. She would not betray the location of the sheltered Lazarists. At the time she was already weakened by the chronic illnesses of diabetes and heart disease. The authorities transferred her from Nitra to Bratislava on 19 March 1952.

After 10 months in pre-trial confinement which included beatings, she was sentenced to *15 years in prison, fine of 20,000 crowns, forfeiture of property and loss of honorary civil rights for 10 years for the crime of high treason.*

424

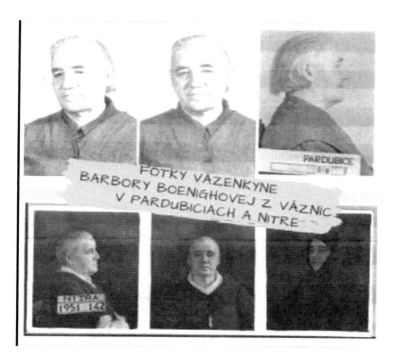

FOTKY VÄZENKYNE
BARBORY BOENIGHOVEJ
V PARDUBICIACH A NITRE

She was imprisoned with sister Vincencia Hanskova, first in Rimavska Sobota in Pardubice, where they met other imprisoned sisters. She was assigned to the knitting factory. Her health continued to deteriorate. She was then transferred to prison no. 2, then to Pankrac prison in Prague. Sister Florina died on January 31, 1956, 8:30 pm, recurrent myocardial infarction.

The nurses learned of her death gradually and it was confirmed when package was returned marked "DIE". Her body dumped in the prison yard until the mortuary service arrived the following day. Snow covered the corpse.

The Sisters found her grave in Prague-Dablice and provided a marker. A lilac grew above the place where it was located. When her prison file was opened, they found that it contained a picture of a child looking at the cross and the Miraculous Medal, which she distributed throughout her life

"Sisters, just pray.
Prayer will save the whole world, including us!"

"I sacrifice it all for you, that you may be faithful and steadfast."

425

References:

1) Hagiography Circle. Slovakia-Sister Florina (Barbora Boenighova).
Accessed 15 May 2022.
http://newsaints.faithweb.com/new_martyrs/Slovakia2.htm

2) Society of Daughters of Christian Love St. Vincenta de Paul. S. Florina
Boenigh. Accessed 15May 2022.
https://www.vincentky.sk/100-rokov-slovenskej-provincie/medailony-o-vyni
mocnych-sestrach/s-florina-boenighova/. (Source of Photo)

426

Sister Izabela (Zofia Luszczkiewicz) (Poland) (1898-1957)

Daughter of Charity,[1]
Nurse during the:Bolshevik War,
Soviet Invasion of Poland,
World War II,
Soviet Occupation of Poland

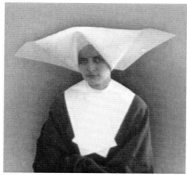

Sister Izabela - Zofia Luszczkiewicz
Source: histroia.tvp.pl

Zofia Luszczkiewicz was born on April 23, 1898 in Krakow, Poland, the first child of Michal and Kazimiera nee Lakocinski. Her father was an attorney. She served as a volunteer nurse during the Polish-Bolshevik War (1919-1920).

In 1923, she entered the Congregation of the Sisters of Mercy in Krakow. Her postulant year was in the house of St. Kazimierz in Lviv. She received the habit and took the name Sister Izabela. She attended the novitiate at the Mother House in Paris, from September 3, 1923 to August 30, 1924. She studied nursing at the College of Nursing in Paris in 1926. Sister Izabela was fluent in French, German, English and Latin

Sister Izabela served as the Headmistress of the School of Nursing at the Lviv General Hospital. She collaborated extensively with the school in Paris to improve the nursing education standard in Lviv. She attended nurses' meetings in various countries: Paris 1937, London, Vienna, Vilnius, New York-1939. Sister Izabela even obtained a cinema operator's license in USA & purchased film equipment using audiovisual aids to assist with occupational therapy. She was an amateur photographer and had driver's license to drive both a car and truck. Sister Izabela had a beautiful voice which enriched the liturgy. She also played piano

She traveled to the United States for an intership which she shortened due to the threat of World War II. After the Soviets invaded Poland, she was sought after by NKVD. During World War II (1938-1945), Sister Izabela cooperated with Home Army and Peasants' Battalions as an emissary. Monitored radio station, delivered weapons and aided in hiding Jews. Once she was rescued

427

from the Nazi Gestapo by Poland's national resistance. Following the war, during the Soviet occupation, she cooperated with WiN (Wolnosci I Niezawislosc = Freedom and Independence), a Polish Underground which operated between 1944-1963.[2] She was arrested and persecuted under the communists. She lost three front teeth under torture; refused to speak against Church leaders; was forced to spend nights naked and doused with water in her prison cell; and threatened to be killed each night. Eventually her death sentence was commuted to Life in prison.

In 1956, she was released conditionally due to poor health. She was ill with tuberculosis of the bone and suffered a tumor in the jaw. Sister Izabela died on August 8, 1957 at the provincial house in Krakow, Poland. She was buried in the tomb of the Sisters of Mercy in Rakowicki Cemetery.

On December 12, 1993, the Provincial Court in Warsaw overturned the convictions of 1949-1950 and ruled that the activities of Sr. Izabela was a fight for the independent existence of the Polish State.[3]

References

1) Hagiography Circle: An Online Resource on Contemporary Hagiography. Poland. Accessed 15 April 2022. http://newsaints.faithweb.com/new_martyrs/Poland2.htm

2) Freedom and Independence - Wolnosc I Niezawislosc, WiN: Polish Underground Socilers 1944-1963 - The Untold Story. Accessed 11 April 2022. https://freedomandindependence.com/

3) Muzeum Pielegniarstwa Polskiego. Sr. Izabela Zofia Luszczkiewicz 1898-1957. Accessed 15 May 2022. http://www.wmpp.org.pl/pl/wzorce-osobowe/%C5%82uszczkiewicz-izabela-zofia-s.html

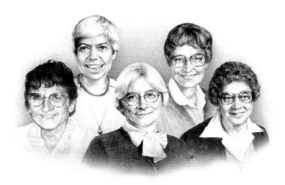

In 1969 a priest, after being turned down by several other religious orders, invited the provincial leader of the Adorers of the Blood of Christ in Ruma, Illinois to work in Liberia, West Africa. The community agreed and the first group of sisters departed for Liberia in 1971. They staffed schools, parishes, clinics and hospitals. The sisters loved the people and served there for more than twenty years despite the civil unrest and other challenges. In 1991, the Liberian Civil War made daily life increasingly dangerous so the five sisters based in Liberia returned to the United States due to safety concerns. A year later they decided to return.

On October 20, 1992 Sister Barbara Ann Muttra and Mary Joel Kolmer were ambushed and killed by gunmen along a dirt road they travels to return a worker to his home. Three days later, on October 23, soldiers shot and kills Sisters Kathleen McGuire, Agnes Mueller and Shirley Kolmer in front of their convent in Gardenersville. The other occupants of the house notified the bishop in Bonga, Bomi County, Liberia. It was not until October 31, 1992 that the sisters in Ruma, Illinois received notification. At that time their mission in Liberia abruptly ended.

Authorities investigated their killing. His Holiness Pope St. John Paul II declared the five Martyrs of Charity. The Sisters erected a sculpture of the martyrs in Ruma, Illinois. In Liberia, clinics, schools and babies were named for the Martyrs of Charity. These five sisters committed their life to charitable works in Liberia. All gave generously. Below is a brief summary of information on the two who were nurses:

Sister Barbara Ann Muttra, (USA/Liberia) (1923-1992), Martyr
Surgical nurse; Worked for Catholic Relief Services in Vietnam
Ran Clinic; Trained midwives and Health Care Workers in Liberia

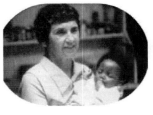

Barbara Ann Muttra was born in 1923. After nursing school, advanced training in surgical nursing, and jobs in hospitals, an orphanage and a nursing home, she signed up with Catholic Relief Services, which needed nurses at the height of the Vietnam War. She served there from 1968-1971, working with orphans, shuttling food and medicine by boat to thousands of refugees, and picking shrapnel from bodies in the operating room.

Before she left Vietnam, she has signed up for the Adorers' mission in Liberia, where she ran clinics, trained midwives and health care workers, and improved the infant mortality. Her trademark smiley-face next to her signature on letter reflected her eternal optimism. Of all the Adorers who went to Liberia, Barbara Ann stayed the longest 21 years from 1971 until her murder, at age 69, on October 20, 1992 on the road between Gardensville and Barnersville. Liberia.

Sister Agnes Mueller, (USA/Liberia) (1930-1992), Martyr
Nurse, spending 15 years in this ministry

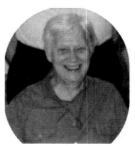

Agnes Mueller was born in 1930. She grew up during the Depression, the fifth of nine children. From the family home, it was an easy walk to the Adorers' residence at their parish school in Bartelso. She visited frequently, so no one was surprised when Agnes said she wanted to become a sister. She yearned to become a missionary and wondered if the Adorers could provide that opportunity.

She joined anyway and became a nurse spending 15 years in the ministry. But it wasn't enough. She hungered for more and kept searching. She studied theology, did parish work, and cared for her aging mother.

Six months after her mom's death, in 1987, she left for

Liberia. She found her most fulfilling ministry there, helping Liberian women become more financially independent and bringing them more fully into the church. She started with the basics: teaching them to read. She taught other classes, worked in a clinic and met with young women interested in spirituality. She was shot to death with two of her sisters on October 23, 1992, outside of the sisters' residence in Gardnersville, Liberia. She was 62.

References:

1) Adorers of the Blood of Christ, United States Region. Martyrs of Charity. https://adorers.org/about-us/history/martyrs/ Accessed 5 June 2022.

2) Hagiography Circle: Liberia. Accessed 5 June 2022. http://newsaints.faithweb.com/new_martyrs/Liberia.htm

APPENDICES

Country of Birth, Mission or Death

Algeria
Bl. Paul-Helene Saint Raymond, martyr
Bl. Denise Leclerc (Sr. Bibiane), martyr
Bl. Esther Paniagua Alonso, martyr

Argentina
St. Nazaria Ignacia March y Mesa
Bl. Maria Crescencia Perez
Bl. Francisca Pons Sarda (Sr. Gabriella of St. John of the Cross), martyr

Austria
Bl. Maria Restituta Helena Kafka, martyr

Belgium
St. Juliana of Mont-Cornillon
Bl. Edward Joannes Maria Poppe

Bolivia
St. Nazaria Ignacia March y Mesa

Brazil
Ven. Noeme Cinque (Sister Serafina)

Canada
Venerable Jeanne Mance

Canary Islands
St. Pedro de San Jose de Betancur

Chile
Bl. Maria Crescencia Perez

Congo, Democratic Republic of the (Zaire / Belgium Congo)
Venerable Luigia Rosina Rondi (Sr. Floralba)
Venerable Alessandra Ghilardi (Sr. Clarangela)
Venerable Anna Maria Sorti (Sr. Danielangela)
Venerable Teresa Santa Belleri (Sr. Dinarosa)
Venerable Celeste Maria Ossoli (Sr. Annelvira)
Venerable Maria Rosa Zorza (Sr. Vitarosa)

Cuba
Bl. Jose Olallo Valdes

Czech Republic (Czechoslovakia)
Bl. Maria Restituta Helena Kafka, martyr

Ecuador
Bl. Maria Troncatti

England
Venerable Magdalen of the Sacred Heart (Frances Margaret Taylor)
Venerable Mary Jane Wilson (Sister Maria de St. Francis)

Ethiopia
Bl. Liduina Meneguzzi

France (the eldest daughter of the Church)
St. Radegund
St. Bertille
St. Elzear of Sabran & Bl. Delphina of Glandeves
St. Roch (St. Rocci) (Kingdom of Majorca)
St. Jeanne (Jane) Antide Thouret
St. Bernadette of Lourdes
Bl. Marie-Catherine de Saint-Augustine
Bl. Olga Perez-Monteserin Nunez, martyr
Bl. Paul-Helene Saint Raymond, martyr
Bl. Denise Leclerc (Sr. Bibiane), martyr
Venerable Jeanne Mance

Germany
St. Radegund (Thuringia)
St. Marianne Cope
Bl. Lukarda of Oberweimar (Thuringia), stigmatic
Bl. Jutta of Thuringia
Bl. Maria Euthymia Uffing
Bl. Anna Ellmerer (Sr. M. Felicitas), martyr

Guatemala
St. Pedro de San Jose de Betancur
Servant of God Barbara Samulowska (Sr. Stanislawa)

Hungary
St. Stephen of Hungary
St. Elizabeth of Hungary

India
Venerable Mary Jane Wilson (Sister Maria de St. Francis)

Italy
St. Fabiola (Rome)
St. Amato Ronconi
St. Margaret of Cortona
St. Elzear of Sabran & Bl. Delphina of Glandeves
St. Roch (St. Rocci)
St. Catherine of Siena
St. Frances of Rome
St. Camillus de Lellis
St. Aloysius (Luigi) Gonzaga
St. Jeanne (Jane) Antide Thouret
St. Vincenza Gerosa
St. Giuseppina Vannini
St. Maria Domenica Mantovani
St. Agostina Livia Pietrantoni
St. Mary Elizabeth Hesselblad
St. Maria Bertilla Boscardin
Bl. Teuzzo of Razzuolo
Bl. Benvenute de Gubbio
Bl. Maria Domenica Brun Barbantini

435

Italy (cont'd)
Bl. Gertrude Prosperi
Bl. Giovannina Franchi
Bl. Luigi Maria Monti
Bl. Enrico Rebuschini
Bl. Maria Troncatti
Bl. Maria (Corsini) Beltrame Quattrocchi
Bl. Aurelia Mercede Stefani (Sister Irene)
Bl. Liduina Meneguzzi
Bl. Leonella Sgorbati, martyr
Venerable Giovanni Nadiani
Venerable Enrica Beltrame Quattrocchi
Venerable Luigia Rosina Rondi (Sr. Floralba)
Venerable Alessandra Ghilardi (Sr. Clarangela)
Venerable Anna Maria Sorti (Sr. Danielangela)
Venerable Teresa Santa Belleri (Sr. Dinarosa)
Venerable Celeste Maria Ossoli (Sr. Annelvira)
Venerable Maria Rosa Zorza (Sr. Vitarosa)

Japan
St. Michael Kozaki

Kenya
Bl. Aurelia Mercede Stefani (Sister Irene)
Bl. Leonella Sgorbati, martyr

Liberia
Sister Barbara Ann Muttra, martyr
Sister Agnes Mueller, martyr

Majorca, Kingdom of (Spain)
St. Roch (St. Rocci) (Kingdom of Majorca)

Mexico
St. Maria de Jesus Sacramentado Venegas de La Torre
St. Nazaria Ignacia March y Mesa

Poland
Bl. Maria Luisa Merkert (Silesia)
Bl. Marta Wiecka (Prussia)
Bl. Hanna Chrzanowska
Bl. Maria Magdalena Jahn (Sr. M. Paschalis) (Silesia), martyr
Bl. Marta Rybka (Sr. M. Melusja Rybka), martyr
Bl. Juliana Kubitzki (Sr. M. Edelburgis), martyr
Bl. Klara Schramm (Sr. M. Adela), martyr
Bl. Jadwiga Topfer (Sr. M. Adelheidis), martyr
Bl. Helena Goldberg (Sr. M. Acutina), martyr
Bl. Anna Ellmerer (Sr. M. Felicitas), martyr
Bl. Elfrieda Schilling (Sr. M. Rosaria), martyr
Bl. Anna Thienel (Sr. M. Sabina), martyr
Bl. Luczja Heymann (Sr. M. Sapientia/Lucia Emmanuela), martyr
Venerable Rozalia Celakowna
Servant of God Barbara Samulowska (Sr. Stanislawa)
Servant of God Sr. Magdalena Maria Epstein, OP
Servant of God Stanislawa Leszczynska
Servant of God Janina Woynarowska
Anna Sonsalla (Sr. Maria Herais), martyr
Sister Florina (Barbora Boenigh), martyr
Sister Izabela (Zofia Luszczkiewicz), martyr

Portugal
St. John of God
Venerable Mary Jane Wilson (Sister Maria de St. Francis)

Slovakia
St. Elizabeth of Hungary (Slovakia/Hungary)
Bl. Zdenka Cecilia Schelingova, martyr
Martyr Sister Florina (Barbora Boenigh), martyr

Somalia
Bl. Leonella Sgorbati, martyr

Spain
St. Didacus
St. John of God
St. Nazaria Ignacia March y Mesa
Bl. Bonaventure of Barcelona
Bl. Maria Rafols Bruna
Bl. Francisco Garate Aranguren
Bl. Josep Tarrats Comaposada, martyr
Bl. Francisca Pons Sarda (Sr. Gabriella of St. John of the Cross), martyr
Bl. Benito Solana Ruiz-martyr
Bl. Juan Bautista Egozcuezabal Aldaz, martyr
Bl. Juan Agustin Codera Marques, martyr
Bl. María Isabel López García (Sr. Mary of Peace), martyr
Bl. Vicenta Achurra Gogenola (Sr. Daniela of San Barnaba), martyr
Bl. Octavia Iglesias Blanco, martyr
Bl. Maria Pilar Gullon Yturriaga, martyr
Bl. Olga Perez-Monteserin Nunez, martyr
Bl. Esther Paniagua Alonso, martyr
Ven. Coloma Antonia Marti y Valls

Sweden
St. Bridget of Sweden
St. Mary Elizabeth Hesselblad

Ukraine
Bl. Marta Wiecka (Prussia)

United States of America (USA)
St. Marianne Cope, O.S.F.
St. Mary Elizabeth Hesselblad
Sister Barbara Ann Muttra, martyr
Sister Agnes Mueller, martyr

Memorial - Feast Day

January
23-St. Marianne Cope

February
2-St. Maria Domenica Mantovani
6-St. Michael Kozaki
22-St. Margaret of Cortona
23-Bl. Giovannina Franchi
23-St. Giuseppina Vannini
28-Martyrs, Who Died in the Great Pestilence in Alexandria

March
7-Bl. Jose Olallo Valdes
8-St. John of God
9-St. Frances of Rome
22-Bl. Lukarda of Oberweimar (Thuringia), stigmatic

April
6-St. Juliana of Mont-Cornillon
16-St. Bernadette of Lourdes
25-St. Pedro de San Jose de Betancur
28 - Bl. Hanna Chrzanowska
29-St. Catherine of Siena

May
5-Bl. Jutta of Thuringia
8-Bl. Marie-Catherine de Saint-Augustine
8-Bl. Paul-Helene Saint Raymond, martyr
8-Bl. Denise Leclerc (Sr. Bibiane)
8-Bl. Esther Paniagua Alonso
10-Bl. Enrico Rebuschini
11-Bl. Maria Magdalena Jahn (Sr. M. Paschalis), martyr
11-Bl. Marta Rybka (Sr. M. Melusja Rybka), martyr
11-Bl. Juliana Kubitzki (Sr. M. Edelburgis), martyr
11-Bl. Klara Schramm (Sr. M. Adela), martyr
11-Bl. Jadwiga Topfer (Sr. M. Adelheidis), martyr
11-Bl. Helena Goldberg (Sr. M. Acutina), martyr

11-Bl. Anna Ellmerer (Sr. M. Felicitas), martyr
11-Bl. Elfrieda Schilling (Sr. M. Rosaria), martyr
11-Bl. Anna Thienel (Sr. M. Sabina), martyr
11-Bl. Luczja Heymann (Sr. M. Sapientia/Lucia Emmanuela),
martyr
15-St. Amato Ronconi
20-Bl. Maria Crescencia Perez
22-Bl. Maria Domenica Brun Barbantini
23-St. Jeanne (Jane) Antide Thouret
30-Bl. Marta Wiecka

June
4-St. Mary Elizabeth Hesselblad
10-Bl. Edward Joannes Maria Poppe
21-St. Aloysius (Luigi) Gonzaga
28-St. Vincenza Gerosa
29-Bl. Benvenute de Gubbio

July
6-St. Nazaria Ignacia March y Mesa
14-St. Camillus de Lellis (16th in USA)
25-Bl. Benito Solana Ruiz
29-Bl. Juan Bautista Egozcuezabal Aldaz
30-St. Maria de Jesus Sacramentado Venegas de La Torre
31-Bl. Zdenka Cecilia Schelingova
31-Bl. Francisca Pons Sarda (Sr. Gabriella of St. John of the Cross
31-Bl. Vicenta Achurra Gogenola (Sr. Daniela of San Barnaba),
martyr

August
7-Bl. Teuzzo of Razzuolo
13-St. Radegund
16-St. Roch (St. Rocci)
25-Bl. Maria Troncatti
26-Bl. Maria (Corsini) Beltrame Quattrocchi
30-Bl. Maria Rafols Bruna

September
2-St. Stephen of Hungary
9-Bl. Francisco Garate Aranguren
9-Bl. Maria Euthymia Uffing
11-Bl. Bonaventure of Barcelona
12-Bl. Gertrude Prosperi
17-Bl. Leonella Sgorbati, martyr
25-Bl. Juan Agustin Codera Marques-martyr
26-St. Elzear of Sabran & Bl. Delphina of Glandeves
28-Bl. Josep Tarrats Comaposada, martyr

October
1-Bl. Luigi Maria Monti
8-St. Bridget of Sweden
20-Maria Bertilla Boscardin
30-Bl. Maria Restituta Helena Kafka
31-Bl. Aurelia Mercede Stefani (Sister Irene)

November
5-St. Bertille
6-Bl. Octavia Iglesias Blanco
6-Bl. Maria Pilar Gullon Yturriaga
6-Bl. Olga Perez-Monteserin Nunez
13-St. Didacus
13-St. Agostina Livia Pietrantoni
14-Bl. Maria Luisa Merkert
17-St. Elizabeth of Hungary
20-Bl. María Isabel López García (Sr. Mary of Peace), martyr

December
1-Bl. Liduina Meneguzzi
27-St. Fabiola

441

LIST OF PATRON SAINTS OF NURSES FOR HEALTH CONDITIONS AND HEALTHCARE

Patron Saints of Nurses

Raphael the Archangel
One of three archangels mentioned in Sacred Scripture. In the Book of Tobit, Raphael travelled with Tobit's son Tobias and cured a man's blindness. Name means "God heals." Memorial September 29.

St. Margaret of Antioch (Syria) (unknown)
Margaret was born in Antioch. She was a virgin and martyr whose father was a pagan priest and mother did when she was an infant. She was raised by a Christian woman who adopted her after her father disowned her. She converted and consecrated herself and her virginity to God. She refused the advanced of a Roman prefect and he denounced her as a Christian. At trial she refused to sacrifice to the pagan gods. Many attempts to kill her by burning or boiling in a large cauldron failed. She was then beheaded. Date of beheading is unknown. Relics are in several locations. Memorial: 20 July; 14 July in the Eastern Church.

St. Agatha (Sicily) (d. 251)
Agatha was born to a wealthy and powerful family in Catania, Sicily, as a young woman, Agatha refused offers of marriage desiring to live a life of a virgin consecrated to God. Quintian attempted to persuade Agatha to marry him and when she refused he had her arrested and brought before a judge. He threatened her with torture and possibly death. She continued to refuse his advances. Quintian then sent her to a brothel where for a month she was assaulted and humiliated. Continuing to refuse his advances, he sent her to prison. St. Agatha continued to profess her faith in Jesus Christ so he had her beaten, imprisoned, tortured and her breasts were crushed and cut off. She was visited by a vision of St. Peter who came to care for her and healed her wounds completely. She was again tortured, rolled on live coals.[1]

Her last prayer, *"Lord, my Creator, You have always protected me from the cradle; you have taken me from the love of the*

442

world and given me the patience to suffer. Receive my soul."
Following this prayer, St. Agatha died. She was martyred in 250 at
Catania, Sicily. She was buried in the Abbey of St. Agatha in
Catania and is incorrupt. St. Agatha is one of seven women,
including the Blessed Virgin Mary, who is commemorated in the
Canon of the Mass.

St. Agatha is the patron saint of those with breast cancer,
fire prevention, nurses, rape and sexual assault victims, and against
natural disasters and volcanic eruptions. She is the patron saint of
nurses because of her vision of St. Peter coming to her aid and
nursing the wounds she received from being tortured.

St. Catherine of Alexandria (Egypt) (d. 305)

Catherine of Alexandria was of noble birth. She was
persecuted under Maximinus. She debated and converted many
pagan philosophers, the empress and the leaders of the army of
Maximus with her knowledge of science, Christianity and her
oratory ability. Maximus ordered her to be broken on the wheel
which broke when she touched it. She was beheaded and her body
whisked away by angels. (Memorial November 25).

St. Catherine of Siena (Italy) (1347-1380)

Nurse. Her mission to serve the poor and sick
(See saints' section for a description).

St. Alexius of Rome (d. early 5th century) (Italy)

Alexius was the only son of a Christian Roman senator who
wanted to devote himself to God against the wishes of his parents
who had arranged a marriage. On his wedding day, his fiancee
agreed to release him to follow his vocation. He lived near a Church
in Syria and lived the life of a beggar. He returned to Rome and
through the generosity of his parents, who did not recognize him, he
was given a place to live under their stairs. Proclaimed 'The Man of
God,' he spent his time praying and teaching catechism to small
children. At the time of his death, his family realized the man under
the stairs was their son who had lived a life of penance for the love
of God. Memorial 17 July Western calendar; 17 March Eastern
Calendar.[2] St. Alexius of Rome is the patron saint of Alexians,
beggars, belt makers, nurses, pilgrims, and travelers.

443

St. John of God (Spain) (1495-1550)
Nurse. His followers formed the Brothers Hospitallers of St. John of God, a world-wide Catholic religious institute dedicated to the care of the poor, sick and those suffering from mental disorders.[3] Declared a patron of nurses and nursing associations by Pope Pius XI in 1930. (See saints section for a description).

St. Camillus de Lellis (Italy) (1550-1614)
Nurse & Priest. Established an order known initially as "Servants of the Sick," then "Order of the Ministers of the Infirm" or now simply the "Camillians." Cared for the sick both in hospital and home. Declared a patron of nurses and nursing associations by Pope Pius XI in 1930.

Any and all of the Nurses in this Text

References:
1) "Saint Agatha of Sicily". CatholicSaints.Info. 12 November 2021. Web. 10 December 2021. <https://catholicsaints.info/saint-agatha-of-sicily/>

2) "Saint Alexius of Rome". CatholicSaints.Info. 31 August 2021. Web. 10 December 2021. <https://catholicsaints.info/saint-alexius-of-rome/>

3) Catholic Online. St. John of God. Accessed 6 June 2022. https://www.catholic.org/saints/saint.php?saint_id=68

Index of Saints for Health Conditions

A

Abandoned Children - St. Jerome Emiliani
Abuse victims - St. Monica
Child Abuse Victim - St. Alodia
Academics - St. Thomas Aquinas
Adopted Children - St. Clotilde, St. Thomas More
Victims of Adultery - St. Monica
AIDS Sufferers - St. Peregrine, St. Therese of Lisieux, St. Aloysius Gonzaga
Alcoholics - St. Monica, St. John of God
Alcoholism - St. Martin of Tours
Amputees - St. Anthony of Padua
Arthritis sufferers - St. James the Apostle

B

Babies - St. Brigid, St. Philomena
Barren Women - St. Anthony of Pauda, St. Felicity
Against Battles - St. Florian
Those in Battle - St. Michael, Archangel
Birth - St. Margaret
Against Bleeding - Rita
Blindness - St. Lucy, Virgin, Martyr; St. Odilia; St. Raphael
Blood Banks - St. Januarius
Bodily Ills - St. Angela Merici, St. Philomena, St. Teresa of Avila, St. Therese of Lisieux
Against Bowel Disorders - St. Bonaventure of Potenza
Breast Cancer - St. Agatha
Against Breast Diseases - St. Agatha
Breast Feeding - St. Giles
Against Broken Bones - St. Stanislaus Kostka

C

Cancer - St. Peregrine
Cancer patients/victims - St. Peregrine, St. Bernard of Clairvaux
Captives - St. Joan of Arc, St. Mark, the Evangelist
Casket Makers -St. Stephen, First Martyr
Catholic Schools - St. Thomas Aquinas

Catholic Youth - St. Aloysius Gonzaga
Chastity - St. Agnes, Thomas Aquinas
Child Abuse Victims - St. Alodia
Childbirth - St. Gerard of Majella, St. Raymond Nonnatus
Against Childbirth Complication - St. Ulric
Against Childhood Illnesses - St. Aldegund, St. Pharaildis
Children - Infant Jesus of Prague, St. Nicholas, St. Philomena,
Nicholas of Myra, Maria Goretti
Sick Children - St. Beuno
Disappointing children - St. Monica
School children - St. Benedict
Children whose parents are not married - St. Brigid
Against Chills - St. Placid
Against Cholera - St. Roch, Confessor
Against Colds - St. Maurus
Colic - St. Charles Borromeo
Colleges - Infant Jesus of Prague
Convulsions - St. John the Baptist
Against Coughs - St. Quentin
Against Cramps - St. Pancras

D
Recently Dead - St. Gertrude of Nivelles
Deaf - St. John Neumann, St. Francis de Sales
Death Row Inmates - St. Dismas
Against Sudden Death - St. Andrew Avellino
Dentists - Saints Cosmas and Damian
Desperate Situations - St. Jude, St. Gregory of Neocaesarea; St. Rita
A Happy Death - St. Joseph
Holy Death - St. Ursula
Death of children - St. Elizabeth of Hungary, St. Elizabeth A. Seton
Desperate causes - St. Philomena
Desperate situation - St. Jude the Apostle, St. Rita of Cascia, widow
Against Diabolic Possession - St. Quirinus; St. Bruno, St. Dymphna
Divorced People - St. Helen
Doctors - St. Raphael the Archangel, St. Luke, Apostle
Drowning - St. Florian
Drug Addiction - St. Maximilian Kolbe
Dying people - St. Benedict

446

E

Engaged Couples - St. Agnes, St. Valentine
Epilepsy - St. Dymphna, St. Genesius of Rome, St. John the Baptist, St. Valentine
Expectant mothers - St. Raymond
Eyes - St. Clare, Abbess
Eye disease - St. Raphael the Archangel
Eye problems - St. Lucy, Virgin, Martyr

F

Fainting - St. Valentine
Falsely accused - St. Dominic Savior, St. Elizabeth of Hungary, St. Gerard of Majella
Families - St. Joseph, St. Maximilian Kolbe
Fever - St. Benedict
Forgotten causes - St. Jude the Apostle

G

Against Gout - St. Andrew the Apostle

H

Handicapped - St. Angela Merici
Headaches - St. Teresa of Avila
Healing Wounds - St. Rita of Cascia, widow
Health - Infant Child of Prague
Healthcare workers - St. Dymphna
Hemorrhage - St. Lucy, Virgin, Martyr
Homeless people - St. Elizabeth of Hungary
Homemakers - St. Monica
Hospital Administrators - St. Frances Xavier
Hospital Workers - St. John of God, St. Jude the Apostle, St. Vincent de Paul
Hospitals - St. Camillus de Lellis, St. Jude the Apostle, St. Vincent de Paul
Housewives - St. Martha

I

Illness - St. Bernadette, St. Catherine of Siena
Against impenitence - St. Mark, the Evangelist

Impossible causes - St. Jude the Apostle, St. Philomena
Incest victims - St. Dymphna
Infants - St. Philomena, St. Raymond
Infertility - St. Philomena
Intestinal disorders - St. Charles Borromeo, St. Timothy
Invalids - St. Roch, Confessor

K
Kidney disease - St. Benedict

L
Woman in Labor - St. Anne, St. Brigid
Laundry Workers - ST. Veronica
Lepers - St. George, St. Vincent DePaul
Loneliness - St. Rita of Cascia
Loss of parents - St. Angela Merici, St. Elizabeth Ann Seton, St.
Kateri Tekakwitha, St. Margaret Mary, St. Teresa of Avila

M
Young Maiden - St. Catherine of Alexandria
Difficult Marriages - St. Helen
Happy Marriage - St. Valentine
Married Couples - St. Joseph
Married Women - St. Monica
Martyrs - St. Agatha, St. Dymphna, St. Joan of Arc, St. Sophia
Mental Illness - St. Dymphna, St. Raphael the Archangel
Midwives - St. Brigid, St. Dorothy, Virgin, Martyr; St. Raymond
Miscarriages - St. Catherine of Siena
Mothers - St. Gerard of Majella, St. Monica

N
Neck Problems - St. Andrew Apostle
Newlyweds - St. Dorothy, Virgin, Martyr
Against Nightmares-St. Raphael the Archangel
Nurses - Raphael the Archangel, St. Margaret of Antioch, St.
Agatha, St. Catherine of Siena, St. Alexius of Rome, St. Camillus de
Lellis
Nursing Associations - St. Camillus de Lellis, St. John of God

448

O
Oppressed people - St. Anthony of Padua
Opticians - St. Hubert
Orphans - St. Frances Xavier, St. Ursula

P
Penitent Men - St. Mary Magdalene
Pharmacists - Saints Cosmas and Damian; St. James the Apostle, St. Mary Magdalene, St. Raphael the Archangel
Physically Challenged - St. Angela Merici
Physicians - Saints Cosmas and Damian, St. Luke, Apostle; St. Raphael the Archangel
Plague - St. Roch, Confessor
Plague epidemics - St. Francis Xavier
Poisoning - St. Benedict
Against Polio - St. Margaret Mary
Polio Patients - St. Margaret Mary
Against Poverty - St. Martin of Tours
Poverty - St. Bernadette
Pregnant Women - St. Gerard of Majella
Prisoners - St. Brigid, St. Joan of Arc, St. Maximilian Kolbe
Pro-Life - Our Lady of Guadalupe
Pro-Life Movement - St. Maximilian Kolbe

R
Radiologist - St. Michael, the Archangel
Rape victims - St. Agnes, St. Dymphna, St. Joan of Arc
Runaways - St. Dymphna

S
Sexual temptation - St. Catherine of Siena
Sick - St. Camillus de Lellis, St. John of God, St. Angela Merici
Sickness - St. Angela Merici
Sick people - St. Peregrine, St. Teresa of Avila
Single women - St. Emily
Skin disease - St. George, St. Peregrine, St. Roch, Confessor
Against sores - St. Clare, Abbess
Against starvation - St. Anthony of Padua
Stomach diseases - St. Timothy

Students - St. John Bosco, St. Gregory the Great, St. Ursula
Students, female - St. Catherine of Alexandria
Students - St. Aloysius Gonzaga
Surgeons - Saints Cosmas and Damian
Syphilis - St. George

T
Teachers - St. Gregory the Great, St. Ursula
Healthy Throats - St. Blaise
Torture victims - St. Julia
Tuberculosis - St. Therese of Lisieux
Those suffering from Tumors - St. Rita of Cascia, Widow

U
Against Ulcers - St. Charles Borromeo

W
Wet Nurses - St. Agatha
Widows - St. Elizabeth of Hungary, St. Elizabeth Ann Seton, St. Sophia, St. Monica
Women in Labor - St. Anne, St. Brigid
Wounds, Healing - St. Rita of Cascia, Widow

Y
Young Maiden - St. Catherine of Alexandria
Youth, Catholic - St. Aloysius Gonzaga

Index of Healthcare Patron Saints

A

St. Alodia - Child Abuse Victims

St. Agatha - Bell ringers, Breast Cancer, Against Breast Diseases, Bakers, Against Fire, Nurses, Wet Nurses, Martyrs

St. Agnes - Chastity, Young girls, Girl Scouts, Engaged Couples, Rape Victims

St. Aldegund - Against Childhood Illnesses

St. Aloysius Gonzaga - Young Students

St. Andrew, the Apostle - Fisherman, Sailors, Against Gout, Neck Problems

St. Andrew Avellino - Against Sudden Death

St. Angela Merici - Bodily Ills, Handicapped, Loss of Parents, Sick, Sickness, Physically Challenged

St. Anne - Grandmothers, Mothers, Housewives, House Keepers, Woman in Labor

St. Anthony of Padua - Lost Articles, Oppressed people, Against starvation, Amputee, Barren Women

B

St. Benedict - Against witchcraft, Temptations, Poisoning, Dying people, Monks, Kidney disease, Fever, Civil engineers, School children

St. Bernadette (Apr 16) - Illness, Poverty, Lourdes, France

St. Bernard of Clairvaux - Cancer Victims

St. Beuno - Sick Children

St. Blaise (Feb 3)- Healthy throats, Builders, Construction workers, Veterinarians, Animals

St. Bonaventure of Potenza - Against Bowel Disorders

St. Brigid (Feb 1) - Babies, Blacksmiths, Chicken farmers, Children whose parents are not married, Dairy workers, Ireland, Midwives, Poor, Prisoners, Scholars, Travelers

St. Bruno - Against Diabolical Possession

C

St. Camillus de Lellis - Sick, Nurses, Nursing Groups, Hospitals

St. Catherine of Alexandria (Nov 25) - Philosophers, Preachers, Young maidens, Female students

St. Catherine of Siena - Nurses, Against fire, Firefighters, Illness, Sexual temptation, Miscarriages

St. Charles Borromeo (Nov 4) - Against ulcers, Apple orchards, Bishops, Catechists, Colic, Catechumens, Intestinal disorders

St. Clare, Abbess (Aug 11) - Embroiderers, Television, Against sores, Eyes, Goldsmith

St. Clotilde - Adopted Children

Sts. Cosmas and Damian (Sep 26) - Physicians, Surgeons, Pharmacists, Dentist, Barbers

D

St. Dismas - Death Row Inmates

St. Dominic Savio - Choirboys, Falsely accused

St. Dorothy, Virgin, Martyr (Feb 6) - Brewers, Brides, Florists, Gardeners, Midwives, Newlyweds

St. Dymphna - Mental illness, Healthcare workers, Martyrs, Epilepsy, Rape victims, Incest victims, Runaways, Against Diabolical Possession

E

St. Elizabeth of Hungary - Homeless people, death of children, bakers, widows, those in exile, falsely accused, brides.

St. Elizabeth Ann Seton - death of children, in-law problems, Loss of parents, Opposition of Church authorities, People ridiculed for their piety, Diocese of Shreveport, Louisiana, Widows

St. Emily - Single women

F

St. Felicity - Barren Women

St. Florian - Against battles, Against fire, Barrel-makers, Brewers, Chimney sweeps, Coopers, Drowning, Fire prevention, Firefighters, Floods, Harvests

St. Francis de Sales - Deaf

St. Frances Xavier - Immigrants, Hospital administrators, Orphans

St. Francis Xavier - African missions, Foreign missions, Navigators, Parish missions, Plague epidemics, Propagation of the faith

452

G
St. Genesius of Rome - Actors, Secretaries, Epilepsy and Comedians
St. George - Boy scouts, Field workers, Lepers, Skin diseases, Soldiers, Shepherds, Syphilis, Agricultural workers, Farmers
St. Gerard of Majella - Pregnant women, Mothers, Falsely accused, Childbirth
St. Gertrude of Nivelles - Recently Dead
St. Giles - Breast Feeding
St. Gregory Neocaesarea - Desperate Situations
St. Gregory the Great - Musicians, Singers, Students, Teachers

H
St. Helen - Difficult marriages, Divorced people, Converts, Archeologists
St. Hubert - Hunters, Mathematicians, Opticians, Metalworkers

I
Infant Child of Prague - Children, Colleges, Good finances, Health

J
St. James the Apostle - Arthritis sufferers, Pharmacists, Veterinarians, Laborers, Pilgrims
St. Januarius - Blood Banks
St. Jerome Emiliani - Abandoned Children
St. Joan of Arc - Martyrs, Captives, Prisoners, Rape victims, France
St. John Bosco - Apprentices, Boys, Editors, Laborers, Students, Young people
St. John of God - Booksellers, Hospital workers, Printers, the Sick, Alcoholics
St. John the Baptist - Baptism, Bird dealers, Epilepsy, Convulsions
St. John Neumann - Authors, Deaf
St. Joseph - Families, Carpenters, Married Couples, Laborers, House Seekers, The Universal Church, A Happy Death
St. Jude the Apostle - Desperate situation, Forgotten causes, Hospital workers, Hospitals, Impossible causes
St. Julia - Corsica, Livorno, Torture victims

K

St. Kateri Tekakwitha - Ecology, Environment, Loss of parents, People in exile

L

St. Lucy, Virgin, Martyr - Eye problems, Blindness, Hemorrhage, Lamplighter

St. Luke, apostle - Doctors, Physicians, Glass makers, Butchers, Sculptors

M

St. Margaret - Birth

St. Margaret Mary - Against polio, Polio patients, Devotees to the Sacred Heart, Loss of parents

St. Maria Goretti - Children

St. Mark, the Evangelist - Attorneys, Barristers, Captives, Against impenitence, Notaries, Stained glass workers

St. Martha - Housewives, Cooks, Restaurants, Hosts

St. Martin of Tours - Against poverty, Alcoholism, Soldiers, Tailors, Cavalry, Innkeepers, Hotel
 keepers

St. Mary Magdalene - Pharmacists, Perfumers, Converts, Hairdressers, Penitent Men

St. Maurus - Against Colds

St. Maximilian Kolbe - Drug Addiction, Families, Journalists, Prisoners, Pro-Life Movement

St. Michael, Archangel - Policemen, Knights, Paratroopers, Grocers, Those in Battle, Radiologist

St. Monica - Abuse victim, Alcoholics, Homemakers, Married Women, Mothers, Victims of adultery, Widows, Disappointing children

N

St. Nicholas - Children, Fishermen, Merchants, Sailors, Bakers, Dock workers

St. Nicholas of Myra - Children

454

O

St. Odilia - Blind

Our Lady of Guadalupe (Dec 12) - Pro-Life; Americas

P

St. Pancras - Against Cramps

St. Peregrine Laziosi - Cancer, Cancer patients/victims, Sick people, AIDS sufferers, Skin disease

St. Pharaildis - Against Childhood Illnesses

St. Philomena - Babies, Bodily ills, Children, Children of Mary, Infants, Infertility, Desperate causes, Impossible causes

St. Placid - Against Chills

Q

St. Quentin - Against Coughs

St. Quirinus - Against Diabolical Possession

R

St. Raphael the Archangel - Against nightmares, Doctors, Pharmacists, Eye disease, Blind, Physicians, Happy meetings, Mental illness, Young people, Travelers

St. Raymond Nonnatus - Child Birth, Expectant Mothers, Midwives, Infants

St. Rita of Cascia, Widow - Desperate Situations, Healing Wounds, Loneliness, Those suffering from tumors, Against bleeding

St. Roch, Confessor - Skin Disease, Plague, Cholera, Invalids

S

St. Sophia - Widows, Martyrs

St. Stanislaus Kostka - Against Broken Bones

St. Stephen, First Martyr - Bricklayers, Builders, Casket Makers, Deacons, Stoneworkers.

T

St. Teresa of Avila - People in need of grace, Headaches, Bodily ills, Sick people, People in religious orders, Loss of parents

St. Therese of Lisieux - African missions, AIDS sufferers, Bodily ills, Tuberculosis

St. Thomas Aquinas - Catholic Schools, Booksellers, Academics, Chastity

St. Thomas More - Adopted Children

St. Timothy - Intestinal disorders, Stomach diseases

U

St. Ulric - Against Childbirth Complications

St. Ursula - Archers, Orphan, Students, Teachers, Holy death

V

St. Valentine - Engaged couples, Bee keepers, Fainting, Epilepsy, Happy Marriage, Love, Lovers, Young people.

St. Veronica - Laundry Workers, Photographers

St. Vincent de Paul - Charities, charitable workers, hospitals hospital workers, lepers, lost articles

Note: Saint in heaven can and do intercede for us. Though Fr. Chad Ripperger below is discussing the role of saints in assisting exorcists, their actions and abilities are also available to the lay faithful through intercessory prayers:

> The human will, much like an angelic will, is capable of moving matter outside the human body by its nature, but due to divine punishment as a result of the fall, God has restricted the will's ability to act only on those faculties of one's own body, as well as the possible intellect. This speculative proposition is not entirely unreasonable. The common experience of exorcists, who petition saints to restrain, punish, and force compliance in the demons during sessions, is to observe the physical effects of those prayer on the energumen.
>
> There is no experienced exorcist who cannot recount numerous occasions in his experience where he has invoked a particular saint to do a particular thing in relationship to the demoniac, and in which the exorcist did not immediately see the effects of his prayers in the saint doing precisely what he asked. What this indicates is that a saint in heaven does not appear to be under this speculative restriction in heaven, since his will is capable of moving the body of the demoniac. We know that the saints in heaven can communicate with us by forming images in our imagination, as is seen when particular saints are petitioned for knowledge in a particular area.[8]

456

The following is an excerpt from the Code of Canon Law Annotated in regards to the cult and veneration of saints.

The Cult of the Saints, of Sacred Images and of Relics[10]
Code of Canon Law, Book IV, Part II, Title IV

Can. 1186 - To foster the sanctification of the people of God, the Church commends to the special and filial veneration of Christ's faithful the Blessed Mary ever, Virgin, the Mother of God, whom Christ constituted the Mother of all. The Church also promotes the true and authentic cult of the other Saints, by whose example the faithful are edified and by whose intercession they are supported.

Can. 1187 - Only those servants of God may be venerated by public cult who have been numbered by ecclesiastical authority among the Saints or the Blessed.
    Explanation 1187: The notion of public cult is expressed in c834, §2. Servants of God who have not yet been canonized or beatified may be venerated in private. Canon 1277, §2 of the CIC/17, made a difference between the saints and the blessed; today, the difference will be made according to liturgical laws. One way to honour the saints consists in making them patron saints. (Cf. S. Congr. For Divine Worship, Norms Patronus of 19-03-1973, AAS 65 [1973] 276-279; CLD 8 [1973-1977] 912-916). For the celebration in honour of a new saint or blessed, cf S. Congr. Of Rites, Instr. *Ad solemnia* of 12-09-1968 (AAS 60 [1968] 602; CLD 7 [1968-1972] 32-33).Cf. The Notification *Il Concilio Vaticano Secondo* on certain aspects of proper calendars and liturgical texts of the Congr. For Divine Worship and the Discipline of the Sacraments of 20-09-1977 (Notitiae 35 [1997] 284-297).

Can. 1188 - The practice of exposing sacred images in churches for the veneration of the faithful is to be retained. However, these images are to be displayed in moderate numbers and in suitable fashion, so that the Christian people are not disturbed, nor is occasion given for less than appropriate devotion.

Can. 1189 - The written permission of the Ordinary is required to restore precious images needing repair: that is, those distinguished by reason of age, art or cult, which are exposed in churches and oratories to the veneration of the faithful. Before giving permission, the Ordinary is to seek the advice of experts.

Can. 1190 - §1. It is absolutely wrong to sell sacred relics.

§2. Distinguished relics, and others which are held in great veneration by the people, may not validly be in any way alienated nor transferred on a permanent basis, without the permission of the Apostolic See.

§3. The provision of §2 applies to images which are greatly venerated in any church by people.

Reference:
Ernest Caparros, Michael Theriault, & Jean Thorn (eds) (1983). *Code of Canon Law Annotated* (2nd ed). The Vatican. Vatican City, 920-922.

THE NURSING APOSTOLATE

His Holiness Pope Pius XI, August 27, 1935. Excerpts from allocution to CICIAMS II World Congress, Rome, Italy at Castel Gandolfo to 2000 Catholic Nurses from around the world

Allocution to Catholic nurses, August 27, 1935, Pope Pius XI

(Words of welcome --- The struggle against paganism.)
Paganism and materialism try to penetrate everywhere. Therefore you must be first and foremost and at all cost, full of the spirit of spirituality, of Christianity, of the Christian supernatural. That is the first thing to be done. That is what is most needed. It is necessary that you do as the good God Himself did, the divine Redeemer, when He thought of sending His apostles into the world to bring to it the treasure of His doctrine, example, and consolation. And what was that He did? He did nought but fill them with the spirit of the Christian supernatural, and make them the bearers of that spiritual and that supernatural. We can never give to others that which we do not ourselves possess... the law remains as inexorable as ever. The measure of the good we do to those with whom we come into contact depends on the abundance of our on riches. And the treasure which your assistance must bring to the infirm is precisely that of spirituality, of the supernatural.

You must also bring material bodily comfort... as did Our Lord Jesus Christ Himself. He commanded His apostles: "Go and bring well-being everywhere, bring health for the body; but above all and before all else, bring salvation to souls. The life of the body, yes; but still more, infinitely more, spiritual life, the life of the soul, of that soul which gives the body its true value. In a word; be what you are, be it always, always more and always better.

(To do honor to Christianity in their profession)
To be outstanding nurses, technically speaking, you have to continue improving on what you do, and keep abreast of all that you ought to know. Yes; for to act, you must know. And not only to act, but also to know what you are capable of doing, to know what it is your duty to do, and at times perhaps to know what it is your duty not to do, or what you can do only under certain conditions and within certain limits. For your activity extends both to the professional and moral field, the assistance of the sick, and the morality of that assistance. We do not wish to repeat here what you know well enough from personal experience and from your participation in this excellent and useful Congress. You comprehend not only the scientific difficulties which beset you, but also the growing requirements of an even

459

broader application which, in the name of science demand your approval and your competence.

You understand, too, the moral difficulties of your profession: you understand them only too well, thanks precisely to this paganism and materialism which insinuate themselves everywhere in order to cast out Christ. They would like to set aside the Christian and leave only the man, pure and simple humanity: this poor, miserable mean humanity, for which the good God was so moved to pity that He gave Himself up to death in order to restore to it those treasures which adorned it when it left the hands of the Creator… this poor human nature, once so rich and now fallen into such poverty and squalor. The world will look only at the man, who must replace the Christian. It is like saying that man must replace the good Lord Himself! In wanting to look no further than the man, that enormous sin is repeated which is condemned in the Old Testament and again in the letters of the apostles by the Holy Spirit: the sin of seeing and recognizing only the creature, and not the Creator.

(The need for unity. -The organization of movements. -The illusion of neutrality. -Necessity of degrees. -Threats of war. -Advantages of peace.)

Reference:
1) The Monks of Solesmes (1960). *The Human Body*, St. Paul Editions. Boston: Daughters of St. Paul, 36-38.

[CICIAMS=The International Catholic Committee of Nurses and Medico-Social Assistants]
[Medico Social Assistant is the title in Asia for Advanced Practice Nurse].

EXCERPT FROM HIS HOLINESS POPE PIUS XI MESSAGE TO CICIAMS III WORLD CONGRESS, LONDON, 1937

The following excerpt from page 25 of the CICIAMS III World Congress report and is what is referred to in the letter below

Reference: —Page 25

. . . The exercise of the profession of nurse is surely one of those which offer the greatest possibility for the apostolate, but we must not forget that the nurse, in the exercise of her profession, has to employ all sorts of technical means, and lives in a materialistic atmosphere, exposed to the danger of a limited interior piety only, dissociated from the profession and exterior practices enjoined by the Church. Furthermore, modern theories seek to penetrate the minds of Catholic nurses and to make them become unconsciously strong agents for the propagation of eugenics and neo-malthusianism. It is necessary, then, to protect them by means of Catholic Action, which has for one of its duties to sustain and fortify them in their professional and Christian formation.

460

LETTER TO THE BISHOPS FROM CARDINAL PIZZARDO
on behalf of His Holiness Pope Pius XI
April 8, 1938

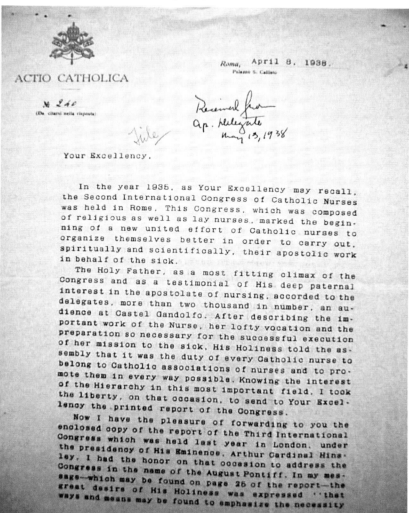

ACTIO CATHOLICA

Roma, April 8, 1938.

Your Excellency,

In the year 1935, as Your Excellency may recall, the Second International Congress of Catholic Nurses was held in Rome. This Congress, which was composed of religious as well as lay nurses, marked the beginning of a new united effort of Catholic nurses to organize themselves better in order to carry out, spiritually and scientifically, their apostolic work in behalf of the sick.

The Holy Father, as a most fitting climax of the Congress and as a testimonial of His deep paternal interest in the apostolate of nursing, accorded to the delegates, more than two thousand in number, an audience at Castel Gandolfo. After describing the important work of the Nurse, her lofty vocation and the preparation so necessary for the successful execution of her mission to the sick, His Holiness told the assembly that it was the duty of every Catholic nurse to belong to Catholic associations of nurses and to promote them in every way possible. Knowing the interest of the Hierarchy in this most important field, I took the liberty, on that occasion, to send to Your Excellency the printed report of the Congress.

Now I have the pleasure of forwarding to you the enclosed copy of the report of the Third International Congress which was held last year in London, under the presidency of His Eminence, Arthur Cardinal Hinsley. I had the honor on that occasion to address the Congress in the name of the August Pontiff. In my message—which may be found on page 25 of the report—the great desire of His Holiness was expressed ''that ways and means may be found to emphasize the necessity of bringing all Catholic nurses within the influence of Catholic Associations of Nurses.'' In accordance with this wish of the Holy Father, it is most desirable, Your Excellency, that the Catholic nurses of the United States be gathered into one national association under the direction of the respective Ordinaries and of the Hierarchy.

The Reverend Father Garesche, S. J., who has given of his time and energy to effect such an organization, now realizing the great good that would ensue if this most important work were carried out under the guidance of the Hierarchy, has signified his intention of retiring from the movement. It is proposed, therefore, in keeping with the wish manifested in the above words of His Holiness; that the Archbishops and Bishops should organize local associations of Catholic nurses according to the needs of their respective dioceses, which in due time, under the guidance of the Hierarchy, might be united to create a National Federation of Catholic Nurses.

In submitting this proposal for your kind consideration, I should be very grateful to Your Excellency if, after full examination, you would give me the benefit of your prudent judgment as to its advisability and as to the most appropriate means of bringing it to realization.

Trusting that I will be favored with an early reply, I am, Your Excellency, with the assurance of my sentiments of high esteem and of cordial regard.

Faithfully yours in Christ,

G. Cardinal Pizzardo

462

NATURE OF THEIR PROFESSION
His Holiness Pope Pius XII, October 29, 1951
Allocution to Midwives

Allocution to midwives, October 29, 1951.

Carefully watch over that silent and dark cradle where God infuses the germ given by the parents with an immortal soul, to lavish your care on the mother and prepare a happy birth for the child she carries within herself: there, beloved daughters, the object of your profession, the secret of its greatness and its beauty.

When one thinks of this admirable collaboration of the parents, of Nature and of God, from which a new human being comes to light in the image and likeness of the Creator (cf. Gn 1, 26-27), how could one not appreciate at its fair value the precious contribution that you bring to such a work? The heroic mother of the Maccabees warned her children: "I do not know in what way you have taken being in my womb; I have not given you the spirit and life, nor have I composed the organism of any of you. Thus, it is the Creator of the Universe who has formed man at his birth" (2 Mac 7, 22).

Therefore, whoever approaches this cradle of the future of life and exercises their activity there in one way or another, must know the order that the Creator wants to be maintained and the laws that govern it. Because it is not a question here of pure physical, biological laws, to which private agents of reason and blind forces necessarily obey, but of laws whose execution and whose effects are entrusted to the voluntary and free cooperation of man.

This order, fixed by the supreme intelligence, is directed to the end desired by the Creator; it understands the external work of man and the internal adherence of his free will; It implies action and omission. Nature makes available to man the entire concatenation of causes from which a new human life will emerge; it is up to man to unleash his living force and his Nature to develop his course and lead it to completion. After man has fulfilled his part and has set in motion the marvelous evolution of life, his duty is to religiously respect its progress, a duty which forbids him to stop the work of Nature or impede the natural development of Nature.

In this way, the part of Nature and the part of man are clearly delimited. Your professional training and your experience put you in a position to know the action of Nature and that of man, as well as the norms and laws to which both are subject; your conscience, enlightened by reason and faith under the guidance of the Authority established by God, teaches you how far the lawful action extends and where, on the other hand, the obligation of omission is strictly imposed.

In the light of these principles, We now propose to present to you some considerations on the apostolate to which your profession commits you. Indeed, every profession willed by God carries a mission, namely: that of realizing in the field of the profession itself, the thoughts and intentions of the Creator, and helping men to understand the justice and holiness of the divine plans and the good that derives for themselves from its fulfillment.

I.
Your professional apostolate is exercised
in the first place through your person

Why are you called? Because you are convinced that you know your art, that you know what mother and child need, to what dangers they are both exposed, how these dangers can be avoided or suppressed. Advice and help are expected of you, naturally, not in an absolute way, but within the limits of knowledge and human power, according to the progress and present state of science and practice in your specialty.

If all this is expected of you, it is because they have confidence in you, and this confidence is, above all, a personal thing. Your person must inspire her. That this trust not be mocked is not only your heartfelt wish, but also a requirement of your trade and your profession and, therefore, a duty of your conscience. That is why you must tend to rise to the apex of your specific knowledge.

But your professional ability is also a requirement and a form of your apostolate. What credit would, in fact, find your word in the moral and religious questions related to your trade if you appeared deficient in your professional knowledge? On the contrary, your intervention in the moral and religious field will have a very different weight if you know how to impose respect with your superior professional capacity. To the favorable opinion that you will have earned with your merit will be added, in the minds of those who turn to you, the well-founded persuasion that Christianity of conviction and faithfully practiced, far from being an obstacle to professional value, is a stimulus and a guarantee on it. You will clearly see that, in the exercise of your profession, you are aware of your responsibility before God; that in your faith in God you find the strongest reason to attend with greater dedication the greater the need; that in the solid religious foundation you find the firmness to oppose to irrational and immoral pretensions (wherever they come from) a calm, but undaunted and irreformable "no".

Esteemed and appreciated as you are for your personal conduct no less than for your science and experience, you will find the care of mother and child willingly entrusted to you, and perhaps without even realizing it you will exercise a deep, often silent , but effective apostolate of lived

464

Christianity. Because as great as the moral authority that is due to properly professional qualities may be, the action of man on man is carried out above all with the double seal of true humanity and true Christianity.

II.
The second aspect of your apostolate is zeal to uphold the value and inviolability of human life

The present world urgently needs to be convinced of this with the triple testimony of intelligence, heart and facts. Your profession offers you the possibility of giving such testimony and making it a duty. Perhaps it is a simple word said opportunely and with tact to the mother or the father; more often it is your whole behavior and your conscious way of acting that discreetly, silently influences them. You are more than others in a position to know and appreciate what human life is in itself and what it is worth before sound reason, before your moral conscience, before civil society, before the Church and, above all, in the eyes of God. The Lord has made all other things on the face of the earth for man, and man himself, as far as he touches his being and his essence, he has been created for God and not for any creature, although in terms of his works he also has obligations towards society. Now, "man" is the child, although he has not yet been born; in the same grade and by the same title as the mother.

In addition, every human being, even if he is a child in the womb, receives the right to life immediately from God, not from parents, nor from any kind of human society or authority. That is why there is no man, no human authority, no science, no medical, eugenic, social, economic, moral "indication" that can exhibit or give a valid legal title to a direct deliberate disposition on an innocent human life; that is, a provision that looks to its destruction, either as an end, or as a means to another end that may not in itself be in any way illegal. Thus, for example, saving the life of the mother is a most noble goal; but the direct death of the child as a means to this end is not lawful. The direct destruction of the so-called "worthless life", born or not yet born, which was practiced a few years ago, on a large scale, can in no way be justified. *(Decr. S. Off. 2 dic. 1940; AAS, val. 32, 1940, p. 553-554)* The life of an innocent person is intangible and any attack or direct aggression against it is a violation of one of the fundamental laws, without which safe human coexistence is not possible. We do not need to teach you in detail the meaning and importance in your profession of this fundamental law, but do not forget that above any human law, any "indication", the law of God rises, inevitably.

The apostolate of your profession imposes on you the duty to also communicate to others the knowledge, esteem and respect for human life that you nurture in your heart out of Christian conviction: to take up, when necessary, courageously, its defense and to protect, when it is necessary and in your power, to the defenseless and still hidden life of the child, relying on the strength of the divine precept: Non occides: you shall not kill (Ex 20, 13). Such a defensive function is sometimes presented as the most necessary and urgent; however, it is not the noblest or the most important part of your mission, because it is not purely negative, but, above all, constructive and tends to promote, build and strengthen.

Instill in the spirit and in the heart of the mother and father the esteem, the desire, the joy, the loving welcome of the newborn from its first cry. The child formed in the womb is a gift from God (Ps 127, 3), who put the care of him to the parents. With what delicacy, with what charm Sacred Scripture shows the gracious crown of the children gathered around the father's table! They are the reward of the just, as barrenness is often the punishment of the sinner. Listen to the divine word expressed with the unsurpassable poetry of the Psalm: "Your wife will be like an abundant vine in the intimacy of your house and your children like olive shoots around your table. Behold how the man who fears God is blessed" (Ps .128, 3-4). While of the wicked, it has been written: "Your offspring be condemned to extermination, and in the next generation even the name may be extinguished" (Ps 109, 13).

From birth, hasten — as the ancient Romans already did — to place the child in the arms of the father, but with an incomparably higher spirit. Among those was the affirmation of paternity and of the authority that derives from it; here it is the homage of recognition towards the Creator, the invocation of divine blessing, the commitment to fulfill with devout affection the office that God has entrusted to them. If the Lord praises and rewards the faithful servant for having made five talents bear fruit (cf. Mt 25. 21), what praise, what reward will He reserve for the father who has guarded and educated for Him the human life entrusted to him, superior to all the gold and all the silver in the world?

But your apostolate is addressed above all to the mother. Without a doubt, the voice of Nature speaks in her and puts in her heart the desire, the joy, the courage, the love, the will to take care of the child; but to overcome the suggestions of pusillanimity in all its forms, that voice needs to be strengthened and to take on, as it were, a supernatural accent. It is up to you to please the young mother, less with words than with your whole way of being and acting, the greatness, the beauty, the nobility of that life that develops, is formed and lives in her womb, that is born of her, which she carries in her arms and nourishes from her breast; make shine in her eyes and in her heart the great gift of God's love towards her and towards her child. Sacred Scripture makes you hear in multiple examples the echo of the supplicant prayer and then that of the songs of recognized joy of so many mothers finally heard, after having long implored with tears the grace of motherhood. Also the pains that, after the original guilt, the mother must suffer in order to give birth to her child, do nothing but tighten the bond that unites them; she will love him all the more the more pain it has cost her. This has been expressed with profound and moving simplicity by the one who molded the hearts of mothers: "A woman, when she gives birth, suffers pain because her hour has come; but when she has given birth to the child, she no longer remembers the anguish for the joy that a man has been born into the world" (John 16:21). And in another passage, the Holy Spirit, through the pen of the apostle Saint Paul, shows once again the greatness and joy of motherhood: God gives the child to the mother, but in giving it makes him cooperate effectively in the opening of the flower whose seed he had placed in his viscera, and this cooperation becomes the path that leads him to his eternal salvation: "the woman will be saved through the generation of children" (Ti 2,15).

This perfect accord of reason and faith gives you the guarantee that you are in the full truth and that you can safely and without doubt continue your apostolate of esteem and love towards the unborn life. If you manage to exercise this apostolate together with the supper where the newborn cries, it will not be too difficult to obtain what your professional conscience, in harmony with the law of God and Nature, imposes on you to prescribe for the good of the mother and child.

We do not need to demonstrate to you, who have experience of it, how necessary this apostolate of esteem and love for the new life is today. However, there are not rare cases in which speaking, even if only with an accent of caution, of children as a "blessing", is enough to provoke contradictions and perhaps even ridicule. Much more frequently the idea and the word of the serious "weight" of the children dominate. How opposed to the thought of Nature is this mentality! If there are conditions and circumstances in which parents, without violating God's law, can avoid the "blessing of children", however, these cases of force majeure do not authorize perverting ideas, depreciating values and vilifying the mother who has had the courage and honor to give her life.

If what we have said up to now refers to the protection and care of natural life, with much greater reason it must be valid for the supernatural life that the newborn receives with baptism. In the present economy there is no other means of communicating this life to the child, who has not yet the use of reason. And yet, the state of grace at the moment of death is absolutely necessary for salvation: without it, it is not possible to reach supernatural happiness and the beatific vision of God. An act of love can be enough for the adult to obtain sanctifying grace and make up for the defect of baptism; to the unborn or newborn child this path is not open. If it is considered, then, that charity towards one's neighbor imposes assisting him in case of need, that this obligation is all the more serious and urgent the greater the good to be procured or the evil to be avoided, and the less the needy is able to help and save himself, then it is easy to understand the great importance to attend the baptism of a child, deprived of all use of reason and who is in serious danger or facing certain death. Undoubtedly, this duty obliges, in the first place, the parents; but in urgent cases, when there is no time to lose and it is not possible to call a priest, it falls to you the sublime office of conferring baptism. Therefore, do not stop rendering this charitable service and exercising this active apostolate of your profession. May the words of Jesus serve as encouragement and encouragement: "Blessed are the merciful, for they shall find mercy" (Mt 5, 7) And what greater and more beautiful mercy than to assure the child's soul — between the threshold of life that has just been born and the threshold of death that is about to pass — the entrance into glorious eternity and beatifying!

III.
A third aspect of your professional apostolate could be called that of assistance to the mother in the prompt and generous fulfillment of her maternal role.

As soon as she had heard the angel's message, the Most Holy Mary responded: "Here is the handmaid of the Lord! Let it be done to me according to your word" (Lk 1, 38). A "fiat", an ardent "yes" to the vocation of mother, virginal Maternity, incomparably superior to any other; but real maternity in the true and proper sense of the word (cf. Gal 4,4). For this reason, when reciting the Angelus Domini, after having recalled Mary's acceptance, the believer immediately concludes: "And the Word became flesh" (Jn 1:14).

It is one of the fundamental demands of the right moral order that the use of conjugal rights corresponds to the sincere internal acceptance of the office and the duty of motherhood. With this condition, the woman walks along the path established by the Creator towards the end that He has assigned to her creature, making her, with the exercise of that function, a participant in his goodness, his wisdom and his omnipotence, according to the proclamation of the Angel: " *Concipies in utero et paries* : you will conceive in your womb and give birth" (cf. Lk 1, 31).

If this is, then, the biological foundation of your professional activity, the urgent object of your apostolate will be: to work to maintain, awaken, stimulate the sense and love of the duty of motherhood.

When the spouses esteem and appreciate the honor of giving birth to a new life, whose sprout they await with holy impatience, your task is very easy: it is enough to cultivate in them this inner feeling: the disposition to welcome and care for that nascent life. But often it is not so; the child is often unwanted; worse still, he is feared. How could readiness for duty exist

468

under such conditions? Here your apostolate must be exercised in an effective and efficient way: first of all, negatively, refusing all immoral cooperation; and positively, directing your delicate care to dissipate prejudices, various apprehensions or pusillanimous pretexts, to remove, as much as possible, the obstacles, even external ones, that can make the acceptance of motherhood painful. If your advice and your help are not used, but to facilitate the procreation of the new life, to protect it and guide it towards its full development, you can without further ado lend your cooperation. But in how many other cases do you resort to preventing the procreation and preservation of this life, without any respect for the precepts of the moral order? Obeying such demands would be lowering your knowledge and your ability, making you accomplices of an immoral action; it would pervert your apostolate. This demands a calm, but categorical "no", which does not allow transgressing the law of God and the opinion of conscience. That is why your profession obliges you to have a clear knowledge of that divine law so that you make it respected, without remaining here or beyond its precepts.

Our Predecessor Pius XI, of happy memory, in his Encyclical *Casti connubii*, of December 31, 1930, once again solemnly proclaimed the fundamental law of the conjugal act and relations: that any attempt by the spouses in the performance of the conjugal act or in the development of its natural consequences, an attack that has the purpose of depriving it of its inherent strength and preventing the procreation of a new life, is immoral; and that no "direction" or necessity can change an intrinsically immoral action into a moral and lawful act (cf. AAS, vol. 22, pp. 559 ff.).

This prescription remains in full force the same today as yesterday, and will be the same tomorrow and always, because it is not a simple precept of human law, but the expression of a natural and divine law.

Let Our words be a sure norm for all the cases in which your profession and your apostolate demand of you a clear and firm determination.

It would be much more than a simple lack of readiness for the service of life if man's attack were not only against a singular act, but if he attacked the organism itself, in order to deprive it, by means of sterilization, of the faculty to procreate a new life. Here too you have for your internal and external conduct a clear norm in the teachings of the Church. Direct sterilization—that is, sterilization that tends, as a means or as an end, to make procreation impossible—is a serious violation of the moral law and, therefore, illicit.

Nor does the public authority have any right here, under the pretext of any kind of "indication," to allow it, much less to prescribe it or have it executed to the harm of the innocent. This principle is already stated in the aforementioned Encyclical of Pius XI on marriage (lc, pp. 564, 565). For

469

this reason, when, now a decade ago, sterilization began to be more and more widely applied, the Holy See found it necessary to expressly and publicly declare that direct sterilization, both perpetual and temporary, and the same of man as of women are illicit by virtue of natural law, from which the Church itself, as you well know, has no power to dispense (Decr. S. Off., February 22, 1940. AAS, 1940, page 73).

Oppose, therefore, as far as you are concerned, in your apostolate, these perverse tendencies and deny them your cooperation.

Furthermore, these days there is the serious problem of whether and to what extent the obligation to be ready for the service of motherhood is reconcilable with the increasingly widespread recourse to times of natural sterility (the so-called agenesis periods of woman), which seems to be a clear expression of the will contrary to that provision.

It is rightly expected of you that you be well informed from the medical point of view of this well-known theory and of the progress that can still be foreseen in this matter, and, moreover, that your advice and your assistance are not based on simple popular publications, but that they are founded on scientific objectivity and on the authorized judgment of conscientious specialists in medicine and biology. It is not the priest's job, but yours, to instruct the spouses, both in private consultations and through publications, on the biological and technical aspect of the theory, but without allowing yourself to be dragged into a propaganda that is neither fair nor convenient. But even in this field your apostolate requires of you, as women and as Christians, that you know and spread the moral norms to which the application of that theory is subject. And in this the Church is competent.

It is necessary, first of all, to consider two hypotheses. If the practice of that theory does not mean anything other than that the spouses can make use of their matrimonial right also on days of natural sterility, there is nothing to oppose; with this, in effect, those do not prevent or harm in any way the consummation of the natural act and its subsequent consequences. Precisely in this the application of the theory of which we speak differs essentially from the abuse mentioned above, which consists in the perversion of the act itself. If, on the other hand, it goes further, that is, the conjugal act is allowed exclusively on those days, then the conduct of the spouses must be examined more closely.

And here again two hypotheses are presented to Our reflection if, already at the celebration of the marriage, at least one of the spouses had the intention of restricting the same matrimonial right and not only its use to times of infertility, so that in the other days the other spouse would not even have the right to demand the act, this would imply an essential defect of the matrimonial consent that would entail the invalidity of the marriage itself, because the right that derives from the marriage contract is a permanent,

470

uninterrupted right, and not intermittent, of each of the spouses with respect to the other.

If instead, that limitation of the act to the days of natural sterility refers, not to the right itself, but only to the use of the right, the validity of the marriage is out of the question; however, the moral legality of such conduct of the spouses would have to be affirmed or denied according to the intention of constantly observing those times, whether or not it was based on sufficient and secure moral reasons.

The reason is because marriage requires a state of life that, in the same way that it confers certain rights, also imposes the fulfillment of a positive work that looks at the state itself. In this case, the general principle can be applied that a positive provision may be omitted if serious reasons, independent of the good will of those who are bound by it, show that such provision is inappropriate or prove that it cannot be fairly sought by the creditor to such provision (in this case the human race).

The marriage contract, which confers on the spouses the right to satisfy the inclination of nature, constitutes them in a state of life, the state of marriage; now, to the spouses who make use of it with the specific act of their state, Nature and the Creator impose the function of providing for the conservation of the human race. This is the characteristic benefit that constitutes the value of its state, the *bonum pholis*. The individual and society, the people and the State, the Church itself, depend for their existence, in the order established by God, on fruitful marriage. Therefore, to embrace the married state, to continually use the faculty that is proper to it and is lawful only in it, and, on the other hand, to always and deliberately evade its primary duty without serious reason, would be to sin against the very meaning of the marriage and of married life.

Serious reasons, such as those that often exist in the so-called medical, eugenic, economic and social "indication" can be exempted from this obligatory positive benefit, even for a long time and even for the entire duration of the marriage. From this it follows that the observance of infertile times can be "lawful" from the moral point of view; and under the conditions mentioned it is really such. But if, according to a reasonable and equitable judgment, there are no such serious personal reasons or reasons deriving from external circumstances, the will to habitually avoid the fertility of the union, even though sensuality continues to be fully satisfied, cannot but derive from a false Appreciation of life and of foreign motives to the straight ethical norms.

Now, perhaps you insist, observing that in the exercise of your profession you sometimes find yourself faced with very delicate cases in which it is not possible to demand that the risk of maternity be run, which must be absolutely avoided, and in which, on the other hand, the observance of the agenesis periods either does not give sufficient security or must be discarded for other reasons. And then you ask how one can still speak of an apostolate at the service of motherhood. If, according to your safe and

471

experienced judgment, the conditions absolutely require a "no"; that is, the exclusion of motherhood, it would be a mistake and an injustice to impose or advise a "yes". Here we are truly dealing with concrete facts and, therefore, not a theological question, but a medical one; that is, therefore, your competence. But in such cases the spouses do not ask you for a necessarily negative medical response, without the approval of a "technique" of conjugal activity, insured against the risk of maternity. And behold, with this you are called once again to exercise your apostolate inasmuch as you do not have to leave any doubt that, even in these extreme cases, any preventive maneuver and any direct attack on the life and development of the germ is prohibited and excluded in conscience and that only one path remains open: that is, that of abstinence from any complete performance of the natural faculty. Here your apostolate obliges you to have a clear and sure judgment and a calm firmness. any preventive maneuver and any direct attack on the life and development of the germ is prohibited and excluded in conscience and that only one path remains open: that is, that of abstinence from any complete action of the natural faculty. Here your apostolate obliges you to have a clear and sure judgment and a calm firmness. any preventive maneuver and any direct attack on the life and development of the germ is prohibited and excluded in conscience and that only one path remains open: that is, that of abstinence from any complete action of the natural faculty. Here your apostolate obliges you to have a clear and sure judgment and a calm firmness.

But it will be objected that such abstinence is impossible, that such heroism is impracticable. You will hear this objection, you will read it frequently even from those who, out of duty and competence, should be in a position to judge very differently. And as proof, the following argument is adduced: "Nobody is obliged to the impossible, and no reasonable legislator is presumed to want to oblige with his law also the impossible. But abstinence for a long period of time is impossible for the spouses. Then they are not obliged to abstinence. The divine law cannot have this meaning."

Thus, from true partial premises a false consequence follows. To be convinced of this, it is enough to invert the terms of the argument: "God does not force the impossible. But God obliges the spouses to abstinence if their union cannot be carried out according to the norms of Nature. Therefore, in these cases, abstinence it's possible." As confirmation of such argument, we have the doctrine of the Council of Trent, which in the chapter on the necessary and possible observance of the commandments, teaches, referring to a passage of Saint Augustine: "God does not command impossible things, but when he commands he warns that do what you can and ask for what you cannot and He helps so that you can" (Conc. Tried., sess. 6, chap. II: Denzinger , no. 804; St. Augustine. De natura et gratia, chap. 43, no. 50: Migne, PL, 44, 271).

For this reason, do not allow yourselves to be confused in the practice of your profession and in your apostolate by therefore speaking of

472

impossibility, neither with regard to your internal judgment, nor with regard to your external conduct. Never lend yourselves to anything that is contrary to the law of God and your Christian conscience! It is an insult to the men and women of our time to consider them incapable of continued heroism. Today, for many reasons—perhaps under the pressure of dire necessity and sometimes even in the service of injustice—heroism is exercised to a degree and to an extent that in times past would have been thought impossible. Why, then, this heroism, if circumstances truly demand it, would it have to stop at the limits marked by the passions and by the inclinations of Nature? It is clear, the one who does not want to dominate himself, he will not be able to either; and whoever thinks he can control himself relying only on his own strength, without sincerely and perseveringly seeking divine help, will be miserably deceived.

Here is what concerns your apostolate to win the spouses to the service of motherhood, not in the sense of a blind slavery under the impulses of Nature, but of an exercise of conjugal rights and duties regulated by the principles of reason and faith.

IV.
The last aspect of your apostolate concerns the defense of the right order of values and the dignity of the human person.

The "value of the person" and the need to respect them is a theme that has been increasingly occupying writers for two decades. In many of his lucubrations, even the specifically sexual act has its place assigned to make it serve the person of the spouses. The proper and deepest meaning of the exercise of conjugal right should be that the union of the bodies is the expression and performance of the personal and affective union.

Articles, chapters, entire books, conferences, especially on the "technique of love", are dedicated to disseminating these ideas, illustrating them with warnings to newlyweds as a guide to marriage so that they do not pass by foolishness or misunderstood modesty or by unfounded scruple what God, who has also created the natural inclinations, offers them. If a new life arises from this complete reciprocal gift of the spouses, this is a result that remains outside, or at most on the periphery of the "values of the person"; results that is not denied, but that is not wanted to be at the center of conjugal relations.

According to these theories, your consecration for the good of life still hidden in the womb, or to favor its happy birth, would have only a minor influence and would go to the second line.

Now, if this relative appreciation did nothing but put the accent on the value of the person of the spouses more than on that of the offspring, one could strictly fail to examine such a problem; but it is, instead, a serious reversal of the order of values and goals set by the Creator himself. We are faced with the propagation of a complex of ideas and affections, directly

473

opposed to the clarity, depth and seriousness of Christian thought. And behold, once again your apostolate has to intervene. It could, in fact, occur to you that you are the confidants of the mother and wife and they interrogate you about the most secret desires and about the intimacies of married life. But how can you then, aware of your mission...

The truth is that marriage, as a natural institution, by virtue of the Creator's will, does not have as its primary and intimate goal the personal improvement of the spouses, but rather the procreation and education of new life. The other ends, although they are also made by Nature, are not in the same degree as the first, much less are they superior to it, but are essentially subordinate to it. This is valid for every marriage, even if it is infertile; As with any eye, it can be said that it is destined and formed to see, although in abnormal cases, due to special internal and external conditions, it is never in a position to lead to visual perception.

Precisely to cut through all the uncertainties and deviations that threaten to spread errors around the scale of the ends of marriage and their reciprocal realizations, We ourselves wrote a few years ago (March 10, 1944) a declaration on the order of those ends, indicating what the very internal structure of the natural disposition reveals, what is the patrimony of the Christian tradition, what the Supreme Pontiffs have repeatedly taught, what later, in due form, has been fixed by the Code of Canon Law (can. 1013 §1). Moreover, shortly after, to correct the opposing opinion, the Holy See, by means of a public decree, declared that the sentence of certain recent authors who deny that the primary purpose of marriage is the procreation and education of offspring cannot be admitted, or they teach that secondary ends are not essentially subordinate to the primary end, but are equivalent to and independent of it (SCS Officii, 1 April 1944: AAS, vol. 36, a. 1944. p. 103).

Does this perhaps mean to deny or diminish how much is good and fair in the personal values resulting from marriage and its practice? No, certainly, because the Creator has destined human beings in marriage, made of flesh and blood, endowed with spirit and heart, and these are called as men, and not as irrational animals, to be the authors of their offspring. To this end, the Lord wants the union of the spouses. Indeed, the Sacred Scripture says of God that he created man in his image and created him male and female (Gn 1,27), and has wanted —as he repeatedly affirms in the sacred books— that "man abandon his father and his mother and be united to his wife and they become one flesh" (Gn 2, 24; Mt. 19.5; Eph 5, 31).

All this is true and willed by God, but it must not be separated from the primary function of marriage; this is from service to a new life. Not only common activity of external life, but also all personal enrichment, the same intellectual and spiritual enrichment, and even everything that is more spiritual and profound in conjugal love as such, has been placed by the will of nature and of the Creator at the service of the offspring. By its nature, the perfect conjugal life also means the total dedication of the parents for the benefit of the children, and conjugal love, with its strength and its tenderness, is itself a postulate of the most sincere care for the offspring and the guarantee of his performance (cf. S. Th , 3 p., q. 29, a. 2. in c.; Suppl., q. 49, a. 2 ad 1).

To reduce the cohabitation of the spouses and the conjugal act to a pure organic function for the transmission of gametes would only be to convert the domestic hearth, family sanctuary, into a simple biological laboratory. For this reason, in our Address of September 29, 1949 to the International Congress of Catholic Physicians, we formally excluded artificial fertilization from marriage. The conjugal act, in its natural structure, is a personal action, a simultaneous and immediate cooperation of the spouses that, by the very nature of the agents and the property of the act, is the expression of the reciprocal gift that, according to the word of the Scripture, effectuates the union "in one flesh."

This is much more than the union of two gametes, which can also take place artificially, that is, without the natural action of the spouses. The conjugal act, ordained and willed by Nature, is a personal cooperation to which the spouses, upon contracting marriage, grant each other the right.

Therefore, when this benefit in its natural form and from the beginning is permanently impossible, the object of the marriage contract is affected by an essential defect. This is what we said then: "Don't forget: only the procreation of a new life according to the will and design of the Creator brings with it, to a stupendous degree of perfection, the realization of the intended ends. This is, at the same time, according to the bodily and spiritual nature and dignity of the spouses, and to the normal and happy development of the child" (AAS, vol. 41, 1949, page 560).

Tell the bride or the newlywed, then, that she comes to talk to you about personal values, which both in the sphere of the body or the senses, as well as in the spiritual, are really genuine, but that the Creator has placed them in the scale of values, not in the first, but in the second degree.

Add another consideration, which runs the risk of being forgotten: all these secondary values of the sphere and of generative activity fall within the scope of the specific job of the spouses, which is to be authors and educators of the new life. High and noble office, but that does not belong to the essence of a complete human being, as if, in the case of not obtaining the natural generative tendency its realization, there would be in a certain way or degree a diminution of the human person. The renunciation of that realization is not —especially if it is done for the noblest reasons— a mutilation of personal and spiritual values. Of this free resignation for love of the kingdom of God, the Lord has said: *Non omnes capiunt verbum istud, sed quibus datum est*: "Not everyone understands this doctrine, but only those to whom it has been granted" (Mt 19, 11).

To exalt beyond measure, as is often done today, the generative function, even in the just and moral form of conjugal life, is therefore not only an error and an aberration; it carries with it the danger of an intellectual and affective deviation, apt to impede and suffocate good and lofty sentiments, especially in youth still devoid of experience and unaware of life's disappointments. Because, finally, what normal man, healthy in body and soul, would want to belong to the number of those deficient in character and spirit?

May your apostolate, wherever you exercise your profession, enlighten minds and inculcate this just order of values so that men conform their judgments and conduct to it!

This exposition of Ours on the function of your professional apostolate would be incomplete if We did not add a brief word on the defense of human dignity in the use of the generative inclination.

The same Creator, who in his goodness and wisdom has wanted for the preservation and propagation of the human race to make use of the cooperation of man and woman by uniting them in marriage, has also arranged that in that function the spouses experience pleasure and happiness in body and spirit. Spouses, therefore, in seeking and enjoying this pleasure do nothing wrong. They accept what the Creator has destined for them.

However, here too the spouses must know how to keep within the limits of just moderation. As in the taste of food and drink, also in the sexual one should not be abandoned without restraint to the impulse of the senses. The correct norm is, therefore, this: the use of the natural generative disposition is morally licit only in marriage, in service and according to the order of the ends of marriage itself. From this it also follows that only in marriage and observing the rule, the desire and enjoyment of that pleasure and satisfaction are lawful. For the enjoyment which is subject to such a reasonable law touches not only the substance, but also the circumstances of the action, in such a way that, even if the substance of the act is saved, one can sin in the manner of carrying it out.

The transgression of this rule is as old as original sin. But in our time there is a danger of losing sight of the same fundamental principle. At present, in fact, the necessary autonomy, the very end and the very value of sexuality and its exercise are usually upheld in words and writings (even by some Catholics), regardless of the purpose of the procreation of a new life. One would like to subject the very order established by God to a new examination and a new norm. One would not want to admit any other brake on the way of satisfying the instinct than observing the essence of the instinctive act. With this, the license to serve blindly and without restraint the whims and impulses of nature would replace the moral obligation to control the passions; which will not be able to less, sooner or later,

If nature had looked exclusively, or at least in the first place, at a reciprocal gift and possession of the spouses in joy, in delight, and if she had arranged that act only to make her personal experience happy in the highest possible degree, and not to stimulate them to the service of life, then the Creator would have adopted another design in the formation and constitution of the natural act. Now, this is, on the contrary and in short, totally subordinated and ordered to that one great law of the generatio et educatio pholis ; that is, to the fulfillment of the primary purpose of marriage as the origin and source of life.

However, incessant waves of hedonism invade the world and threaten to submerge the entire married life in the tide of thoughts, desires and acts, not without serious dangers and serious damage to the primary job of the spouses.

This anti-Christian hedonism often does not blush to erect it as a doctrine, instilling the desire to make the joy in the preparation and execution of the conjugal union ever more intense; as if in matrimonial relations the entire moral law were reduced to the regular fulfillment of the act itself, and as if all the rest, done in any way, were justified with the effusion of reciprocal affection, sanctified by the sacrament of marriage, deserving of praise and reward before God and conscience. Of the dignity of man and the dignity of the Christian, which put a brake on the excesses of sensuality, no care is taken.

The seriousness and sanctity of the Christian moral law do not admit an unrestrained satisfaction of the sexual instinct and thus tend only to pleasure and enjoyment; it does not allow the reasonable man to allow himself to be dominated to such an extent, neither as regards the substance nor as regards the circumstances of the act.

Some would like to argue that happiness in marriage is a direct ratio of reciprocal enjoyment in conjugal relations. No: the happiness of marriage is instead a direct reason for the mutual respect between the spouses even in their intimate relationships; not as if they judge immoral and reject what nature offers and the Creator has given, but because this respect and mutual esteem that He engenders is one of the most effective elements of a pure love, and for that very reason all the more tender.

In your professional activity oppose as much as possible to the impetus of this refined hedonism, devoid of spiritual values, and therefore unworthy of Christian spouses. Show how Nature has given, it is true, the instinctive desire for enjoyment and approves it in legitimate marriage, but not as an end in itself, but ultimately for the service of life. Banish from your spirit that cult of pleasure and do everything you can to prevent the spread of a literature that believes in the obligation to describe in detail the intimacies of married life under the pretext of instructing, directing, and assuring. To calm the timid conscience of the spouses, in general, good sense, natural instinct and a brief instruction on the clear and simple maxims of the Christian moral law suffice.

These Our teachings have nothing to do with Manichaeism and Jansenism, as some want to make believe to justify themselves. They are only a defense of the honor of Christian marriage and of the personal dignity of the spouses.

Serving for this purpose is, especially nowadays, an urgent duty of your professional mission.

With this we have reached the conclusion of what we had proposed to expose to you.

Your profession opens up to you a vast field of apostolate in multiple aspects; apostolate, not so much in word as in action and guidance; an apostolate that you can usefully exercise only if you are perfectly aware of the purpose of your mission and the means to achieve it, and if you are endowed with a firm and resolute will, founded on a deep religious conviction, inspired and enriched by faith and Christian love.

Invoking upon you the powerful help of divine light and divine help, we wholeheartedly impart to you, as a pledge and auspices of the most abundant heavenly graces, Our Apostolic Blessing.

*   AAS 43 (1951) 835 ff.

Reference:

1) Pope Pius XII (1951). Vatican Library. Accessed 7 June 2022. https://www.vatican.va/content/pius-xii/es/speeches/1951/documents/hf_p-xii_spe_19511029_ostetriche.html (in Spanish & Italian).

2) The above is from a google translation. A professional translation is available in English in the EWTN Library online at: https://www.ewtn.com/catholicism/library/allocution-to-midwives-8965

THE NURSING VOCATION
His Holiness Pope Pius XII, May 21, 1952
Allocution to the Nursing Staff of Roman Institutions

We greet you, beloved sons and daughters, with all Our heart, you who have come in such great numbers from the hospitals, homes, clinics, and houses of care of Our diocese to receive the blessing of the Vicar of Christ. Your presence here bears witness to the noble concept you have of your profession, and leads Us to say a few words on the vocation to which you are dedicated.

Yes, a vocation: for whoever embraces the nursing profession, responds to the voice of the love of Christ: "Come, ye blessed of My Father," Jesus will say to you on the day of judgment, "because...I was sick, and you cared for Me...when you did it to one of the least of My sick brethren, you did it to Me." (Mt 25:36-40).

These words of the divine Master, explicit as they are, have formed the charter of every Christian work of mercy. We know from the oldest historians of the Church with what generosity and care the Christians themselves looked after the sick, because they saw in them the brethren of Him Who bore for all men the torments of the passion and cross. Eusebius of Caesarea[19] describes a horrible plague which laid waste Africa shortly after the year 250. During this plague, the Christians, priests and laity, ignoring the danger to their own lives, cared for the sick whom the pagans for fear of contagion drove away and abandoned unburied. Later, on, when the Church was free to grow and develop, there arose the first hospitals. Thus the hospital erected in Caesarea by the great bishop, St. Basil, about the year 370, was a city in itself, cut off from other living areas, a city in which all illnesses were treated, leprosy included.[20]

In this our city of Rome, St. Jerome explicitly attests[21] that **Fabiola** founded the first hospital where she brought and cared for the sick without distinction of illness or malady. She used to carry them upon her own shoulders and washed putrid wounds which others could not even bear to look at. Alongside the two great basilicas of Constantine --- that of the Holy Savior at the Lateran, and of St. Peter at the Vatican,---Rome soon saw the birth of two other institutes: refuges provided by Christian charity for the poor, for pilgrims and for the sick. From one of these there later sprang the famous hospital of the Holy Spirit; from the other, that of the Most Holy Savior. It would take too long to trace the marvelous story of hospitals in Rome in the Middle Ages and subsequent centuries, but these were two names which must be commemorated: those of your holy patrons, **St. John**

---

[19] Hist. Eccl., I, 7, ch. 22. P.G.20, 685-692
[20] St. Greg. Naz., *In laudem Basilii M.*, no. 63. P.G.36. 577-580
[21] *Epist. 77 ad Oceanum, de morte Fabiolae*, 399. P.L.22. 694

of God and **St. Camillus de Lellis.** The former founded that order which has become so well known as the Fatebenefratelli. The other was founder of the Clerics Regular, Ministers of the Sick. On the 23rd of June 1886 the Holy Father Leo XIII proclaimed them heavenly patrons of hospitals and of the sick, and on August 28, 1930, Our venerable Predecessor Pius XI named them patrons of all nurses of both sexes, and of their Catholic associations.[22]

A mention apart is reserved to St. Vincent de Paul, who took the ten revolutionary step of combining with the religious life the special aptitude of women for the care of the sick. The Daughters of Charity inaugurated that magnificent procession of nursing Congregations of Sisters, which today are spread all over the world, even to the most remote mission posts.

Nevertheless, the care of the sick is not the exclusive prerogative of religious, but seeks out from the ranks of the laity a whole army of competent and generous assistants. Just as this care of the sick sprang from the spirit of Christianity, so now it must be fed on and nourished by this spirit.

It is the importance of an office which determines the responsibility of the person who exercises it.[23] Now the nurse must answer not for any material business, but for a man who lives, one whose very life is more or less gravely affected, one who depends, ---often depends completely---on the knowledge, ability, delicacy and patience of doctor and nurse. In fact, under certain aspect, he depends even more on the nurse than on the doctor, as an eminent surgeon once pointed out: "It is to the nurse that the patient is entrusted for the greater part of the day; it is the nurse who receives the patient after the operation, and who, by unobtrusive, modes and effective aid, makes possible the success of the efforts of doctors and surgeons."[24]

Your profession therefore supposes in you qualities over and above the ordinary: a solid professional formation, which means a technical knowledge soundly absorbed and constantly kept up to date, an acute intelligence, capable of constantly grasping developments, applying new methods, and utilizing new instruments and medicines.

Besides this, a calm, competent, attentive, conscientious temperament. You must specialize in self-mastery: a harsh gesture can bring new suffering for the patient, make a doctor feel ill at east, inspire fear in the heart of the sick. The nurse must remain unruffled in receiving unreasonable complaints and requests from patients, and when faced with unforeseen emergencies. The nurse must foresee and prepare in time all that is needed for the care of the sick, a duty which can be quite complicated. Nothing must be forgotten; at the same time, all the precautions imposed by hygiene

---

[22] AAS, 33, 1931, pp. 8-9
[23] *"L'importanza dell'ufficio e misura della responsabilita di chi lo esercita."*
[24] E. Giupponi. *Il chiurgo allo specchio*, 3rd ed. p. 251.

and prudence must be taken. Time table must be faithfully observed, doses scrupulously administered. The nurse must be as well a scrupulous observer, who can make known to the doctor the reactions of the patient and symptoms recognized from experience. Add to these qualities attention in the reception of orders, and promptness in their execution.

The nurse must possess as well a no less imposing array of moral qualities: an unassuming, sensitive and fine tact, which can understand the sufferings of the sick and forestall their needs, which can distinguish what must be said from that which is better left unspoken; tactful too, in the relations with the doctor, whose authority must always be respected and upheld, and with fellow nurses, particularly those who are younger, who must never be embarrassed or shamed, but rather aided when the need arises.

Your profession demands a complete dedication to the patient, be he rich or poor, be he a pleasant person or not. The nurse is not like the clerk in the office, who can leave without a worry at the day's end. You may be called in for urgent cases, and your work promises days so full that there is no possibility of rest or relaxation.

Patience, too, is part of this total dedication. There are some who can rise to great heights now and then in extraordinary circumstance, but who tire and are irritated by the constant small bothers which occur day in and day out.

The crown, finally, of all the moral virtues of the nurse, is discretion. The nurse must observe strictly the professional secret. Nothing the patient has said in confidence or in delirium may be revealed, nor anything which will harm his reputation or family.[25]

There are other nobler virtues, too, on which Christian faith confers a special splendor. We are referring to respect for the sick, truthfulness, and moral firmness:

Respect for him who at times loses many of the qualities which earn our respect: courage, calmness, lucidity. Respect for his body, too, which is the temple of the Holy Spirit, redeemed with the precious blood of Christ, destined to rise again and enjoy eternal life (1 Cor 6:19-20).

Truthfulness in contacts with doctors, with patients, and their families: these must all be able to trust implicitly in the nurse's word. This matter is important not only for the health of the body, but for that of the soul: to delay by reticence a patient's preparation for his passing into eternity could easily be a grave sin.

Finally, moral firmness, especially when the law of God is at stake. What We have on other occasions said on moral problems in medicine, for

---

[25] "Mai non possono essere da lui rivelate le cose dette dal malato in confidenza o nel delirio, null ache possa nuocere alla sua riputazione o arrecar danno alla sua famiglia."

example in Our allocution to the Italian Medical Union of Saint Luke on November 12, 1944, and to Catholic midwives on October 29, 1951 should likewise be applied to nursing.

This, then, beloved sons and daughter, is the outline of that which your profession demands of you. Few enough attain to this ideal, you may say! Could this be true? It is to your honor that We believe We can say rather that a large number among you practice this ideal in its fullness.

Nevertheless, you certainly cannot be equal to the task which your office and your obligations imposed, if you do not possess the moral energies which derive from and are nourished by a deep and living faith. Were you to consider your work in practice simply as an occupation, honorable enough certainly, but a thing purely human, and if you do not draw especially from the Eucharistic Fount, the water of Christian fortitude, you will not be able for long to remain faithful to your duties.

For in your life, there are so many sacrifices to be made, so many danger to be overcome, that it would be impossible without supernatural help, to triumph constantly over human weakness. You must cultivate the spirit of self-denial, purity of heart, delicacy of conscience, so that your service may be truly that act of supernatural charity which the Christian faith asks of you. As We remarked at the very beginning, you must serve Jesus Christ Himself in the sick: it is He Who begs your care, just as one day He begged of the Samaritan woman a glass of water. And to you We repeat those words spoken to her, to lead her to overcome her sense of surprise: "If thou knowest what it is God gives, and Who this is that is saying to you, Give Me a drink, it would have been for thee to ask Him instead, and He would have given thee living water." (Jn 4:7-10)

You well know that today more than ever people go to hospitals, clinics and sanatoria for care, so that the field of your beneficent activity extends wider and wider. One can almost say that you penetrate into every family. For this reason We ardently desire that you should acquire an ever clearer consciousness of your responsibilities, and an ever firmer will to correspond fully to these responsibilities. While entrusting you and your work to the protection and maternal love of the Blessed Virgin, and all Our heart We impart to you Our Apostolic Benediction.

Reference:

1) The Monks of Solesmes (1960). *The Human Body*, St. Paul Editions. Boston: Daughters of St. Paul, 187-193.

2) Available in Italian only on Vatican website at:
https://www.vatican.va/content/pius-xii/it/speeches/1952/documents/hf_p-xii_spe_19520521_personale-ospedaliero.html

INDEX of the Saints, Blesseds, Venerables, Servants of God and Martyrs (Individuals are indexed according to their first and last names and sorted by their title or first name if there is no title [e.g. St., Bl., Ven., Fr., etc.]

485

487

REFERENCES

1) Congregation for the Causes of Saints..
http://www.causesanti.va/it/celebrazioni.html

2) Hagiography Circle. http://newsaints.faithweb.com/index.htm

3) Marion A. Habig, O.F.M. (1979). The Franciscan Book of Saints. Chicago: Franciscan Herald Press. (Also available online at www.roman-catholic-saints.com)

4) Matthew Bunson and Margaret Bunson. (2014). *Encyclopedia of Saints*, 2nd ed. Huntington, Indiana: Our Sunday Visitor Publishing Division.

5) Reverend Alban Butler (1883). *The Lives of the Saints*. Vol I-VII. Re-published by Loreto Publications: Fitzwilliam, New Hampshire, 2020. *(Original texts reproduced with permission)*.

6) Terry Jones. "Saints who were Nurses". CatholicSaints.Info. 21 October 2008. Web. 31 May 2022. <https://catholicsaints.info/saints-who-were-nurses/>

7) "The List of Popes." The Catholic Encyclopedia. Vol. 12. New York: Robert Appleton Company, 1911. 31 May 2022 <http://www.newadvent.org/cathen/12272b.htm>

8) Fr. Chad Ripperger (2022). *Dominion*. Sensus Traditionis Press, Keenesbrg, Colorado, 322-323. https://sentradpress.com/product/dominion-the-nature-of-diabolic-warfare/

9) Various congregations, personal communications, Vatican New Agency, Catholic New Agency etc. (See specific saint for reference)

10) Ernest Caparros, Michael Theriault, & Jean Thorn (eds) (1983). *Code of Canon Law Annotated* (2nd ed). The Vatican. Vatican City, 920-922.

ABOUT THE AUTHOR

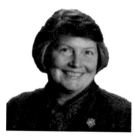

Diana Ruzicka, MSN, MA, MA, PHN, RN is a cradle Catholic. She is the third of six children born to Clarence (Chuck) and Joanna (Huyge) Prunty. She was baptized at St. Paul the Apostle Catholic Church in Tullahoma, Tennessee on December 6, 1959, by Rev. John Nolan Cain. She was raised in Sunnyvale, California where she attended Church of the Resurrection Catholic School for 3rd-8th grade and was a member of the Legion of Mary, praying the rosary daily most of her life. At the parish church she received the Sacrament of Reconciliation and First Holy Communion on April 27, 1967, from Fr. Nicholas Farana. He made a great impression on her life with his R.O.P.E. program (Reach Out to People Everywhere), in which he gave 10% of all collections, before expenses, directly to missionaries around the world, including to Diana when she spent six weeks with the Missionary Sisters of the Immaculate Conception in Peru in 1982, discerning a call to religious life. She perpetually remembers his statement, *"Be a turtle Catholic and stick out your neck for Christ."* His favorite song was, *"What's it all about Alfie."* His dog, named Alfie, and a turtle are at the base of the cross on the stained glass window in the new Church of the Resurrection that he had built in Sunnyvale, California. She received the Sacrament of Confirmation on May 19, 1973 from Archbishop Joseph Thomas McGucken also at the Church of the Resurrection. Her patron saint is St. Catherine of Siena.

Diana graduated from San Jose State University with a bachelor's degree in nursing in December 1982. She was awarded the American Red Cross nursing pin (#348559) in 1985 for her volunteer activities and, following Army retirement, volunteered locally and then worked for ARC National Headquarters for seven years. She served twenty-five years in the United States Army as a registered nurse retiring with the rank of Colonel in 2008, working in: inpatient medical, surgical and pediatric wards, emergency room, outpatient primary care and speciality clinics, oncology, pain management, administration (Clinic Commander and Hospital Chief Nurse). She returned to active duty in 2020 serving six additional months in Public Health Nursing during the corona virus (COVID-19) pandemic. Diana attended the Holy Sacrifice of the Mass daily when she was blessed with a chapel in or in close proximity to the military hospitals and clinics and continues to do so.

Diana has a Master in Nursing from Vanderbilt University in Oncology and Nursing Administration; Masters in Strategic Studies from the Army War College; certificate in Health Care Ethics from the National Catholic Bioethics Center and MA in Theology from Catholic Distance University. Her thesis: *Redemptive Suffering in the Life of the Church: Offering Up Your Daily Suffering to Cooperate with Christ in Redeeming the World*, is available at www.lulu.com (Search Ruzicka).

While on active duty she received various military awards including the Legion of Merit, Order of Military Medical Merit, and the Army Surgeon General's 9A designator for her expertise in Medical Surgical Nursing. Following retirement she was recognized at the Vanderbilt University centennial anniversary celebration as one of the 100 honored graduates and in 2015 she received the Julia Greeley

Award from ENDOW (Educating on the Nature and Dignity of Women). She has served as a nurse on several international flight accompanying special needs pilgrims to the Sanctuary at Lourdes with the North American Lourdes Volunteers. Diana served twice as President of the National Association of Catholic Nurses, U.S.A. (NACN-USA), as a Regional Director, Chair of the Communications & Publicity Committee, Website and Newsletter Editor; Board Member and Newsletter Editor for of the Military Council of Catholic Women, Europe; President, Catholic Women of the Chapel, Hanau Military Chapel; President of the Redstone Arsenal Military Council of Catholic Women; Extraordinary Minister of Holy Communion; Weekly Eucharistic Adoration since 2007 *(with a break during COVID-19 and return to active duty while larger perpetual adoration chapel being built)*; Medical Director, North American Lourdes Volunteers; Health Services Director, Instructor and Disaster Action Team member for the Madison County Chapter, American Red Cross (ARC); State Nurse Liaison for the ARC National Headquarters; Advancement Chair, Hanau Boy Scout Trop #49; Chairperson, School Advisory Council, Hanau High School, Germany; Board Member and Government Relations Committee Chair, Item writer and reviewer for certification exam and contributing author for the core curriculum for the American Society of Pain Management Nurses; Guest Lecturer (Pain Management), Medical Residency Program, Anesthesia Nursing, Obstetrics Nursing and Pediatric Nursing Specialty Courses; Coordinator, Breast Cancer Clinical Pathway; Facilitator, Breast Cancer and Cancer Support Groups.

She is currently a member of The International Catholic Committee of Nurses and Medico-Social Assistants (CICIAMS), NACN-USA, the Diocese of Birmingham in Alabama Council of Catholic Nurses (DBACCN) and the Army Nurse Corps Association. Diana served as a catechist throughout her children's youth and taught adult religious education with her husband following retirement from the U.S. Army.

Diana made her 1st consecration as a Marian Catechist before Raymond Cardinal Burke at the Shrine of Our Lady of Guadalupe in La Crosse, Wisconsin on the Feast of St. James the Great, July 25, 2021 which she renews annually.

Diana has been married 38 years to Alan, her Army Aviator. They celebrated the Sacrament of Matrimony on the Feast of St. Thomas Aquinas, January 28, 1984 at the Fraunkirche (Our Lady's Church) in Nürnberg, West Germany officiated by Fr. Thomas Mullins. Alan and Diana have been blessed with three children and three grandchildren.

Books by the Author:
Our Lady of Fatima, 1917-2022 (2nd ed). March 28, 2022.
www.lulu.com/spotlight/Ruzicka (or search "Ruzicka" at www.lulu.com)
Stations of the Cross of the Holy Face, 2022. lulu.com/spotlight/Ruzicka
Redemptive Suffering in the Life of the Church: Offering Up Your Daily Suffering to Cooperate with Christ in Redeeming the World, 2nd ed., 2016. https://www.lulu.com/spotlight/Ruzicka
Memories, Tributes & History: Francis Patrick Prunty (1890-1971) and Victoria Josephine (Schmit) Prunty (1898-1993), 2016.
Redemptive Suffering in the Life of the Church: Offering Up Your Daily Suffering to Cooperate with Christ in Redeeming the World, 1st ed., 2015.
The Descendants of Abbegail (Kallahan) and Felix Locklin Prunty, 1791-2001, 3rd ed, 2001 and *The Prunty Family Records*, 2nd ed, 1987.

Chapters Authored or Co-Authored
Benefits of Proper Pain Management. In *Core Curriculum for Pain Management Nursing*, 2016.
Benefits of Proper Pain Management. In St. Marie, B. (ed). *Core Curriculum for Pain Management Nursing*, 2008.
Economic Issues & Addiction. In *Pain Management Certification Exam*, 2005.
Patient/Family Education & Counseling, Crisis Management, Evaluation of Understanding/ Comprehension/Competency, In *Guide for the Pain Management Nursing Review Course*, American Society of Pain Management Nurses, 2004.
VHA/DoD Clinical Practice Guidelines for the Management of Post-Operative Pain (Version 1.1). Office of Performance and Quality, Veterans Health Administration, Washington, DC & Quality Management Directorate, U.S. Army Medical Command, July 2001.
Cancer Pain Management. In Gates, R. & Fink, R. (eds). *Oncology Nursing Secrets,* 2nd ed, 2001
Care of the Patient Receiving Epidural Analgesia module produced by Pain Management Service, Tripler Army Medical Center, June 1997.
Cancer Pain Management. In Gates, R. & Fink, R. (eds). *Oncology Nursing Secrets*, 1997

Selected Article(s)
Preserving Consciousness at the End of Life. *Ethics & Medics* 43(9), Philadelphia: National Catholic Bioethics Center, 2018.
Implementing a Pain Management Service at an Army Medical Center, *Military Medicine*, 2001.

Featured In:
Kaiser, Darrel Philip (2013). *Widower: Our story of God's Grace, Mercy and Blessings*. www.DarrelKaiserBooks.com, 82-83.
Kay, David (2000). All You Can Be: A Soldier's reflection on service in the greatest Army the world has ever seen. Puyallup, WA: Valley Press, 349.

Made in United States
North Haven, CT
13 May 2024

52447449R00267